DEPRESSION IN NEUROLOGIC DISEASE

THE JOHNS HOPKINS SERIES IN PSYCHIATRY AND NEUROSCIENCE

CONSULTING EDITORS

Paul R. McHugh, M.D.
Richard T. Johnson, M.D.

DEPRESSION IN NEUROLOGIC DISEASE

Edited by

SERGIO E. STARKSTEIN, M.D., Ph.D.
Raúl Carrea Institute of Neurological Research
Buenos Aires, Argentina

and

ROBERT G. ROBINSON, M.D.
Department of Psychiatry
University of Iowa College of Medicine
Iowa City, Iowa

THE JOHNS HOPKINS UNIVERSITY PRESS
Baltimore and London

To Leonardo, Dobe, Adela, Lucila, Gretchen, Christopher, and Jonathan in appreciation of their unfailing support.

Printed in the United States of America on acid-free paper

The Johns Hopkins University Press
2715 North Charles Street
Baltimore, Maryland 21218-4319
The Johns Hopkins Press Ltd., London

Library of Congress Cataloging-in-Publication Data

Depression in neurologic disease / edited by Sergio E. Starkstein and Robert G. Robinson.
p. cm. — (The Johns Hopkins series in psychiatry and neuroscience)
Includes bibliographical references and index.
ISBN 0-8018-4567-X
1. Depression, Mental—Physiological aspects. 2. Nervous system—Diseases—Psychological aspects. I. Starkstein, Sergio E. II. Robinson, Robert G. (Robert George), 1945– . III. Series.
[DNLM: 1. Depression—diagnosis. 2. Depression—therapy. 3. Nervous System Diseases—complications. WM 171 D4215]
RC537. D4383 1993
616.85′27—dc20
DNLM/DLC
for Library of Congress 92-49732
CIP

CONTENTS

PREFACE

Depression has become a topic of increasing interest and concern among neurologists, psychiatrists, and other health professionals who provide care for patients with neurologic diseases. The reasons for this concern involve both the prevalence of depressive disorders among these patients, as well as the growing recognition of the impact of depression on long-term outcome.

Many of the chapters in this text report frequencies of 25% to 50% for depression among patient groups with disorders as diverse as stroke, Parkinson disease, and multiple sclerosis. Although the prevalence in community surveys may be lower than in these hospital populations, depression appears to be the most common emotional disorder among patients with neurologic disease.

Not only is depression a common accompaniment of neurologic disease, but there is also growing evidence that the existence of depression has a significant negative impact on progression of illness (Chapter 7), recovery from illess (Chapter 3), and even survival (Chapter 4). What has not been established, thus far, is whether the treatment of depression has an ameliorating influence on outcome. It is easy to appreciate, however, why clinicians are concerned with identifying and treating depressive disorders among patients with neurologic disease.

This book is intended to be a resource for neurologists, psychiatrists, and other health professionals to identify depression in patients with neurologic diseases and to see that they receive appropriate treatment for depression. We tried to be both focused and brief. Our goal was to provide the latest available information about depressive disorder in a wide range of neurologic illnesses. Issues of clinical manifestation, prognosis, and treatment are coverd for each neurologic disorder. The cause of depression is a topic addressed in all of the chapters but remains an enigma. It seems almost certain that depression (either major or minor depression) is not a unitary phenomenon and that depressive disorders will have different etiologies both across diseases as well as within each neurologic disease. This means that our search for specific treatments, aimed at etiology, goes on, and that for those of us working in the interface of neurology and psychiatry, there is much left to do.

We are indebted to our many colleagues without whom this work would have been impossible. We are particularly grateful to Thomas R. Price, M.D., Professor of Neurology at the University of Maryland, who inspired and supported this work as early as 1978. He provided patients through his stroke service and was instrumental in recognizing depression as an important clinical entity in patients with stroke. Drs. Preziosi, Leiguarda, Lipsey, Pearlson, Berthier, Parikh, Bolla, Forrester, and Morris also made significant contributions to our work. The editorial assistance from The Johns Hopkins University Press was outstanding and allowed the completion of this book in a timely fashion.

Our preparation of this text was supported in part by the following grants: National Institute of Mental Health MH40355, Research Scientist MH00163 (RGR), National Alliance for Research in Schizophrenia and Affective Disorder New Investigator Award (SES), and a grant from the Instituo Di Tella.

CONTRIBUTORS

Alfredo Ardila, Ph.D., Department of Neuropsychology, Instituto Neurológico de Colombia, Bogotá, Colombia

D. Frank Benson, M.D., Augustus S. Rose Professor, Department of Neurology, University of California School of Medicine, Los Angeles, California

Jeffrey L. Cummings, M.D., Director, UCLA Alzheimer's Disease Center, Associate Professor of Neurology and Psychiatry & Behavioral Sciences, and Chief Behavioral Neuroscience Section, Psychiatry Service, West Los Angeles Veterans Affairs Medical Center

J. Paul Fedoroff, M.D., Division of Forensic Psychiatry, The Clarke Institute of Psychiatry, Toronto, Canada

Marshal F. Folstein, M.D., Professor, Department of Psychiatry, Johns Hopkins University School of Medicine, Baltimore, Maryland

Susan E. Folstein, M.D., Professor, Department of Psychiatry, Johns Hopkins University School of Medicine, Baltimore, Maryland

Steven J. Huber, Ph.D.(deceased), Assistant Professor, Department of Neurology, University of Kansas Medical Center, Kansas City, Kansas

Ricardo E. Jorge, M.D., Department of Psychiatry, University of Iowa College of Medicine, Iowa City, Iowa

David J. Loreck, M.D., Department of Psychiatry, Johns Hopkins University School of Medicine, Baltimore, Maryland

Helen S. Mayberg, M.D., Assistant Professor of Neurology, Psychiatry, and Radiology, Research Imaging Center, University of Texas Health Science Center, San Antonio, Texas

Carol E. Peyser, M.D., Assistant Professor, Department of Psychiatry, VA Medical Center, Menlo Park, CA

Stephen M. Rao, Ph.D., Professor, Section of Neuropsychology, Department of Neurology, Medical College of Wisconsin, Milwaukee, Wisconsin

Howard A. Ring, Raymond Way Lecturer in Neuropsychiatry, Institute of Neurology, London, England

Daniel Rogers, M.R.C.P., M.R.C. Psych., Consultant Neuropsychiatrist, Burden Neurological Hospital, Bristol, England

David L. Sultzer, M.D., Assistant Clinical Professor of Psychiatry & Biobehavioral Sciences, UCLA School of Medicine and Chief, Geriatric Psychiatry Research Unit, Behavioral Neuroscience Section, Los Angeles, California Psychiatry Service, West Los Angeles Veterans Affairs Medical Center

Michael R. Trimble, Raymond Way Reader in Behavioural Neurology, Institute of Neurology, London, England

1

DIAGNOSIS OF DEPRESSION IN NEUROLOGIC DISEASE

Robert G. Robinson, M.D.

Perhaps the most fundamental problem to be addressed in a text entitled *Depression in Neurologic Disease* is how to diagnose depression in a population of patients with another potentially interactive disorder. This issue involves a variety of questions, such as whether a valid diagnosis of depression can ever be made convincingly in a medically ill population, where symptoms fundamental to the diagnosis of depression (e.g., a disturbance of sleep or appetite) may be produced by the neurologic disease itself independent of the depressive disorder. Another question raised by this issue is whether the assessment method of depressive disorder should be altered radically, because some symptoms are nonspecific, as indicated previously, while others may be masked by the neurologic disease, such as by neglect or denial of illness or the patient's inability to express verbally the symptoms (i.e., nonfluent aphasia) or to comprehend the questions that are asked (i.e., fluent or global aphasia).

Given the current state of our research into depressive disorders, these are difficult questions to answer, and the answers are likely to vary with each neurologic disease. Symptoms that are specific for the diagnosis of depression in patients with Parkinson disease, for example, may be different from those in patients with multiple sclerosis; however, this issue has been examined in patients with stroke and Parkinson disease (Starkstein et al. 1990, Fedoroff et al. 1991). The results of these studies are described and suggest that symptoms of depressive disorder, although sometimes nonspecific, are not widespread in patients with acute neurologic disease and that the symptoms of neurologic disease do not appear to interfere frequently with the typical symptoms of depression.

DIAGNOSTIC ISSUES

Before addressing the specificity of the symptoms of depression, a brief review of the diagnostic issues is appropriate. Depressive disorders associated with neurologic disease may fall into one of four different diagnostic categories (Table 1.1). The diagnosis of *major depressive disorder* using *Diagnostic and Statistical Manual of Mental Disorders III-Revised* (DSM-III-R) requires the existence of five of nine possible symptoms, including depressed mood and loss of interest or pleasure, continuously present for at least a 2-week period. *Dysthymic depressive disorder* requires the existence of depressed mood associated with at least two symptoms of depression continuing over a 2-year period without remissions of more than 2 months in duration. Although both major depression and dysthymic depression exclude depressions thought to be related etiologically to an organic factor, numerous studies conducted by our group have demonstrated the importance of distinguishing these two types of depressive disorder (Starkstein et al. 1987, Lipsey et al. 1985). Furthermore, the proposed changes in the *Diagnostic and Statistical Manual of Mental Disorders IV* (DSM-IV) would eliminate the distinction in diagnostic criteria between a depressive disorder that is associated with a known neuropathology (to be termed a *secondary depression*) and one that is unassociated with an underlying neuropathologic disorder (to be termed a *primary depression*). Although we presume that primary depression ultimately will have an etiology based on some neuropathologic disorder, we do not yet know the nature or location of the brain abnormality.

Many have argued that the distinction between major and minor (dysthymic) depression is important, because previous studies conducted in patients with stroke have demonstrated that major (but not minor) depression is associated with the following:

1. left frontal or left basal ganglia lesions (Starkstein et al. 1987),
2. failure to suppress serum cortisol for 24 hours following dexamethasone administration (Lipsey et al. 1985),
3. a global cognitive impairment associated with mood disorder (such as dementia of depression) (Robinson et al. 1986), and
4. an untreated duration of depression between 6 months and 1 year with subsequent spontaneous remission (Robinson et al. 1987).

Although major depression and dysthymic depression have been diagnoses traditionally applied to patients without a known neuropathology, these diagnostic criteria also define depressive disorders that appear to be applicable in patients with neurologic illness.

The third possible depressive diagnosis applicable to patients

Table 1.1. Possible Depression Diagnoses in Patients with Neurologic Disorders

Diagnosis	Major Depression*	Dysthmic (Minor) Depression†	Adjustment Reaction with Depressed Mood	Organic Mood Syndrome
Symptom Criteria	1. Depressed mood and/or 2. Loss of interest plus 3. Weight change 4. Sleep disturbance 5. Agitation or retardation 6. Fatigue or energy loss 7. Worthlessness, guilt 8. Poor concentration 9. Thoughts of death	1. Depressed mood plus 2. Poor appetite or overeating 3. Sleep disturbance 4. Low energy 5. Poor concentration 6. Hopelessness	1. Depressed mood, tearfulness, or hopelessness 2. Impairment in social or occupational activity	1. Depressed mood 2. Mood related to organic factor 3. Without delirium
Duration Criteria	2 weeks or longer	2 years or longer	Occurs within 3 months after known stressor	None

*Five symptoms needed for diagnosis.
†Three symptoms needed for diagnosis.

with stroke is *adjustment disorder with depressed mood*. Adjustment disorder with depressed mood requires that depressed mood, tearfulness, or feelings of hopelessness be present as a reaction to an identifiable stressor that has occurred not more than 3 months previously. This depression is accompanied as well by impairment in either occupational or social activities and social relationships or the existence of symptoms that are markedly in excess of what would be expected for that stressor. The depressive symptoms also cannot be symptoms of a long-standing pattern of overreaction to stress.

The final diagnostic entity appropriate to patients with neurologic disease, and the one that clinically has been used most frequently, is *organic mood syndrome*. A diagnosis of organic mood syndrome requires the existence of a depressed mood associated with a specific organic factor judged to be related etiologically to the mood change. The organic causes may range from pharmacologic agents such as reserpine to endocrine disorders such as hypothyroidism to structural brain diseases such as stroke or trauma. The lack of syndrome specificity of these last two diagnoses, however, makes them appropriate to almost anybody with an acute event such as stroke or trauma who has either depressed mood, tearfulness, or feelings of hopelessness regardless of the severity of these symptoms, the presence or absence of other depressive symptoms (i.e., there is no required syndrome of depressive symptoms), or the duration of the depressive symptoms.

In summary, although there are four possible categories for diagnosing depression in patients with neurologic disease, most research dealing with these depressive disorders has found the diagnostic specificity of major depression versus dysthymic (i.e., minor) depression to be validated by differences in clinical correlates of these two disorders (Starkstein et al. 1987, Robinson et al. 1986). Ultimate validation of the distinction between major and minor depression will require the identification of differences in the depressive mechanisms for each neurologic disorder; in the mean time, the identification of differences in their clinical pathologic correlations or treatment response helps to validate these diagnoses. The validation of diagnostic entities in psychiatry as well as other fields of medicine is an ongoing process, requiring numerous studies, and ends only when differences in the etiology of the disorders are identified.

THE USEFULNESS OF SPECIFIC SYMPTOMS

One investigation of the diagnosis of depressive disorder in patients with stroke included 205 patients with acute stroke (Fedoroff et al. 1991); the only acute stroke patients excluded from this study were those with a decreased level of consciousness or a moderate to severe comprehension deficit. Patients were divided into those who reported a depressed mood (85 patients, or 41%) and those who reported no mood change (120, or 59%). There were no statistically significant differences in demographic or background characteristics between the depressed and nondepressed groups in terms of sex, race, socioeconomic status, marital status, personal or family history of psychiatric disorder, previous medical history, or medications taken at the time of interview. The depressive group, however, was found to be younger than the nondepressed group (mean of 56.5 ± 12 years [depressed group] versus 60.4 ± 14 years [nondepressed]). The depressed patients also had more severe cognitive impairment as evidenced by lower Mini-Mental Scores (22 ± 5.6 versus 24 ± 4.8) and greater impairment in activities of daily living as evidenced by higher scores on the Johns Hopkins Functioning Inventory (7.3 ± 5.7 versus 5.3 ± 5.8). The frequency of eight autonomic symptoms and 13 psychologic symptoms of depression between the depressed and nondepressed groups was then compared, and the autonomic symptoms included autonomic anxiety, anxious foreboding, morning depression, weight loss, delayed sleep, subjective anergia, early awakening, and loss of libido. The psychological symptoms included worrying, brooding, loss of interest, hopelessness, suicidal plans, social withdrawal, self-depreciation, lack of self-confidence, simple ideas of reference, guilty ideas of reference, pathologic guilt, and irritability. All symptoms were highly significantly more frequent in the depressed than the nondepressed group, with the exception of early morning awakening. The depressed patients had an average of 3.6 ± 2.14 SD autonomic symptoms and 4.12 ± 2.82 SD psychologic symptoms; the nondepressed group had an average of 0.96 ± 1.12 SD autonomic and 0.94 ± 1.12 SD psychologic symptoms ($P < .001$ for both comparisons).

Because the autonomic symptoms might be construed as related to the nonspecific effect of an acute medical illness, the frequency of major depression was assessed when one additional autonomic symptom (i.e., the baseline frequency of autonomic symptoms in the nondepressed group) was added to the diagnostic criteria for major depression (Fedoroff et al. 1991). This resulted in a change of diagnosis (i.e., failure to meet diagnostic criteria) in three of 46 patients with major depression (7%). The addition of two more autonomic symptoms reduced the frequency of major depression by five of 46 patients (11%). Thus, in the overall population, a reduction in the number of patients meeting criteria for major depression from 46 to 43 would mean a change in the frequency of major depression from 24% to 22.5%. Fedoroff et al. estimated that use of DSM-III criteria for major depression in a group of patients hospitalized with an acute stroke might falsely elevate the frequency of major depression by 1.5%.

Fedoroff et al. then determined whether patients might be underdiagnosed for major depression because they were unable or unwilling to acknowledge their depressed mood; therefore, they ascertained how many patients failed to meet diagnostic criteria for major depression only because they denied having a depressed mood (i.e., patients who met all of the required diagnostic criteria for major depression except they did not acknowledge feelings of depressed mood). There were 10 such patients of the 205 with acute stroke. Although there were no differences in demographic or any other clinical characteristics between the patients who acknowledged depression and those who did not (even though they otherwise met criteria for major depression), the patients who acknowledged depression had a higher frequency of left hemisphere lesions (54% versus 10%). Thus, if these 10 patients are added to those with major depression who acknowledged a depressed mood, the frequency of major depression would increase from 24% to 29%. It should be stressed, however, that all of the patients who denied a depressed mood acknowledged the presence of other psychologic symptoms of depression, such as loss of interest, feelings of hopelessness, and so on.

Fedoroff et al. concluded that both autonomic and psychologic depressive symptoms are strongly associated with the presence of a depressed mood even among patients with acute stroke. If altered diagnostic criteria were used, most of these patients with "modified" major depression still were identified using the standard DSM-III diagnostic criteria. Altering the diagnostic criteria to account for the baseline rate of autonomic symptoms would have resulted in less than a 2% decrease in the frequency of major depression; similarly, less than 5% of the acute-stroke population in this study may have had a "masked depression" (i.e., all necessary symptoms for major depression except depressed mood). Although this study does not answer the question of whether the diagnostic criteria for major depression identify a specific entity (this validation requires multiple studies and has not been fully accomplished even for patients without neurologic disease), its results suggest that depressive symptoms are not highly prevalent among nondepressed patients with acute stroke, and that accounting for false-positive as well as false-negative diagnoses changes the frequency of the diagnosis to a relatively small degree (i.e., from a low of 22.5% to a high of 29%).

Starkstein et al. (1990) conducted a similar study examining the specificity of psychologic and autonomic symptoms of depression in patients with Parkinson disease. This study included 33 patients who reported a depressed mood compared with an identical number of nondepressed patients who were matched for Hoehn and Yahr stage of Parkinson disease, duration of illness (± 2 years), age (± 2 years), and education (± 2 years). All patients were attending an outpatient follow-up clinic, and the mean duration of illness was 10.6 years. There were no significant between-group differences in the symptoms of Parkinson disease, levodopa dosage, or frequency of "on–off" phenomenon. After Present State Examination (PSE) items were clustered into autonomic and affective symptoms of depression (using the same autonomic and psychologic symptoms as in Fedoroff et al. 1991), a two-way ANOVA (factor 1: group [depressed versus nondepressed], factor 2: PSE cluster [autonomic versus affective]) showed a significant effect of group ($F = 138.7$, $df = 1, 28$, $P < 0.00001$) but no significant group by PSE cluster interaction (the depressed group did not have more psychologic than autonomic symptoms). On individual autonomic symptom comparisons, the depressed group showed a significantly higher frequency of autonomic anxiety, loss of appetite, initial insomnia, middle insomnia, and loss of libido. The two autonomic symptoms for which there were no significant between-group differences were early morning awakening (24% nondepressed versus 45% depressed) and anergia and retardation (58% nondepressed versus 76% depressed). All of the psychologic symptoms of depression (including worrying, brooding, loss of interest, suicidal ideation, social withdrawal, self-depreciation, and ideas of reference) were significantly different between groups. In summary, among patients with chronic Parkinson disease, all depressive symptoms (including "vegetative" symptoms) were more frequent in the depressed than the nondepressed group, with the exception of early morning awakening and loss of energy. Also, although it is not surprising that anergia and retardation might be similarly frequent in nondepressed as in depressed patients with Parkinson disease because of akinesia (a defining characteristic of Parkinson disease), all the other symptoms were significantly more common in the depressed than the nondepressed patients.

Taking the findings from the studies of stroke and Parkinson disease together, there are three significant conclusions. First, each neurologic disease needs to be investigated independently to determine which symptoms can be used in the diagnostic criteria for depressive disorders. Thus, studies that investigate depressive disorders in neurologic diseases should define the criteria for diagnosis and demonstrate that these symptoms are significantly associated with depressed mood and are not symptoms of the underlying neurologic disorder. Second, depressive symptoms are not rampant among patients with acute or chronic neurologic disease; symptoms such as loss of appetite, difficulty in falling asleep, loss of libido, and anxiety with palpitations or light headedness are not found in all patients, even those with acute neurologic disease. These symptoms can be used to define a syndrome cluster that is highly significantly associated with the existence of a depressed mood. Third, attempts at clinical differentiation between nonspecific symptoms that are secondary to the hospital routine or the patient's chronic neurologic illness and symptoms that are related to depressive disorders are unnecessary. The futility of trying to make this clinical differentiation is illustrated by a patient who may complain of a loss of appetite, attribute it to eating hospital food, and not recognize that this symptom is related to his or her low mood; symptoms such as loss of appetite, difficulty in concentrating, or middle insomnia should be regarded as a part of the syndrome cluster of depressive disorder if they exist in concert with other depressive symptoms, even if the patient attributes these vegetative disturbances to hospital routine or nonspecific affects of the neurologic disease.

THE DIAGNOSIS OF DEPRESSIVE DISORDER

Another related issue is how the treating physician should go about making a diagnosis of depressive disorder in patients with neurologic disease. As indicated by our previous studies, depressive symptoms are not affected greatly by the existence of chronic or acute neurologic disease; thus, the way to determine the existence of depressive disorder in patients with neurologic disease is to conduct a mental status examination in which the specific symptoms of depressive disorder are systematically evaluated. Patients should be asked specifically about the existence of each symptom included in the diagnostic criteria for major and minor (dysthymic) depression (Table 1.1). Patients who meet the diagnostic criteria for major or minor depression can be expected to respond to antidepressant treatments and, without treatment, to show a characteristic natural course of the disorder. Although they are often convenient and may be an adjunct to diagnosis, depression rating scales are not a substitute for a systematic mental status examination that leads to a diagnosis based on the existence of a syndromic symptom cluster.

Depression rating scales are used widely to rate the severity of depressive disorder and often are appropriate as screening instruments to determine the likelihood of the existence of depression. Although a number of depression rating scales have been used with cutoff scores to define the presence or absence of depression, a score above an arbitrary cutoff point only can be considered suggestive that a depression may exist. The "gold standard" for the existence of depression remains diagnostic criteria elicited through clinical interview. Studies evaluating the relationship between depression based on depression rating scale cutoff score and that based on clinical interview with diagnostic criteria consistently have found cases of major or minor depression that did not meet the cutoff criteria on the depression rating scale and, similarly, cases that met the cutoff criteria on the depression rating scale but did not fulfill the diagnostic criteria for depressive disorder. Although these types of studies generally have been applied to patients with functional depressive disorder, Parikh et al. (1988) conducted one in patients with depression following stroke and compared the Center for Epidemiological Studies Scale for Depression (CES-D) (Radloff et al. 1977) with DSM-III criteria for a major depression based on a structured psychiatric interview. In this study, 180 patients were given the CES-D and a structured psychiatric interview with DSM-III diagnostic criteria. Using a cutoff score of 16 or greater on the CES-D, the specificity of that cutoff score for major or minor depression was 90%; sensitivity was 86% with a positive predicted value of 80%. Increasing the cutoff score to 21 or greater increased the specificity to 94% but decreased the sensitivity to 72% with a positive predicted value of 85%. The correlation between DSM-III diagnosis for major or minor depression and CES-D in-hospital score was 0.53 using a Spearman rank correlation coefficient.

The question then arises why patients with major depression are missed by depression rating scales? The answer involves two issues. One is the appropriateness of the symptoms evaluated by the depression rating scale, which might falsely elevate the depression score. The second is failure to evaluate symptoms that are essential to the diagnosis. For example, as indicated by the previous studies of depressive disorders in Parkinson disease and stroke, the frequency of early morning awakening was not significantly different between depressed and nondepressed patients with those disorders; thus, the inclusion of symptoms in a depression rating scale that do not differentiate depressed from nondepressed patients detracts from the ability of the instrument to distinguish depressed from nondepressed patients. In addition, there are symptoms included in depression rating scales that are not integral to the diagnostic criteria for depressive disorder and, therefore, can falsely elevate or decrease the depression rating score without contributing to the diagnosis of depression.

Some of the most widely used depression rating scales include the Hamilton Depression Scale (Hamilton 1960), an interviewer-rated scale; the Beck Depression Inventory (Beck et al. 1961), a self-rated questionnaire; the Zung Depression Scale (Zung 1965), a self-rated scale; the General Health Questionnaire (Goldberg and Hiller 1979), a self-rated scale that involves several areas of assessment besides depression; the CES-D, another self-rated scale; and the Montgomery-Asberg Depression Rating Scale (Montgomery and Asberg 1979), an interviewer-rated scale. Each of these instruments contains different questions about depression, and the relevance of these questions to the neurologic condition varies. The Hamilton Depression Scale evaluates the patient's capacity to carry on usual work and activities; the most severe rating for depression (a rating of 4) is based on the patient's stopping working because of the present illness. Rating this item in a patient who has had a stroke or other neurologic illnesses producing a physical impairment requires some judgement. Similarly, the Hamilton Scale evaluates the severity of retardation, which includes slowness of thought and speech that can be complicated by aphasia in stroke patients or bradykinesia because of Parkinson disease. Symptoms related to somatic anxiety, gastrointestinal or genital symptoms, and hypochondriasis also may be complicated by the existence of a neurologic condition. This problem of the applicability of rating-scale symptoms for depression in neurologic disease is also true of the Beck Depression Inventory, which includes a question about self-appearance where the most severe rating (a rating of 3) is based on the patient's belief that they "look ugly." This obviously could be complicated by physical impairments produced by the neurologic disorders; similarly, ratings of "capacity to work" and "worries about health" also may be influenced by the existence of a neurologic condition. Decisions about scoring each of the items on the rating scale must be interpreted in relationship to the physical or cognitive effects of the neurologic condition, and they could either increase or decrease the score depending on the judgement made. Although some modifications of the Hamilton Depression Scale have been made to account for the effects of the neurologic conditions (particularly with regard to somatic symptoms, hypochondriasis, work, and activities), these scales may not accurately reflect the severity of the depression. The Hamilton Depression Scale and the Beck Depression Inventory, however, have been the most widely used rating scales to assess the severity of depressive symptoms in patients with neurologic disorders.

In summary, depression rating scales may be useful either for screening patients for depressive disorder in neurologic conditions or for determining the relative severity of depressive symptoms. They particularly may be helpful in quantifying the improvement of depressive symptoms with treatment or in differentiating the relative severity of depression from one patient to the next. All of these scales, however, fail to identify some patients with major depression who do not reach the cutoff criteria for the depression rating scale; they also identify some patients as depressed who do not meet criteria for major depressive disorder. The only fully accurate way of determining the existence of depressive disorder is to examine the patient by clinical interview and determine whether they meet the diagnostic criteria for major (or minor) depressive disorder.

THE ETIOLOGY OF DEPRESSIVE DISORDER

A discussion about diagnosis would not be complete without a consideration of the issue of etiology. For example, depressions that are seen as understandable psychologic responses to an acute neurologic disease or the change in life circumstances associated with a chronic physical or cognitive impairment may be regarded as "reactive" depressions that either will improve on their own or require psychotherapeutic intervention to deal with the underlying psychologic issue. On the other hand, severe depressions that involve physiologic changes, such as early morning awakening, diurnal mood variation (i.e., more severe depression in the morning as compared with the evening), or loss of appetite or libido, may be regarded as "biochemical" depressions, which require pharmacologic or other physical treatment. While these kinds of consideration are helpful in directing therapeutic efforts, one should remember that we do not know the etiologic mechanism of any depressive disorder at present. When drawing etiologic inferences about depressive disorders in patients with neurologic disorders, physicians should be cognizant that patients with chronic or acute neurologic disorders almost always have an understandable explanation for their depression. The idea that "anybody would be depressed in that circumstance" has an empathic appeal and may sometimes be valid; that kind of explanation, however, may lead a clinician to overlook a major depressive disorder that could respond to antidepressant treatment. As a general guideline, even if a patient has an understandable explanation for her or his depression and some of the symptoms appear to be attributable to the medical illness or hospital routine, any patient who meets diagnostic criteria for a major depressive disorder or dysthymic disorder should be regarded as having a clinically significant depression that is potentially treatable. Treatment of the depressive disorder or referral to a psychiatric specialist should be considered.

CONCLUSIONS

The diagnosis of depressive disorder in patients with neurologic disease requires a clinical mental status examination that specifically elicits the symptoms of both major and dysthymic depression. Depressive symptoms are not rampant among nondepressed patients with either acute stroke or chronic Parkinson disease, and although the specificity of depressive disorder symptoms needs to be investigated for each neurologic condition, studies so far have indicated that most depressive symptoms occur in the context of a depressed mood. Preconceptions about the etiology of depressive disorder tend to inhibit the examination of patients for specific syndromes of major or minor depression, but patients should be evaluated for the existence of a syndromic cluster of major or minor depression and, if it exists, evaluated for possible treatment. The mainstay of the treatment of depressive disorders in patients with neurologic disease has been the tricyclic antidepressants; however, the chapters that follow provide detailed descriptions of the kinds of condition in which depressive disorders frequently are encountered as well as the special issues that are relevant to the understanding and treatment of depression in each of these disorders.

REFERENCES

Beck AT, Ward CH, Mendelson M, et al. 1961. An inventory for measuring depression. *Arch Gen Psychiatry* 4:551–571.

Fedoroff JP, Starkstein SE, Parikh RM, et al. 1991. Are depressive symptoms non-specific in patients with acute stroke? *Am J Psychiatry* 148:1172–1176.

Goldberg DP, Hiller VF. 1979. A scaled version of the General Health Questionnaire. *Psychol Med* 9:139–198.

Hamilton M. 1960. A rating scale for depression. *J Neurol Neurosurg Psychiatry* 23:56–62.

Lipsey JR, Robinson RG, Pearlson GD, et al. 1985. Dexamethasone suppression test and mood following stroke. *Am J Psychiatry* 142:318–323.

Montgomery SA, Asberg M. 1979. A new depression scale designed to be sensitive to change. *Br J Psychiatry* 134:382–389.

Parikh RM, Eden DT, Price TR, et al. 1988. The sensitivity and specificity of the Center for Epidemiologic Studies depression scale as a screening instrument for post-stroke depression. *Int J Psychiat Med* 18:169–181.

Radloff LS. 1977. The CES-D Scale, a self-report depression scale for research in the general population. *Appl Psychol Meas* 1:385–401.

Robinson RG, Bolduc P, Price TR. 1987. A two year longitudinal study of post-stroke depression. Diagnosis and outcome at one and two year follow-up. *Stroke* 18:837–843.

Robinson RG, Bolla-Wilson K, Kaplan E, et al. 1986. Depression influences intellectual impairment in stroke patients. *Br J Psychiatry* 148:541–547.

Starkstein SE, Preziosi TJ, Forrester AW, et al. 1990. Specificity of affective and autonomic symptoms of depression in Parkinson's disease. *J Neurol Neurosurg Psychiatry* 516:127–131.

Starkstein SE, Robinson RG, Price TR. 1987. Comparison of cortical and subcortical lesions in the production of post-stroke mood disorders. *Brain* 110:1045–1059.

Zung WWK. 1965. A self-rating depression scale. *Arch Gen Psychiatry* 12:63–70.

2

FUNCTIONAL DEPRESSION VIEWED AS NEUROLOGIC DISEASE

Daniel Rogers, M.R.C.P., M.R.C.Psych.

Consider the following two statements:

> Depression in Parkinson disease may result from a putative neurophysiologic dysfunction or from a psychologic reaction to the burden of the physical symptoms.
>
> Today it is either raining or it is Wednesday.

These two statements are equivalent, and they both contain the same logical flaw. The flaw is not so obvious in the first statement, but it is equally severe. The apparent alternatives that are offered are not true alternatives; they are not mutually exclusive. The apparent alternatives in the first statement result from the two paradigms, one neurologic and the other psychologic, that we have available for making sense of psychiatric disorder. There are not two types of depression in Parkinson disease, but rather two ways of making sense of it. Equally, "functional depression" can be viewed from a psychologic or a neurologic paradigm.

The term *depression* was introduced by Adolph Meyer at the beginning of this century. It replaced the previous term, *melancholia*, that had been a category of mental disorder since the ancient Greeks, with various connotations. By the end of the nineteenth century, melancholia meant a psychiatric disorder whose chief symptoms were a sad change of mood as well as slowing of ideation or inhibition of thought. Some, such as Carl Wernicke, attributed a primary significance to the retardation of thought. After the turn of the century, however, a psychologic conception of psychiatric disorder became the predominant paradigm, and mood change came to be regarded as the central feature of the disorder now called depression.

Interest in a neurologic perspective of depressive disorder waned after that, until the resurgence of a neurologic approach to psychiatric disorder in the 1960s. Since then, there have been increasing numbers of neurologic studies concerning functional depression and increasing appreciation of depression's overlap with known neurologic disorders.

COGNITIVE DEFICITS

In elderly people, depressive illness can be associated with cognitive deficits comparable to those in dementing illnesses such as Alzheimer disease. Thirty or forty years ago, a considerable advance was made when depressive disorder in elderly patients was separated from dementing illnesses, because depression is treatable. The associated cognitive disorder is reversible, with improvement in the affective disorder. Because at this time the psychologic paradigm was in the ascendant and cognitive disorder was a hallmark of cerebral disorder, the cognitive deficits of depression were explained away as "pseudodementia," with the implication that it did not represent cerebral disorder. Kiloh, for example, writing in 1961 on pseudodementia, warned against such clinical features of psychomotor retardation as a slow, shuffling gait that could create the "illusion" of central nervous system involvement.

After the 1960s, views concerning a cerebral basis for depressive disorder began to change. Donnelly et al. (1972), for example, compared the performance on neuropsychologic tests from the Halstead-Reitan battery of patients with affective disorder and patients with temporal lobe epilepsy. On the basis of their results, 69% of the patients with affective disorder were scored as having "mild to severe brain damage." The authors suggested that affective disorder might be associated with cerebral dysfunction, which, unlike brain damage, could be reversible.

In 1975, Miller published the first comprehensive review of cognitive disorder in depression. Severe depression often was associated with marked degrees of cognitive impairment, and even subjects who were mildly depressed could manifest severe deficits on some tests. The cognitive deficit was not in any way pathognomonic of depressive illness; it seemed to be reversible with improvement in clinical state. In keeping with the new approach, it was renamed *the dementia syndrome of depression* (Folstein and McHugh 1978). In a further review, McAllister (1981) felt that the most consistent features of this cognitive disorder were the impairment of memory, speed of performance, and decision making. He supported the suggestion that cognitive deficits associated with depressive disorder should be viewed as a reversible, organic brain syndrome.

This cognitive disorder could be associated with structural brain disorder. In a computerized tomography (CT) study of the brains of elderly patients that compared a group with DSM-III major depression, a group with probable Alzheimer disease, and normal controls (Pearlson et al. 1989), measures of atrophy for the patients with depression lay between those of both patients with Alzheimer disease and normal controls. Values for the patients with depression and cognitive disorder clustered near those of patients with Alzheimer disease. The pattern of cognitive deficits as well as the correlation of cognitive measures with CT attenuation values were similar in patients with Alzheimer disease and those with "the dementia syndrome of depression." The contrast between these two groups came when patients were reassessed 2 years after initial testing; where only one of 11 patients with the dementia syndrome of depression had undergone cognitive decline, all of the patients with Alzheimer disease had declined significantly. Again, the authors (Rabins et al. 1991) suggested that poor cognitive performance during depression results from structural and functional brain changes.

Coffman et al. (1990) reported significant levels of diffusely represented cognitive impairment in 30 patients from 20 to 50 years of age with a DSM-III diagnosis of bipolar affective disorder (all currently well enough to be out of the hospital) compared with controls. The degree of this impairment correlated significantly with reduction in midsagittal areas of brain structures measured on magnetic resonance imaging (MRI) scans.

IMAGING STUDIES

The first modern imaging studies of the brain were performed with CT scanning. In 1980, Jacoby and Levy reported a study of cerebral CT scans in elderly patients with affective disorder, and they described a subgroup with enlarged ventricles. Soon after, Pearlson and Veroff (1981) reported cerebral atrophy on CT scans of younger patients with manic-depressive disorder. Many other studies of depression followed, showing that this was a consistent finding. Shima et al. (1984), for example, showed that 46 patients from 25 to 77 years of age with DSM-III major affective disorder had increased ventricular:brain ratios on CT brain scans compared with those age-matched normal controls. Also, Dolan et al. (1985) reported increased cerebral ventricular size on CT brain scans in 101 patients with depression (mean age, 55.2 years) compared with 52 age-matched normal control subjects.

In a study of brain-tissue density measured by CT scanning, Jacoby et al. (1983) compared 37 elderly patients with depression, 23 patients suffering from senile dementia, and 36 healthy controls.

Low brain-tissue density values were associated with ventricular dilatation, a one-way ANOVA showed that the patients with depression constituted a significant intermediate group between those with dementia and healthy controls. As a group, the patients with depression resembled those with dementia more than the controls.

The structural brain abnormalities demonstrated by these studies were related to both aging and the clinical features of the illness. Schlegel et al. (1988) correlated CT brain-scan measurements with depression ratings from a variety of different scales in 44 patients with a DSM-III major depressive episode while controlling for age-related CT scan changes. The common psychopathologic features of the scales that correlated with measures of mild brain atrophy on CT scan were psychomotor retardation and emotional blunting.

In a recent study, Andreasen et al. (1990) measured the ventricle:brain ratio on CT brain scans of 24 patients with DSM-III bipolar disorder (mean age, 36.5 years), 27 patients with unipolar disorder and major depression (mean age, 37.3 years), and 75 age-matched normal controls. The male patients with bipolar disorder had significantly larger ventricles, but the patients with unipolar disorder did not. The authors suggested that ventricular enlargement during bipolar disorder could reflect some pathologic process independent of aging, whereas when found in patients with unipolar disorder, it was associated with aging.

Magnetic resonance imaging has both confirmed and added to the findings of CT-scan studies. Krishnan and Fiegel (1989) performed MRI brain scans on 60 patients over 45 years of age who satisfied DSM-III criteria for a major depressive episode with no history or clinical evidence of dementia. Fourteen patients had lesions of the basal ganglia characterized by punctate or multipunctate foci of increased signal intensity on the T_2-weighted scans, mostly in the dorsolateral part of the caudate nucleus. Twenty-one of the remaining patients showed subcortical white-matter hyperintensities, cortical atrophy, or ventricular enlargement.

Other studies have found the same. Zubenko et al. (1990) studied 128 elderly patients admitted over a 3-year period to one center who met DSM-III criteria for dementia (61 patients) or major depression (67) and 44 elderly control subjects. All underwent MRI brain scan. Patients with dementia had more cortical atrophy and infarction than controls and more cortical atrophy than the patients with depression, but those patients had more cortical infarctions and leukoencephalopathy than controls. Rabins et al. (1991) also compared the MRI brain scans of 21 patients aged 60 years or older having major depression with 14 age-matched controls; the patients with depression had greater cortical and subcortical atrophy and more basal ganglia lesions than the control subjects.

Swieten et al. (1991) showed that diffuse white-matter lesions shown on MRI scans of elderly patients most probably are caused by arteriosclerosis. This suggests that cerebrovascular disease could be responsible for the MRI changes that have been described and could contribute to depressive disorder in elderly patients.

Abnormalities are not confined to elderly patients, however. Swayne et al. (1990) compared the MRI brain scans of 46 patients (mean age, 33.9 years) with bipolar affective disorder and 47 age- and education-matched normal controls; the male patients with bipolar disorder showed a trend toward larger ventricular size and a significant increase in the number of focal signal hyperintensities. Also, Altschuler et al. (1991) showed significantly smaller bilateral temporal lobe volumes on MRI scans of 10 patients, aged from 30 to 58 years with a Research Diagnostic Criteria diagnosis of bipolar disorder compared with 10 age-, sex-, and education-matched normal controls.

In positron-emission tomography studies (Schwartz et al. 1987), currently depressed patients with bipolar disorder have shown a reduction in the local cerebral metabolic rate for glucose of all supratentorial structures, whereas the rate for currently hypomanic patients with bipolar disorder did not differ significantly from that of normal controls. When scanning was performed on the same patients during different mood states, their cerebral metabolic rate increased during the more euphoric mood. Glucose hypometabolism on positron-emission tomography studies in patients with depression has been confirmed in other studies, with a suggestion of left prefrontal emphasis to the hypometabolism (Baxter et al. 1989, Martinot et al. 1990).

CEREBROSPINAL FLUID STUDIES

Hunter et al. (1969) examined the cerebrospinal fluid (CSF) of 256 psychiatric inpatients. Thirty-five patients (14%) had elevated CSF total protein; eight of these 35 had major depression. Pitts et al. (1990) examined the CSF of 24 patients with major depression and 17 healthy controls, and nine (38%) of the depressed patients and no normal controls had an elevation of CSF protein that was not attributable to medication. Elevation of CSF protein, therefore, is a nonspecific marker of central nervous system dysfunction. Also, neurochemical investigations of patients with depressive illnesses have shown relationships between individual symptoms such as that between increased levels of homovanillic acid and 5-hydroxyindoleacetic acid with delusions (Aberg-Wistedt et al. 1985) and decreased levels of homovanillic acid with psychomotor retardation (Praag et al. 1975, Banki 1977).

ELECTROENCEPHALOGRAM STUDIES

No consistent abnormalities in the waking electroencephalogram (EEG) of patients with depression have been established, even with quantitative assessment of the EEG. The situation is different for sleep recordings, however, where consistent abnormalities have been demonstrated, typically in rapid-eye-movement (REM) sleep. In a recent study, Lauer et al. (1991) compared EEG sleep recordings from 74 patients with major depression and 51 healthy volunteers from 18 to 65 years of age. This showed increased eye movements during REM sleep in patients with major depression at any age as well as an earlier onset of REM in such patients, but only after the age of 35 years.

Several types of event-related cortical evoked potentials have been found to accompany depressive illness (Ashton et al. 1988). The contingent negative variation consistently has been reported to be smaller than normal, and some patients with depression show an abnormally prolonged postimperative negative variation. Hendrickson et al. (1979) recorded the averaged cortical evoked responses to auditory stimuli in 35 patients with depression, 27 patients with dementia, and nine with both diagnoses among those admitted to the psychogeriatric unit at Bethlem Royal Hospital as well as in 30 elderly, healthy control subjects. The latency of the auditory response was significantly longer in the patients with dementia than in the control subjects. The patients with depression had intermediate latencies, similar but less severe than those of the patients with dementia, and patients with both dementia and depression had latencies between those of patients with dementia or depression alone. On repeat testing, the abnormality in the patients with depression did not return to normal after recovery.

COMPARISON WITH EPILEPSY

Silberman et al. (1985), in what may come to be regarded as a classic study, found transient sensory, cognitive, affective, and motor phenomena (classically accompanying complex partial seizures) in patients with major affective illness. Their findings had never been reported before, chiefly because no one had asked the appropriate questions. Silberman et al. interviewed 44 patients with affective illness, 37 with complex partial seizures, and 30 hypertensive controls. No patient with affective illness had an EEG suggesting an epileptic process, and both the affective and epileptic groups reported many symptoms, either during or between episodes of mania or depression in the patients with affective illness, or seizures in the patients with epilepsy.

Symptoms reported significantly more often in both patients with affective illness and epilepsy than by the hypertensive control subjects included illusions of significance (mystical or religious), derealization, formed auditory hallucinations, olfactory hallucinations, epigastric hallucinations, altered sound intensity, altered odor intensity, altered color intensity, distortions of size and shape; distortions of distance, jumbled thoughts, and amnesic episodes. Symptoms significantly more common in patients with affective illness than in either patients with epilepsy or controls were speeded thoughts in mania and slowed thoughts in depression; sudden, intense, unexplained fear; sudden, intense, unexplained depression; sudden, intense, unexplained pleasurable sensations; sudden, unexplained sexual sensations; altered sound quality; autoscopic states; and formed visual hallucinations.

The number of episode-related symptoms did not differ between the affective and epileptic groups. Interestingly, in the patients with affective illness, a greater number of reported symptoms was associated with a better response to lithium and tricyclic antidepressants. The authors speculated that subtle electrophysiologic abnormalities in the temporal and limbic cortex might underlie the symptoms in the affective as well as the epileptic groups.

MOTOR DISORDER

Motor disorder is the most striking sign of neurologic dysfunction in affective disorder. Psychomotor retardation is the most consistent feature of major depression (Nelson and Charney 1981), and it was well described in the early literature. For a long time, however, interest was focused on psychologic interpretations of this disorder. Views such as McCurdy's (1925) were typical: painful thoughts are slow, and retardation was an expression of mental pain. Neurologic investigations of this motor disorder only recently have started again.

Clinical descriptions of psychomotor retardation have remained consistent. Widlocher (1983) described a general slowing down of motor activity in the limbs and trunk. The patient rarely moves his trunk or limbs, especially proximally; in stupor, the most severe form of psychomotor retardation, there is almost no movement. The amplitude of movements is reduced. The shoulders droop, and the patient stares toward the floor. The gait is impaired, with smaller, shuffling steps and loss of associated movements, and the face is immobile and blank. Speech is slowed, with a weak, monotonous voice. Psychic activity is slowed as well. Responses are slow and brief, and there is impoverishment of ideas, with ruminative thinking and difficulty moving on to a new idea. There also is difficulty with concentration and memory because of impaired recall. Both motor and mental slowing generally are felt as fatigue in everyday life and are not improved, and even worsened, by rest. Not all activities are equally affected, however; the slowing can vary through the day, typically being worse first thing in the morning, and is sensitive to environmental change.

Widlocher argues that psychomotor retardation and not mood should be regarded as the central feature of depressive illness, thus returning to the view held at the end of the last century. The issue of whether mood or psychomotor retardation is the central feature of depression cannot be resolved by experimental findings; it is a conceptual issue.

For a long time, studies showed patients with depression as having slower reaction times than controls. Martin and Rees (1966) showed that this objective measure of slowness is related closely to clinically observed retardation. Many of their patients were slow to grasp instructions and said they had difficulty in summoning the required effort, but when told that their responses were slow and urged to try again, they could improve considerably.

Szabadi et al. (1976) used a technique developed for measuring periodicity of speech in parkinsonism and showed that pause times (the silent intervals between audible portions of speech) during automatic speech, such as counting, was prolonged significantly in four unmedicated patients with depression compared to healthy subjects, but not after treatment and recovery from their depressive illness. This retardation of speech was present even when trained clinicians were unable to detect motor retardation. The association of objectively assessed speech pause time with psychomotor retardation in patients suffering depression as well as its return to normal with clinical improvement was confirmed by subsequent studies (Teasdale et al. 1980, Greden et al. 1981, Godfrey and Knight 1984, Hardy et al. 1984, Hoffmann et al. 1985), but not all studies agree (Nilsonne 1988). This prompted Greden and Carroll (1981) to suggest that the speech disturbance in depressive illness was caused by the same dysfunction of mesolimbic/nigrostriatal dopamine projection systems that had been demonstrated in Parkinson disease.

Byrne (1976) studied a three-choice reaction-time task in 125 patients who were neurotically depressed, 15 who were psychotically depressed, and 15 normal controls. The task allowed differentiation of the "decision" and "movement" components of the reaction time, and both decision and movement times were increased in both depression groups compared with the normal controls. Lapierre and Butter (1980) compared mean visual, auditory, and tactile reaction times as well as movement times in 20 agitated and 20 retarded, depressed psychiatric patients and controls; the measures were significant discriminators between the control subjects and the retarded, but not the agitated, depressed groups. Also, Knott and Lapierre (1987) examined cortical-evoked potentials and the integrated myogram from the dominant forearm extensor muscles during psychomotor task performance in 21 women with significant depressive illness and 21 controls. The patients with depression in this study showed a slower reaction time overall than did the controls, and analysis of this showed that both the central processing and the motor response time contributed to this slowing.

In a recent study comparing patients with Parkinson disease and those with primary depressive illness (Rogers et al. 1987), both groups showed a comparable slowing in the performance of a computerized digit-symbol substitution test compared with age- and education-matched normal control subjects. Use of a simpler cognitive task, a matched choice reaction time test involving the same motor responses, allowed estimation of the relative contributions of the motor and cognitive elements in the digit-symbol test; both motor and cognitive slowing contributed to the slowing of the response times in both groups.

OVERLAP WITH PARKINSONISM

One of the most significant areas of overlap between affective and neurologic disorder is between parkinsonism and depression. This was first noted over 100 years ago (when depression was still called melancholia) by France's first professor of psychiatry: "An invisible weight seems to crush the intellect and slow down perception, movement and ideas . . . The present case is obviously one of paralysis agitans with dementia, but one cannot help, on observing these symptoms, but think of certain cases of melancholic stupor, such as one sees in our mental asylums" (Ball 1882). The author here is discussing what later came to be called *bradyphrenia,* or *subcortical dementia,* in Parkinson disease (Rogers 1986), comparing it with the psychomotor retardation of affective disorder. Bradyphrenia first was described in the wake of the epidemic of encephalitis lethargica in the 1920s, but the obvious resemblance between this new concept and the psychomotor retardation of depressive illness did not prompt further study for a considerable time, however, because of the conceptual separation of neurology and psychiatry.

Micrographia is a classic sign of parkinsonism. Court (1964) administered a battery of tests, including four writing tasks, to 44 consecutively admitted, short-term psychiatric patients at intervals during their stay and to 34 normal controls. Quite considerable changes in the size of handwriting were associated with changes in mood, with decreases in size related to depressive states and increases related to states of excitement. Writing size increased as patients who had been depressed improved in mood; conversely, patients who were in states of excitement or admission produced smaller writing as they improved clinically. The analogy with parkinsonian micrographia was not mentioned in this paper.

In our study comparing Parkinson disease and primary depressive illness (Rogers et al. 1987), there was a significant overlap between the affective and motor disorder found in both groups. Thirty patients with depression showed a significant clinical motor impairment compared with normal controls at the beginning of the study, with significant improvement on retesting when their depression had improved. Motor disorder was comparable to that in the patients with Parkinson disease though not as severe; motor impairment was measured with the Webster rating scale for extrapyramidal disorder (1968), which is normally used to assess the severity of parkinsonism. In both the patients with depression and Parkinson disease, this measure correlated with the mean response times on the two computerized reaction-time tests performed by the patients after the clinical ratings.

Each of the 10 individual items of the Webster scale (1968) contributed to the total rating in the patients suffering depression, with the highest ratings for arm swing, facial expression, and speech impairment. The only items with a mean rating per patient in the parkinsonian group of over twice that in the depressed group were tremor, rigidity, self-care, and bradykinesia. One of the patients with depression had been admitted initially to a neurologic ward when he was noted to have a resting tremor, increased tone, and difficulty initiating movements when his only medication was a benzodiazepine; treatment of his depressive psychosis with an antidepressant and neuroleptic resulted in improvement of his symptoms, including motor signs. The highest Webster rating was made on a patient in depressive stupor.

Almost every study of stupor in psychiatric disorder has emphasized its equivalence to the neurologic state of akinetic mutism. Williams and Parsons Smith, investigating thalamic activity in stupor (1951), commented that comparison showed the clinical state called *stupor* by psychiatrists and that called *akinetic mutism* by neurologists was one and the same. Smith (1959), describing 27 patients presenting psychiatrically with immobility and muteness without loss of consciousness or "organic paralysis" (12 of whom had a final diagnosis of depressive reaction), agreed that the term akinetic mutism was used by neurologists to describe the stupor described by psychiatrists. Joyston-Bechal (1966) reviewed 100 of the 250 cases of stupor (defined as akinesis, mutism, and relative preservation of consciousness) admitted to the Bethlem and Maudsley hospitals between 1948 and 1961, 25 of whom had a diagnosis of depression made after recovery from the stupor. Joyston-Bechal felt, again, that akinetic mutism was equivalent to stupor.

Akinesia, defined as difficulty with the initiation, efficient execution of, and persistence with purposive movement, now is regarded as one of the major motor symptoms of parkinsonism. The concept of akinesia was a psychiatric one until the end of the nineteenth century, when the word *akinesia* was coined by Wernicke. It replaced the older term *abulia*, denoting lack or weakness of will. The use of the term akinesia by neurologists only became current in the wake of the epidemic of encephalitis lethargica, and even then it was regarded by many as a simple corollary of muscular rigidity. Only after the introduction in the 1960s of levodopa, which had a dramatic effect on the symptoms of parkinsonism and especially akinesia, did akinesia become accepted as a symptom in its own right and, now by some, even as the core symptom of parkinsonism. An identical symptom is one of the commonest symptoms in different psychiatric disorders, including affective disorder, but because of the historical division of neurologic and psychiatric disorders is not recognized as such and is not compared to its counterpart in neurologic disorder such as parkinsonism.

CONCLUSIONS

For a long time, the neurologic aspects of functional depression were either ignored or played down because of a conceptual separation of neurology and psychiatry at the end of the last century; however, these two disciplines are now coming together again. An increasing number of recent studies have shown that affective disorder in both elderly and younger patients is associated with cognitive deficits; structural and functional cerebral disorder shown on CT, MRI, and positron-emission tomography scans; and abnormalities in CSF and EEG studies. These recent studies also show a significant clinical overlap between primary affective disorders and neurologic disorders such as complex partial epilepsy and parkinsonism.

There are not two mutually exclusive types of depressive disorder, "functional" and "organic," but rather two mutually exclusive ways of regarding depressive disorder, psychologic and neurologic. Both are valid. The most appropriate perspective can vary according to circumstance; for example, when faced with an acute bereavement reaction, one does not say here is a person suffering from an acute brain disorder even though brain function must be disturbed, and possibly disturbed severely. We make sense of the disorder in psychosocial terms, and our immediate management is rightly based on this way of viewing the disorder. On the other hand, when faced with a severe, chronic, depressive psychotic disorder, viewing it as neurologic disorder with appropriate investigation and treatment makes sense. Needless to say, this does not alter the understanding and support a patient expects from his physician, whether psychiatrist or neurologist.

The depression associated with known neurologic disorders and considered in this book can shed considerable light on the neurologic mechanisms underlying all depressive disorders. There is one feature that remains a major challenge, however. Psychosocial factors can precipitate depression, including major depressive disorder (Lloyd 1980, Hirschfeld et al. 1985), and such factors equally can precipitate neurological disorders. The term *psychic trauma* was introduced by the German neurologist Albert Eulenburg in 1878 (Hart & Brown 1990). He suggested that sudden psychic trauma caused "actual molecular concussion" of the brain like the "commotio cerebri" of physical trauma; today we would postulate neurotransmitter disturbance as the most likely mechanism involved. Future effort needs to be directed at the cerebral mechanisms that underlie the precipitation by psychosocial factors of neurologic disorder including functional depression.

REFERENCES

Aberg-Wistedt A, Wistedt B, Bertilsson L. 1985. Higher CSF levels of HVA and 5-HIAA in delusional compared to nondelusional depression. *Arch Gen Psychiatry* 42:925–926.

Altschuler LL, Conrad A, Hauser P, et al. 1991. Reduction of temporal lobe volume in bipolar disorder: a preliminary report of magnetic resonance imaging. *Arch Gen Psychiatry* 48:482–483.

Andreasen NC, Swayze V, Flaum M, et al. 1990. Ventricular abnormalities in affective disorder: clinical and demographic correlates. *Am J Psychiatry* 147:893–900.

Ashton H, Golding JF, Marsh VR, et al. 1988. Cortical evoked potentials and clinical rating scales as measures of depressive illness. *Psychological Med* 18:305–317.

Ball B. 1882. De l'insanite dans la paralysie agitante. *l'Encephale* 2:22–32.

Banki CM. 1977. Correlation between cerebrospinal fluid amine metabolites and psychomotor activity in affective disorders. *J. Neurochem* 28:255–257.

Baxter LR, Scwartz JM, Phelps ME, et al. 1989. Reduction of prefrontal cortex glucose metabolism common to three types of depression. *Arch Gen Psychiatry* 46:243–250.

Byrne DG. 1976. Choice reaction times in depressive states. *Br J Soc Clin Psychiatry* 15:149–156.
Coffman JA, Bornstein RA, Olson SC, et al. 1990. Cognitive impairment and cerebral structure by MRI in bipolar disorder. *Biological Psychiatry* 27:1188–1196.
Court JH. 1964. A longitudinal study of psychomotor functioning in acute psychiatric patients. *Br J Medical Psychol* 37:167–173.
Dolan RJ, Calloway SP, Mann AH. 1985. Cerebral ventricular size in depressed subjects. *Psychological Med* 15:873–878.
Donnelly EF, Dent JK, Murphy DL. 1972. Comparison of temporal lobe epileptics and affective disorders on the Halstead-Reitan test battery. *J Clin Psychol* 28:61–62.
Folstein MF, McHugh PR. 1978. Dementia syndrome of depression. In: Katzman R, Terry RD, Bick KL, eds. *Alzheimer's Disease: Senile Dementia and Related Disorders* (*Aging, Vol.* 7). New York: Raven Press, pp 87–96.
Godfrey HPD, Knight RG. 1984. The validity of actometer and speech activity measures in the assessment of depressed patients. *Br J Psychiatry* 145:159–163.
Greden JF, Carroll BJ. 1981. Psychomotor function in affective disorders: an overview of new monitoring techniques. *Am J Psychiatry* 138:1441–1448.
Greden JF, Albala AA, Smokler IA, et al. 1981. Speech pause time: a marker of psychomotor retardation among endogenous depressives. *Biological Psychiatry* 16:851–859.
Hardy P, Jouvent R, Widlocher D. 1984. Speech pause time and the retardation rating scale for depression (ERD). *J Affective Disord* 6:123–127.
Hart O, Brown P. 1990. Concept of psychological trauma. *Am J Psychiatry* 147:1691.
Hendrickson E, Levy R, Post F. 1979. Averaged evoked responses in relation to cognitive and affective state of elderly psychiatric patients. *Br J Psychiatry* 134:494–501.
Hirschfeld RMA, Klerman GL, Andreasen NC, et al. 1985. Situational major depressive disorder. *Arch Gen Psychiatry* 42:1109–1114.
Hoffman GMA, Gonze JC, Mendlewicz J. 1985. Speech pause time as a method for the evaluation of psychomotor retardation in depressive illness. *Br J Psychiatry* 146:535–538.
Hunter R, Jones M, Malleson A, et al. 1969. Abnormal cerebrospinal fluid total protein and gamma-globulin levels in 256 patients admitted to a psychiatric unit. *J Neurological Sciences* 9:11–38.
Jacoby RJ, Levy R. 1980. Computed tomography in the elderly. 3. Affective disorder. *Br J Psychiatry* 136:270–275.
Jacoby RJ, Dolan RJ, Levy R, et al. 1983. Quantitative computed tomography in elderly depressed patients. *Br J Psychiatry* 143:124–127.
Joyston-Bechal MP. 1966. The clinical features and outcome of stupor. *Br J Psychiatry* 112:967–981.
Kiloh LG. 1961. Pseudo-dementia. *Acta Psychiatr Scand* 37:336–351.
Knott VJ, Lapierre YD. 1987. Electrophysiological and behavioural correlates of psychomotor responsivity in depression. *Biological Psychiatry* 22:313–324.
Krishnan KRR, Figiel GS. 1989. Neurobehavioral changes with caudate lesions. *Neurology* 39:1410–1411.
Lapierre YD, Butter HJ. 1980. Agitated and retarded depression, a clinical psychophysiological evaluation. *Neuropsychobiology* 6:217–223.
Lauer CJ, Riemann D, Wiegand M, et al. 1991. From early to late adulthood

changes in EEG sleep of depressed patients and healthy volunteers. *Biological Psychiatry* 29:979–993.
Lloyd C. 1980. Life events and depressive disorder reviewed. II. Events as precipitating factors. *Arch Gen Psychiatry* 37:541–548.
Martin I, Rees I. 1966. Reaction times and reactivity in depressed patients. *J Psychosomatic Res* 9:375–382.
Martinot JL, Hardy P, Feline A, et al. 1990. Left prefrontal glucose hypometabolism in the depressed state: a confirmation. *Am J Psychiatry* 147:1313–1317.
McAllister TW. 1981. Cognitive functioning in affective disorders. *Comparative Psychiatry* 22:572–586.
McCurdy JT. 1925. *The Psychology of Emotion*. London: Willey.
Miller WR. 1975. Psychological deficit in depression. *Psychological Bull* 82:238–260.
Nelson JC, Charney DS. 1981. The symptoms of major depressive illness. *Am J Psychiatry* 138:1–13.
Nilsonne A. 1988. Speech characteristics as indicators of depressive illness. *Acta Psychiatr Scand* 77:253–263.
Pearlson GD, Veroff AE. 1981. Computerised tomographic scan changes in manic-depressive illness. *Lancet* ii:470.
Pearlson GD, Rabins PV, Kim WS, et al. 1989. Structural brain CT changes and cognitive deficits in elderly depressives with and without reversible dementia ('pseudodementia'). *Psychological Med* 19:573–584.
Pitts AF, Carroll BT, Gehris TL, et al. 1990. Elevated CSF protein in male patients with depression. *Biological Psychiatry* 28:629–637.
Praag HM, Korf J, Lakke JPWF, et al. 1975. Dopamine metabolism in depressions, psychoses and Parkinson's disease: the problem of the specificity of biological variables in behaviour disorders. *Psychological Med* 5:138–146.
Rabins PV, Pearlson GD, Aylward E, et al. 1991. Cortical magnetic resonance imaging changes in elderly inpatients with major depression. *Am J Psychiatry* 148:617–620.
Rogers D. 1986. Bradyphrenia in parkinsonism: a historical review. *Psychological Med* 16:257–265.
Rogers D, Lees AJ, Smith E, et al. 1987. Bradyphrenia in Parkinson's disease and psychomotor retardation in depressive illness: an experimental study. *Brain* 110:761–766.
Schlegel S, Maier W, Philipp M, et al. 1988. The association between psychopathological aspects and CT measurements in affective disorders. *Pharmacopsychiatry* 21:416–417.
Schwartz JM, Baxter LR, Mazziotta JC, et al. The differential diagnosis of depression. Relevance of positron emission tomography studies of cerebral glucose metabolism to the bipolar-unipolar dichotomy. *JAMA* 258:1368–1374.
Shima S, Shikano T, Kitamura T, et al. 1984. Depression and ventricular enlargement. *Acta Psychiatr Scand* 70:275–277.
Silberman EK, Post RM, Nurnberger J, et al. 1985. Transient sensory, cognitive and affective phenomena in affective illness. A comparison with complex partial epilepsy. *Br J Psychiatry* 146:81–89.
Smith S. 1959. An investigation and survey of akinesis with mutism (stupor). *J Mental Sci* 105:1088–1094.
Swayne VW, Andreasen NC, Alliger RJ, et al. 1990. Structural brain abnormalities in bipolar affective disorder. *Arch Gen Psychiatry* 47:1054–1059.

Swieten JC, Hout JHW, Ketel BA, et al. 1991. Periventricular lesions in the white matter on magnetic resonance imaging in the elderly. *Brain* 114:761–774.
Szabadi E, Bradshaw GM, Besson JAO. 1976. Elongation of pause-time in speech: a simple, objective measure of motor retardation in depression. *Br J Psychiatry* 129:592–597.
Teasdale JD, Fogarty SJ, Williams JMG. 1980. Speech rate as a measure of short-term variation in depression. *Br J Social Clin Psychiatry* 19:271–278.
Webster DD. 1968. Clinical analysis of the disability in Parkinson's disease. *Mod Treatment* 5:257–282.
Widlocher DJ. 1983. Psychomotor retardation: clinical, theoretical, and psychometric aspects. *Psychiatr Clin North Am* 6:27–40.
Williams D, Parsons-Smith G. 1951. Thalamic activity in stupor. *Brain* 74:377–398.
Zubenko GS, Sullivan P, Nelson JP, et al. 1990. Brain imaging abnormalities in mental disorders of late life. *Arch Neurol* 47:1107–1111.

3

DEPRESSION IN CEREBROVASCULAR DISEASE

Sergio E. Starkstein, M.D., Ph.D.,
Robert G. Robinson, M.D.

Stroke is one of the leading causes of death and disability in elderly people. While the incidence of stroke has declined recently, the prevalence of stroke has remained constant because of increased long-term survival (Millikan et al. 1987).

Depression is one of the most frequent neurobehavioral sequelae of stroke, and during the past several years, we have examined systematically depressive disorders among patients with stroke who are capable of giving reliable responses to a verbal interview. In this chapter, we examine several issues related to post-stroke depression (PSD). First, we discuss methodologic issues in the diagnosis of PSD; next, we examine the prevalence and course of PSD among both in- and outpatients. We also consider the relationship of PSD to lesion location and impairment variables and also examine the relationship of PSD to premorbid risk factors and biologic markers. Finally, we discuss the possible biologic underpinnings of PSD and the most useful treatment modalities.

THE DIAGNOSIS OF POST-STROKE DEPRESSION

Chapter 1 addressed the issue of the specificity of symptoms used in the diagnosis of PSD. Our study, which examined the frequency of autonomic and psychologic symptoms of depression in 205 patients with and without depression with acute stroke, was presented. This study found that all depressive symptoms (with the exception of morning awakening) were significantly more common among patients with depression (Fedoroff et al. 1991). Altering the diagnostic criteria to account for the rate of nonspecific vegetative symptoms among the patients without depression would have reduced the frequency of major depression by only 1.5%, from 24.0% to 22.5%. Thus, the diagnostic criteria included in the DSM-III and DSM-III-R (American Psychiatric Association 1980, 1987) (see Table 1.1) appear to be applicable to patients with acute stroke.

We also use DSM-III diagnostic symptom criteria for dysthymic depression to define minor depression. We use the term *minor depression*, because the dysthymic depression diagnosis requires a duration of 2 years and we make the diagnosis in patients with acute stroke. Our studies have found some validation for these major and minor depression categories. Specifically, only major depression shows a specific association with lesion location (Starkstein et al. 1987b) and produces a dementia of depression (Bolla-Wilson et al. 1989) as well as a failure to suppress serum cortisol following dexamethasone administration (Lipsey et al. 1985). Moreover, major depression spontaneously remits 1 to 2 years after the stroke, while minor depression lasts more than 2 years (Robinson et al. 1987).

A related question that remains unanswered, however, is whether PSD is phenomenologically similar to functional (i.e., no known neuropathology) depression. In a study specifically designed to address this issue, we found that the depressive syndrome profiles for 43 patients with major PSD were very similar to those found in 43 age-comparable patients with functional major depression (Lipsey et al. 1986). The only symptoms that were significantly different between these groups included slowness and psychomotor retardation, which were more common in the patients with stroke, and difficulty with concentration, which was more frequent in the patients with functional depression.

In conclusion, the evidence suggests that DSM-III diagnostic criteria can be used to make the diagnosis of depression among patients with stroke. Major PSD depression also is phenomenologically similar to "functional" depression in terms of clinical symptoms; however, minor PSD fulfills the diagnostic symptom criteria for dysthymic disorder and is distinguished from major depression in terms of cognitive impairment, duration, biologic markers, and response to treatment.

THE PREVALENCE OF POST-STROKE DEPRESSION

The prevalence of PSD has been studied in several settings. We examined this prevalence among patients attending an outpatient stroke unit who were from 1 month to more than 10 years after stroke; we found that 30% of the 103 consecutive patients examined were depressed (Robinson and Price 1982). Similar frequencies were reported by Feibel and Springer (1982), who found a 26% prevalence of depression in 91 stroke outpatients who were studied 6 months after their stroke. In a consecutive series of patients with stroke admitted to a general hospital, Ebrahim et al. (1987) reported that 23% of these patients had mild or moderate depressions, while another 23% had a severe depression.

Two community studies were reported recently as well. Wade et al. (1987) found 22% of patients were depressed 3 weeks after stroke, while another 11% were "probably" depressed. In the second study, Sharpe et al. (1990) examined 60 patients from a community-based stroke register and found that 18.3% had DSM-III-R diagnoses of depression and 13% a diagnosis of anxiety disorder.

Among patients referred to a rehabilitation unit, reported frequencies of depression also were quite high. Eastwood et al. (1989) found a frequency of depression (major or minor) of 54%, and Sinyor et al. (1986b) reported the prevalence of mild, moderate, and severe depression to be 17%, 23%, and 9%, respectively.

In conclusion, cross-sectional studies of patients admitted to either acute stroke units, general hospitals, or rehabilitation centers have demonstrated that approximately 30% to 50% of patients with stroke have a clinically significant depression. The same is true for community studies as well.

THE LONGITUDINAL EVOLUTION OF POST-STROKE DEPRESSION

We recently reported a prospective, longitudinal, 2-year follow-up study that included 103 patients who were hospitalized for an acute stroke (Robinson et al. 1987). At the time of the acute event, 27% of the patients had a symptom cluster of major depression, and 20% showed symptoms of minor (dysthymic) depression. At the 1-year follow-up, 60% of those with in-hospital major depression who were available for interview were still depressed (20% with major and 40% with minor depression) (Fig. 3.1). However, only one patient had a major depression by the time of the 2-year follow-up, and only 2 patients had a minor depression. Among patients with an in-hospital diagnosis of minor depression, 57% had depression (28.5% major and 28.5% minor depression) at the 1-year follow-up, and 60% had depression at the 2-year follow-up (30% major and 30% minor depression). At the 1-year follow-up, 20% of the patients originally without depression were depressed (8% with major and 12% with minor depression), and at the 2-year follow-up, 34% of the patients originally without depression were depressed (19% with major and 15% with minor depression) (Fig. 3.1). This study demonstrates the prolonged nature of both major and minor depression; in addition,

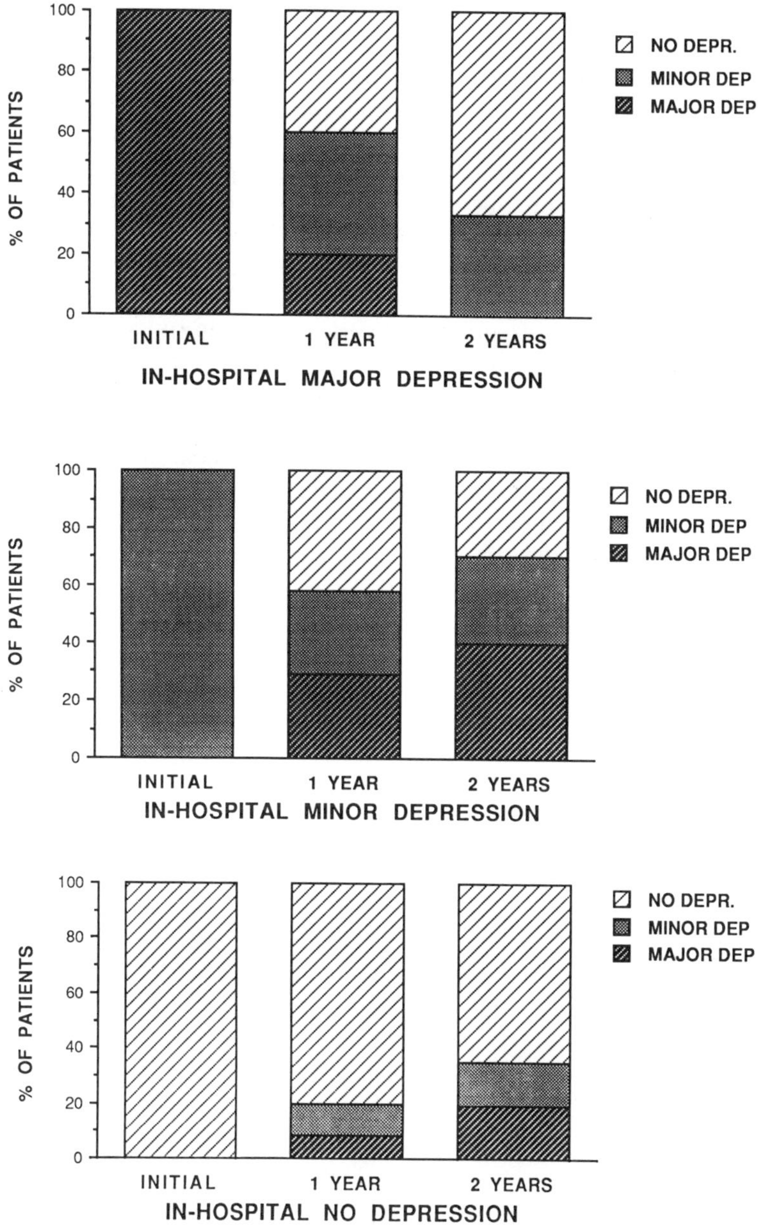

Figure 3.1. Outcome of depression at 1 and 2 years of follow-up for patients with in-hospital major depression (Major dep) (*upper panel*), in-hospital minor depression (Minor dep) (*middle panel*), and no depression (No depr.) in-hospital (*lower panel*). Major depression was no longer present in the majority of cases at 1 year, while more than half the patients with minor depression were still depressed (approximately half had developed major depression) at 2 years of follow-up. Some patients with no depression in-hospital developed a "delayed onset" major or minor depression during the 2 years of follow-up.

the absence of depression at the time of the acute stroke does not mean that patients will not develop depression at a later time.

To determine which factors contribute to the duration of depression, we compared patients who had developed PSD in the acute stage after the lesion but were not depressed 6 months after the stroke ($n = 6$) and patients with acute PSD who still remained depressed ($n = 10$) 6 months after the stroke (Starkstein et al. 1988e). We found that patients who had not recovered from depression had a significantly higher frequency of cortical lesions and a significantly greater degree of physical impairments; however, patients who did recover from the depression had a significantly higher frequency of subcortical or brainstem/cerebellar lesions. In a recent study that included a large population of patients with cerebellar/brainstem lesions, we confirmed this shorter duration of depressions produced by cerebellar/brainstem strokes as compared with depressions produced by lesions in the middle cerebral artery (MCA) territory (Starkstein et al. 1988c) (Fig. 3.2).

In conclusion, major depression lasts for approximately 1 year, while minor depression lasts for more than 2 years. Lesion location is an important factor influencing the duration of PSD, and patients

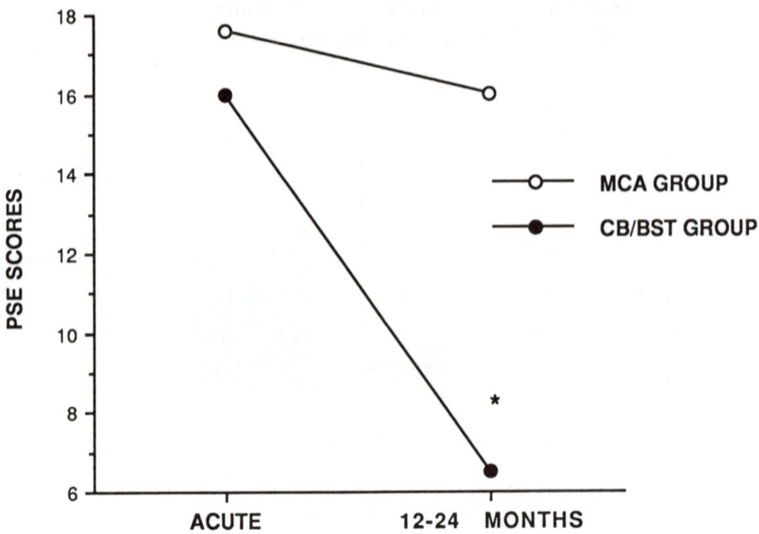

* Group × Trial $F(1,23) = 6.14$, $P < 0.01$

Figure 3.2. Severity of depression during 12 or more months of follow-up, measured by total PSE score in patients with stroke. Depressive symptoms improved significantly during follow-up in patients with cerebellar–brainstem (*CB/BST*) lesions compared with those having middle cerebral artery (*MCA*) lesions.

with subcortical or cerebellar/brainstem lesions have significantly briefer depressions than patients with lesions in the MCA territory.

LESION VARIABLES IN POST-STROKE DEPRESSION

THE IMPORTANCE OF LESION LOCATION

In several independent studies, we have demonstrated that lesion location is an important factor in the production of PSD. Patients with lesions in the left frontal cortex show a significantly higher frequency of depression than patients with more posterior lesions within the left hemisphere or patients with either anterior or posterior right hemisphere lesions. Moreover, we have found a significant correlation between distance from the lesion's anterior border to the frontal pole and depression scores (i.e., the more anterior the lesion, the more severe the depression).

Several investigators have tried to replicate these findings, and four have used methods comparable to ours. Both Sinyor et al. (1986b) and House et al. (1990) found a significant correlation between the distance of the lesion from the frontal pole and depression scores for patients with either left or right hemisphere lesions; however, no significant differences in the frequency of depression were found between patients with either left or right anterior lesions. In a study that used a similar methodology, Eastwood et al. (1989) found a significant correlation between lesion location and depression scores only in patients with left hemisphere lesions. So, while all five groups demonstrated that, among patients with left hemisphere lesions, the more anterior the lesion the more severe the depression, a similar correlation for right hemisphere lesions was not replicated consistently.

In a recent study that included a large number of patients with right hemisphere lesions, we examined this issue in more detail (Starkstein et al. 1989b). We studied a consecutive series of 94 patients with acute, single, right hemisphere lesions, and analysis of lesion location with CT scans demonstrated that six of nine patients (66%) with major depression and five of eight patients (63%) with minor depression had lesions involving the parietal lobe, compared with nine of 25 patients (36%) without mood changes and one of 12 patients (2%) with "undue cheerfulness" ($X^2 = 9.6$, df $= 2$, $P < 0.05$). Moreover, in a study using a different sample of patients with right hemisphere lesions, we found a significant correlation between the posterior border of the lesion to the occipital pole and depression scores ($r = 0.76$, $P < 0.01$) (i.e., more severe depressions were associated with more posterior lesions) (Robinson et al. 1984a). A similar association between posterior right hemisphere lesions and PSD also was reported by Finset et al. (1989).

In several prospective longitudinal studies, we found that the association between lesion location and depression is not static; it is dynamic. For example, we found that during the first 6 months after stroke, there was a changing association between right hemisphere lesions and depression scores. While immediately after the stroke lesion the closer the right hemisphere lesion was to the occipital pole the more severe the depression, the correlation was reversed by the sixth month of follow-up, and more anterior lesions correlated significantly with more severe depressions ($r = 0.63$, $P < 0.05$) (Robinson et al. 1984b). Both Sinyor et al. (1986b) and House et al. (1990), who examined their patients between the third and sixth month after the stroke lesion, reported a similar finding as well. Thus, the time since onset is a critical variable in the study of lesion location and depression in patients with right hemisphere strokes. The discrepancies between some of the studies described may lie in time-since-stroke differences when the patients were examined.

Glucose metabolic studies carried out in patients with functional depression provide additional evidence for the importance of the left anterior dysfunction in the production of depression. Baxter et al. (1989) reported that patients with functional depression had significantly lower metabolic activity in the left anterolateral prefrontal cortex than patients without depression who had other psychiatric conditions. They also found a significant correlation between frontal metabolic activity and depression scores (lower frontal metabolic activities were associated with more severe depressions).

SUBCORTICAL LESIONS AND POST-STROKE DEPRESSION

We also examined the importance of subcortical lesions in the production of PSD in two different studies. In the first, patients with left anterior subcortical lesions (mainly in the basal ganglia) had a significantly higher frequency of depression than patients with either left posterior subcortical lesions or patients with right anterior or right posterior subcortical lesions (Starkstein et al. 1987b); moreover, there was a significant correlation between the distance of the left subcortical lesion to the frontal pole and depression scores (i.e., more anterior lesions correlated with more severe depressions). In the second study, we examined the location of subcortical lesions in more detail, and patients with lesions in the left basal ganglia (mainly the head of the caudate) had a significantly higher frequency of major depression than patients with either right basal ganglia or right or left thalamic lesions (Starkstein et al. 1988b). These findings not only demonstrate that patients with subcortical lesions have the same lateralization of mood disorders as patients with cortical lesions, they also show that small subcortical lesions of the left hemisphere may produce a frequency of depression similar to that in patients with more extensive cortical lesions.

POSTERIOR CIRCULATION LESIONS AND POST-STROKE DEPRESSION

We recently examined the frequency, phenomenology, and course of depression after lesions in the posterior circulation territory (i.e., strokes involving primarily the cerebellum and/or brainstem) as well. While the phenomenology of PSD in patients with either posterior circulation or MCA lesions was similar, patients with posterior circulation lesions showed a significantly lower frequency of depression than patients with MCA lesions at both 6 months and 1 to 2 years after the stroke lesion (Starkstein et al. 1988c) (Fig. 3.3). As already mentioned, another significant difference was that the duration of PSD in patients with posterior circulation lesions was significantly shorter than in patients with MCA lesions. These findings

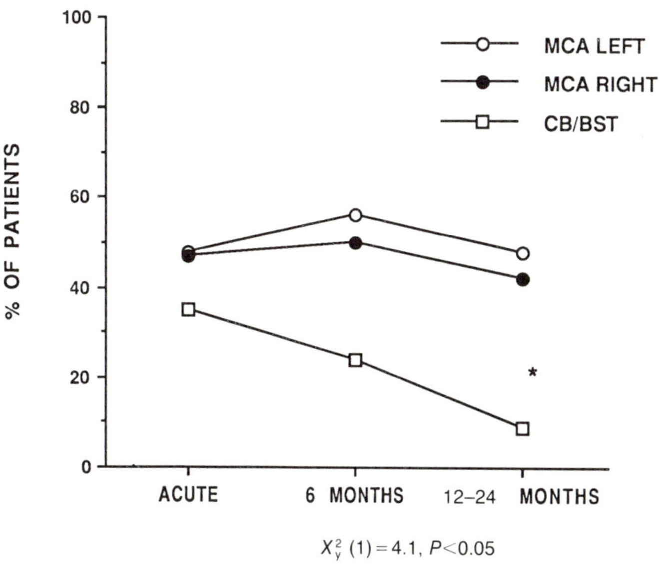

Figure 3.3. Frequency of depression (major plus minor) during 12 or more months of follow-up among patients with cerebrellar–brainstem (*CB/BST*) infarctions or left (MCA left) or right (MCA right) middle cerebral artery (*MCA*) infarctions. Patients with CB/BST lesions showed a lower frequency, which reached statistical significant at 12 months of follow-up.

suggest that the mechanism of depression after posterior circulation or MCA lesions may be different.

BRAIN ASYMMETRIES AND POST-STROKE DEPRESSION

Because most patients included in our studies were right-handed, the finding of a significant association between PSD and the side of the lesion (i.e., a significantly higher frequency of major depression in patients with left anterior lesions) may be related to handedness. To examine empirically this hypothesis, we studied a consecutive series of 30 left-handed patients with acute stroke lesions for the presence of depression (Robinson et al. 1985). While 10 of 18 left-handed patients with left hemisphere lesions were depressed, only one of the 12 left-handed patients with right hemisphere lesions was depressed ($X_y^2 = 5.7$, df = 1, $P < 0.05$). Moreover, the proximity of the anterior border of the left lesion to the frontal pole correlated significantly with depression scores (i.e., the closer the lesion to the frontal pole, the more severe the depression). These findings are similar to our own findings among right-handed patients with stroke lesions, and they demonstrate that brain specialization for handedness does not appear to be a major determinant in the lateralization of PSD.

Several authors have demonstrated that the left occipital area in normal human subjects is larger than the right, while the opposite is true for frontal areas. We examined the association between PSD and the pattern of brain asymmetries in a study that included a consecutive series of patients with a single acute stroke lesion (Starkstein et al. 1991b); based on CT scan measurements, patients were divided into those with typical or reversed frontal and/or occipital brain asymmetries. Among patients with a typical occipital asymmetry (n = 39), those with left anterior lesions showed a significantly higher frequency of major depression (seven of eight patients [88%]) than patients with a similar lesion location and a reversed occipital asymmetry (0 of four) (Fisher test, $P < 0.025$) or patients with a typical occipital asymmetry and lesions in other left posterior or right anterior or posterior brain areas (five of 31 [16%]) (Fig. 3.4). There was no significant association, however, between left anterior lesions and PSD among patients with a *reversed* occipital asymmetry (Fig. 3.4). Similar findings were observed when patients were divided into those with typical or reversed frontal plus occipital asymmetries; thus, this study empirically demonstrated that the significant association between major PSD and lesion location is restricted to patients with a typical, but not reversed, occipital asymmetry. (We will speculate later on the importance of this finding for the mechanism of PSD.)

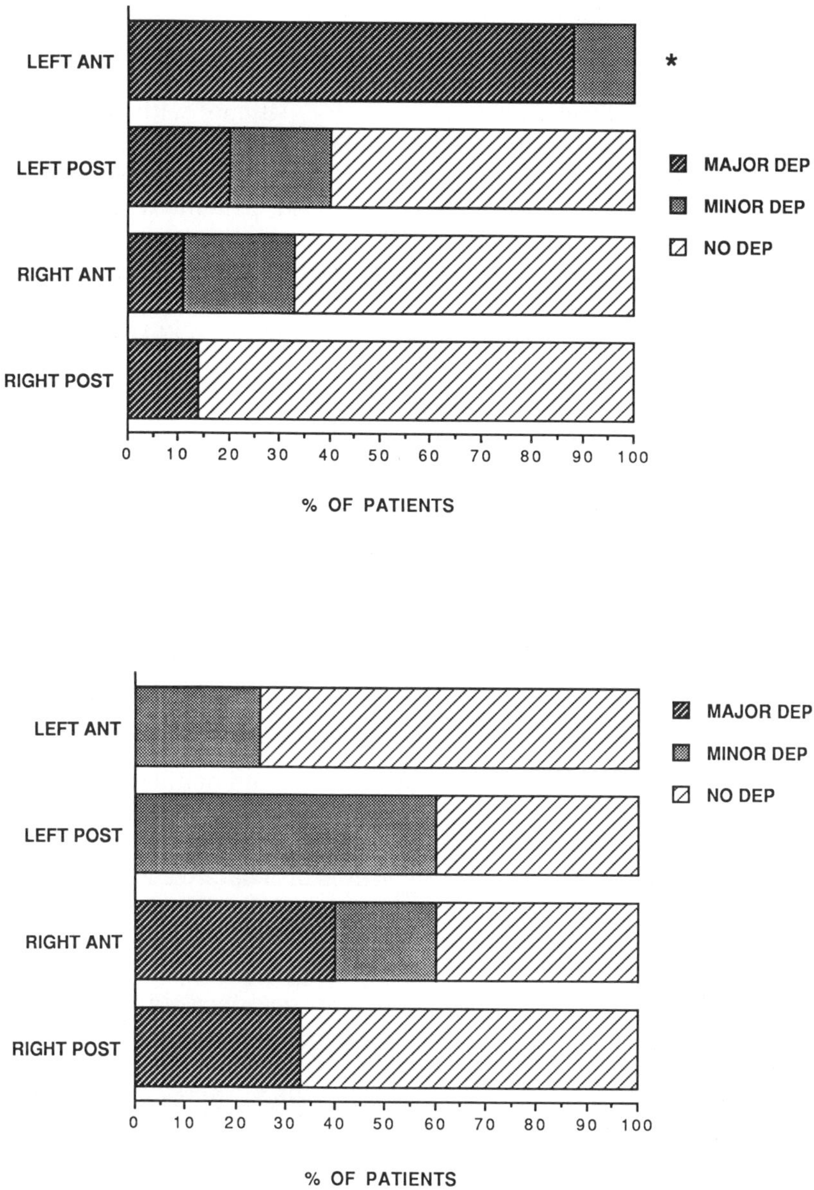

Figure 3.4. Among patients with typical occipital asymmetries (*top panel*), those with left anterior (*ANT*) lesions showed a significantly higher frequency of depression (*DEP*) than patients with any other lesion location. However, patients with reversed occipital asymmetries (*bottom panel*) did not show a significant association between frequency of depression and lesion location. The left anterior lesion groups (i.e., typical versus reversed pattern) were significantly different in their frequency of major depression. *Note:* POST = posterior.

In conclusion, lesion location is an important variable underlying the production of PSD. Several independent studies have found that the closer the lesion is to the frontal pole, the more severe the depression, and this correlation is stronger for patients with left hemisphere lesions. Patients with left frontal cortical or left basal ganglia lesions showed a significantly higher frequency of depression than patients with any other lesion location. Also, patients with cerebellar or brainstem lesions not only showed a significantly lower frequency of depression than patients with MCA lesions, but the depression was significantly shorter than in patients with MCA-related depressions. Finally, the association between PSD and lesion location is independent of handedness but is present only among patients with typical brain asymmetries.

POST-STROKE DEPRESSION AND RELATED VARIABLES

ASSOCIATION WITH OTHER PSYCHIATRIC DISORDERS

Anxiety and Post-Stroke Depression. Because anxiety is a common finding among patients with functional depression, we examined its frequency and correlates among patients with PSD in a prospective longitudinal study that included a consecutive series of patients with acute stroke in a 2 × 2 design (i.e., patients with major depression and anxiety, patients with depression but no anxiety, patients with anxiety but no depression, and patients with neither depression nor anxiety) (Starkstein et al. 1990a). The first important finding was that 23 of 47 patients (49%) with major PSD also met slightly modified (i.e., more restrictive) DSM-III criteria of generalized anxiety disorder; however, only six of 98 patients met DSM-III criteria for this disorder in the absence of depression.

The second finding was that 16 of 19 patients (84%) in the group with both anxiety and depression had cortical (mainly left frontal) lesions, compared with seven of 15 patients (47%) with depression only ($X^2 = 5.40$, df = 1, $P < 0.05$) and 13 of 27 (48%) with no mood disorders ($X^2 = 6.22$, df = 1, $P < 0.05$). Eight of 15 patients with major depression without anxiety, however, had subcortical (mainly basal ganglia) lesions compared with only two of 19 patients with anxious-depression ($X^2 = 7.40$, df = 1, $P < 0.01$).

Bipolar Disease after Stroke Lesions. Longitudinal studies of PSD have demonstrated that depression may occur at any time following stroke, ranging from immediately post-stroke to years after the acute event, and may last for months to years. We recently studied a small group of patients with a post-stroke bipolar disorder (Starkstein et al. 1991b), and this group consisted of seven patients with a depression immediately after the stroke who then developed one or more manic episodes. All seven patients had subcortical lesions in the right hemisphere (two with lesions of the caudate head, three with thalamic lesions, one with a pituitary tumor, and one with both cortical and subcortical right hemisphere damage). Other distinctive features of these patients were the presence of a significantly higher frequency of psychiatric disorders in their families compared with families of patients having no mood disorder following stroke, and significantly more subcortical atrophy as evidenced by enlarged ventricular:brain ratios (Starkstein et al. 1987a). Thus, post-stroke bipolar disorders may be quite rare, because they require a right hemisphere subcortical lesion in the presence of either a genetic vulnerability for affective disorder or a pre-existing subcortical brain atrophy.

PHYSICAL IMPAIRMENTS AND POST-STROKE DEPRESSION

Several studies have examined the importance of physical impairments in the production of PSD. While PSD has been considered by some as secondary to the physical impairments, most empiric studies have demonstrated a weak correlation between the severity of physical impairments and the severity of depression (Starkstein and Robinson 1989a). Three recent studies, however, demonstrated that depression influences the rate of recovery from physical impairments.

In a study that included patients with stroke admitted to a rehabilitation unit, Sinyor et al. (1986a) found that while patients without depression had a slight increase or no change in functional state over the first month following stroke, patients with depression had a significant decrease in function during this period. We followed a consecutive series of 25 patients with stroke having depression (major or minor) and 38 patients with stroke without depression for a 2-year period (Parikh et al. 1990); while both groups had similar impairments in the activities of daily living during the acute stage after stroke, the 2-year follow-up evaluation showed that patients with depression improved significantly less than patients without depression. Malec et al. (1990) also examined patients who were admitted to a rehabilitation clinic within the first 6 weeks after stroke and found that patients with depression were discharged significantly earlier than patients without depression.

In conclusion, several empiric studies have demonstrated that impairment in the activities of daily living is a poor predictor of PSD. Once PSD developed, however, this was an important variable in the recovery from physical impairments of patients with stroke, and patients with more severe depression showed less recovery in their activities of daily living.

COGNITIVE IMPAIRMENTS AND POST-STROKE DEPRESSION

Cognitive impairments are a frequent finding among elderly patients with depression, and recent studies have demonstrated this also is true for patients with PSD. We examined 53 patients with stroke using a comprehensive neuropsychologic battery (Bolla-Wilson et al. 1989). Ten patients with major PSD after a left hemisphere lesion had significantly more-severe cognitive impairments on five of nine cognitive domains than 16 patients with left hemisphere lesions but no depression. Deficits were most severe in tasks assessing orientation, language, visuoconstructional ability, executive motor functions, and frontal lobe tasks; however, no significant differences in cognitive performance were found between eight patients with major depression after right hemisphere lesions and 19 patients with a similar lesion location but no depression.

In another study, we examined the influence of PSD on the recovery from cognitive impairments (Robinson et al. 1986). After 6 months of follow-up, patients with in-hospital PSD showed significantly less recovery from cognitive impairments than patients without depression.

In conclusion, several studies demonstrated that PSD is associated significantly with cognitive impairments. This association is stronger for patients having major depression with left hemisphere lesions.

SOCIAL FUNCTIONING AND POST-STROKE DEPRESSION

The role of psychosocial factors in the production of PSD has not been examined extensively. Morris et al. (1990), however, recently found that among a group of 76 elderly patients (mean age, 71 years) in a rehabilitation hospital, the perception of a lack of support from a spouse caregiver was associated significantly with an increased frequency of major or minor depression (eight of 11 patients) compared with patients having strong spousal support (10 of 27) ($X^2 = 4.0$, $P < 0.05$). In addition, patients with poor social support had an average duration of depression of 40.8 weeks compared with 14.3 weeks for those with strong social support ($P = 0.04$).

Schulz et al. (1988) examined a consecutive series of patients with an acute stroke lesion as well as their primary social supports. They found that while some primary-support persons had high depression levels immediately after the stroke that decreased over the following 6 months, others had depression scores that increased from normal to clinically significant levels during the same period. Within the first 2 months after stroke, the most important predictors of depression in primary-support persons were stroke-related variables, such as stroke severity, and concern about future care; however, at 7 months after the stroke, demographic variables such as health, income, and age were the most important predictors. Among patients with stroke, overall analysis of the longitudinal data showed that increases in depression were related significantly to a decrease in reciprocal confiding relationships with intimate-network members and to a decrease in satisfaction with social concepts.

To summarize, evidence exists that psychosocial factors may play an important role in the development of PSD; in addition, depression in primary caregivers may have a direct impact on the psychologic well-being of stroke patients. (This aspect of PSD has not been extensively studied, but it deserves further investigation.)

RISK FACTORS OF POST-STROKE DEPRESSION

As indicated in the section on lesion variables, patients with left anterior stroke lesions have a significantly higher frequency of major depression than patients with lesions in any other brain area. Not every patient with a left anterior lesion, however, will develop depression; thus, we looked for potential risk factors that may predispose patients to develop PSD. Comparing 13 patients with and 13 without major PSD and matching them for age as well as lesion size and location (Starkstein et al. 1988d), we found no between-group differences in demographic characteristics or neurologic findings. Patients with depression, however, had significantly more subcortical atrophy (as evidenced by increased ventricular:brain ratios) than patients without depression. Because CT scans were performed within the first week after the brain lesion, and the increased ratios were found in the lateral ventricle contralateral to the lesions, atrophy probably existed before the brain injury. That 11 of the 13 pairs of patients had a left hemisphere lesion limits the finding of subcortical atrophy as a risk factor for the production of PSD to patients with left hemisphere lesions.

In another recent study, we examined the presence of risk factors for PSD among 93 patients with right hemisphere lesions (Starkstein et al. 1989b). Patients with major depression had a significantly higher frequency of familial history of mood disorders (i.e., approximately one third) than either patients without depression having right hemisphere lesions or patients with major depression after left hemisphere lesions (Fig. 3.5).

In conclusion, we found two important risk factors for the production of PSD. Subcortical atrophy was significantly more severe in depressed patients with left hemisphere lesions compared with patients having exactly the same lesions but without major depres-

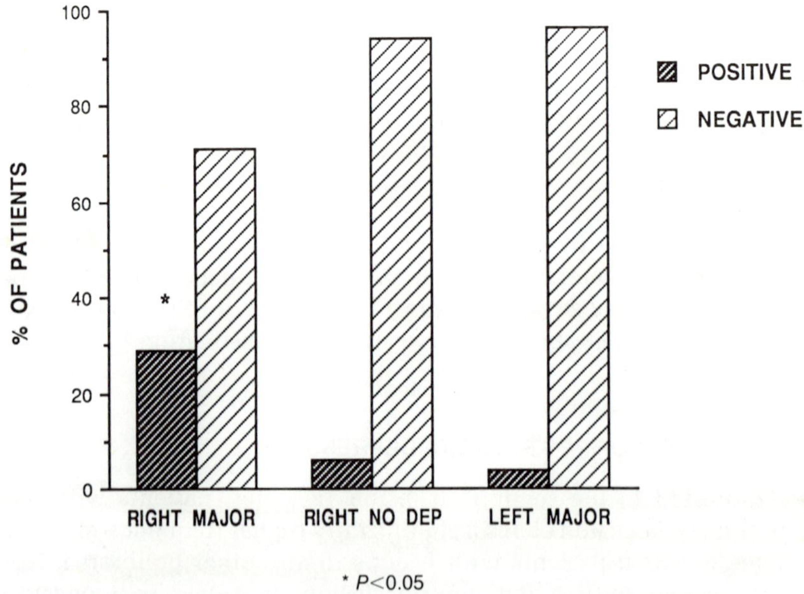

Figure 3.5. Patients with major depression after a right hemisphere stroke (n = 17) showed a significantly higher frequency of positive family history of psychiatric disorders (i.e., approximately 30%) than patients with either no depression after a right hemisphere stroke (n = 46) (i.e., approximately 5%) or patients with major depression after a left hemisphere lesion (n = 27) (i.e., approximately 3%).

sion. A genetic marker for depression was significantly more frequent in depressed patients with right hemisphere lesions.

BIOLOGICAL MARKERS OF POST-STROKE DEPRESSION

One of the unresolved problems of studying patients with stroke is how to diagnose depression in cases with moderate to severe comprehension impairment. Lim and Ebrahim (1983) reported that aphasic patients received significantly less antidepressant treatment than nonaphasic patients with stroke, even though on formal assessment they had similar frequencies of depression. One way to deal with this limitation would be to find a biologic depression marker of at least moderate sensitivity and high specificity for PSD. The dexamethasone suppression test (DST) was found to be a sensitive biologic marker of depression among patients with functional melancholic depression, and several studies have examined it as a biologic marker of PSD.

Finklestein et al. (1981) found a significant association between abnormal DST results and the presence of moderate to severe depression, loss of appetite, and sleep disturbances. In a study that included 65 patients with a recent or remote stroke, we found that 67% of patients with major depression, 25% of those with minor depression, and 32% of those without depression had an abnormal DST (i.e., they did not suppress the secretion of serum cortisol during the 24 hours after dexamethasone administration) (Lipsey et al. 1985). Thus, while the sensitivity of DST for major PSD was 67%, the specificity was only 70%. Another recent study included patients with chronic stroke, and the specificity of DST for PSD was found to be somewhat higher (83%) (Bauer et al. 1983).

In a study of 62 patients with acute strokes, Olsson et al. (1989) found a significant association between abnormal DST and proximity of the lesion to the frontal pole. Patients with left hemisphere lesions had a significantly higher frequency of major depression in this study.

Two investigators have reported a significant association between DST nonsuppression and lesion size, but the direction of this association is unclear. Lipsey et al. (1985) found a significantly higher frequency of abnormal DSTs in patients with large lesions; Olsson et al. (1989) reported a higher frequency of abnormal DSTs in patients with small lesions. Our previous studies showed that patients with small lesions in the left basal ganglia have the same frequency of depression as patients with large cortical lesions involving the dorsal lateral left frontal cortex; therefore, it is important to control for anterior–posterior distance when large and small lesions are compared. For example, patients with large left frontal cortical lesions may show more depression and abnormal DSTs than patients with small, more posterior, thalamic lesions (i.e., significant association between large lesions and abnormal DSTs). Patients with small lesions in the left head of the caudate (i.e., anterior), however, may show more depression and abnormal DSTs than patients with large left posterior cortical lesions (i.e., significant association between small lesions and abnormal DSTs). Thus, the significant interaction between anterior–posterior lesion location and depression must be controlled before the effect of lesion size on DST response can be assessed.

Barry and Dinan (1990) demonstrated a blunted growth-hormone response to desipramine in patients with functional depression. They examined this method as a biologic marker of PSD and found a specificity of 75% and sensitivity of 100% in such patients.

In conclusion, DST has not proved to be a useful biologic marker of PSD, because its specificity is only moderate. Future studies may demonstrate whether the GH response to desipramine is a more useful diagnostic test.

THE MECHANISM OF POST-STROKE DEPRESSION

The high prevalence of PSD among patients with left anterior lesions suggests that left anterior brain structures may play an important role in the mechanism of PSD. We previously suggested that lesions near the frontal pole and head of the caudate may damage the ascending biogenic amine pathways that run through the ventral striatum as well as anteriorly to posteriorly through the deep layers of the cortex (Starkstein et al. 1987b). These lesions, being more proximal to the cell bodies of monoaminergic nuclei, may disrupt significantly more fibers ascending to the cortex than do more caudal lesions.

While this hypothesis may explain the significant association between anterior lesions and PSD, it does not explain why left hemisphere lesions produce significantly more PSD. Significant asymmetries in subcortic biogenic amine innervation, however, have been described in both laboratory animals and human primates. We demonstrated in rats that brain lesions may produce a different behavior, depending on whether the lesion is in the left or right anterior cortex or ventral striatum (Starkstein et al. 1988a); lesions of the right frontal cortex of the right nucleus accumbens septi produce locomotor hyperactivity in rats, while similar lesions of the left hemisphere do not. Moreover, right (but not left) frontal lesions in rats produce bilateral depletions of cortical and brainstem norepinephrine as well as a bilateral decrease in cortical serotonergic ($5HT_2$) receptors (Mayberg et al. 1990). Using positron-emission tomography in patients with stroke, we also found lateralized change in serotonergic ($5HT_2$) receptors in the temporal and parietal cortex depending on the side of lesion (Mayberg et al. 1988).

In conclusion, the mechanism of PSD may involve the disruption of biogenic amine circuits produced by strategically located lesions. Also, the significant association between PSD and left hemisphere lesions may be related to a lateralized biogenic amine response to unilateral brain lesions.

THE TREATMENT OF POST-STROKE DEPRESSION

Although depression is one of the most readily treatable complications of stroke, relatively few studies have examined different treatment modalities prospectively. We conducted a randomized, double-blind, placebo-controlled study of the tricyclic drug nortriptyline in the treatment of PSD (Lipsey et al. 1984); the active group was treated with 20 mg for 1 week, 50 mg for 2 weeks, 75 mg for 1 week, and 100 mg for weeks 5 and 6. By the end of the study, all patients had achieved therapeutic (i.e., between 50 and 150 ng/ml) serum nortriptyline blood levels. Eleven of the 17 patients on active treatment completed the study. Three of six patients who did not finish the study experienced delirium; one had a sudden syncopal episode of unknown etiology, one complained of dizziness, and one complained of oversedation. Of the 22 patients who were on placebo, one developed mania, two refused interview, two died of recurrent cardiovascular disease, and two were lost to follow-up. The active and placebo groups were comparable in terms of demographic variables and neurologic, cognitive, and psychiatric deficits. By the end of the trial, patients on active treatment had significantly lower Hamilton Depression scores than patients who received placebo; moreover, patients with serum nortriptyline concentrations of approximately 100 ng/ml had significantly lower Hamilton Depression scores than patients with serum nortriptyline concentrations below this level. Finally, patients who received active treatment for 6 weeks showed significantly lower depression scores than patients who were treated for 4 weeks, and these findings suggest there may be an interaction between the duration of treatment and the serum concentration of nortriptyline, with either higher drug levels or longer duration of treatment providing optimal outcome.

Reding et al. (1986) conducted another double-blind treatment study of PSD using trazodone hydrochloride. The active drug was started at a dose of 50 mg/day at night, then increased by 50 mg every 3 days until a total dose of 200 mg was achieved. Patients with an abnormal DST who were on trazodone showed a significantly greater improvement in their scores of activities of daily living than did patients on placebo. The authors concluded that abnormal DST results may define a subgroup of patients with stroke and depression who are most likely to improve in their activities of daily living following treatment with antidepressant drugs.

A third study, although retrospective, also found that PSD may improve after treatment with a variety of antidepressant drugs (Finklestein et al. 1987). Moreover, it showed a significant relationship between improvement in both depression and ADL scores.

Tricyclic drugs should be used cautiously in elderly patients. Possible contraindications for their use include cardiac conduction abnormalities, recent myocardial infarction, urinary outlet obstruction, and narrow-angle glaucoma. Medications such as diuretics, β-blockers, and hypnotics may interact with tricyclic drugs and produce orthostatic hypotension and sedation. The most frequent side effects in the post-stroke population are delirium and sedation.

Electroconvulsive therapy is another useful treatment modality for PSD. In a retrospective study, Murray et al. (1987) found that 12 of 14 patients with PSD showed a marked improvement of depression after electroconvulsive therapy. In some patients, depression-related problems such as cognitive deficits and delusions also improved.

Other therapeutic modalities such as cognitive therapy also may be useful. The relative efficacy of these treatment modalities compared with tricyclic antidepressants, however, needs to be established through prospective controlled studies.

CONCLUSIONS

Post-stroke depression is one of the most frequent complications of brain injury, and approximately 40% of patients with an acute stroke lesion will show either a major or a minor depression. DSM-III symptom criteria for major or dysthymic (minor) depression appear to be valid criteria for the diagnosis of PSD. Depending on the site of lesion and the type of depression, PSD may last from 3 months to 1 or 2 years. Several studies have demonstrated a significant association between PSD and lesions in anterior areas of the left hemisphere (frontal cortex and head of the caudate), and half of the patients with PSD also will have a generalized anxiety disorder. Patients with anxious-depression are more likely to have cortical lesions than patients with depression only, who tend to have basal ganglia lesions. Several risk factors for PSD also have been identified; among patients with left hemisphere lesions, a mild degree of subcortical brain atrophy may predispose to depression, while among patients with right hemisphere lesions, those with a positive familial history of mood disorder may be at a greater risk to develop PSD. Patients with PSD also may show depression-related deficits, such as cognitive impairments and less recovery from their physical impairments. Finally, PSD may respond to tricyclic antidepressants or electroconvulsive therapy. Our hypothesis that PSD results from the disruption of asymmetric biochemical pathways will need further study.

ACKNOWLEDGMENTS

This work was supported in part by the following National Institute of Mental Health grants: MH40355, Research Scientist Award, MH00163 (RGR), as well as a Young Investigator Award from the National Alliance for Research in Schizophrenia and Depression; a grant from Institute of Neurological Investigation Raúl Carrea; and a grant from the Sandoz Foundation for Gerontological Research.

REFERENCES

American Psychiatric Association. 1980. *Diagnostic and Statistical Manual of Mental Disorders, 3rd Edition (DSM-III)*. Washington D.C.: American Psychiatric Press.

American Psychiatric Association. 1987. *Diagnostic and Statistical Manual of Mental Disorders 3rd Ed. Revised*. Washington D.C.: American Psychiatric Press.

Barry S, Dinan TG. 1990. Alpha-2 adrenergic receptor function in post-stroke depression. *Psychological Med* 20:305–309.

Bauer M, Gans JS, Harley JP, et al. 1983. Dexamethasone suppression test and depression in a rehabilitation setting. *Arch Phys Med Rehabil* 64:421–422.

Baxter LR, Schwartz JM, Phelps ME, et al. 1989. Reduction of prefrontal cortex glucose metabolism common to three types of depression. *Arch Gen Psychiatry* 46:243–250.

Bolla-Wilson K, Robinson RG, Starkstein SE, et al. 1989. Lateralization of dementia of depression in stroke patients. *Am J Psychiatry* 146:627–634.

Eastwood MR, Rifat SL, Nobbs H, et al. 1989. Mood disorder following cerebrovascular accident. *Br J Psychiatry* 154:195–200.

Ebrahim S, Nouri F. 1987. Affective illness after stroke. *Br J Psychiatry* 151:52–56.

Fedoroff JP, Starkstein SE, Price TR, et al. 1991. Are depressive symptoms non-specific in patients with acute stroke? *Am J Psychiatry* 148:1172–1176.

Feibel JH, Springer CJ. 1987. Depression and failure to resume social activities after stroke. *Arch Phys Med Rehabil* 68:772–776.

Finklestein S, Benowitz LI, Baldessarini. 1981. Mood, vegetative disturbance, and dexamethasone suppression test after stroke. *Ann Neurol* 12:463–468.

Finklestein SP, Weintraub RJ, Karmouz N. 1987. Antidepressant drug treatment for poststroke depression: retrospective study. *Arch Phys Med Rehab* 68:772–776.

Finset A, Goffeng L, Landro NI, et al. 1989. Depressed mood and intrahemispheric location of lesion in right hemisphere stroke patients. *Scand J Rehab Med* 21:1–6.

House A, Dennis M, Warlow C, et al. 1990. Mood disorders after stroke and their relation to lesion location. A CT scan study. *Brain* 113:1113–1130.

Lim ML, Ebrahim SBJ. 1983. Depression after stroke: a hospital treatment survey. *Postgrad Med J* 59:489–491.

Lipsey JR, Robinson RG, Pearlson GD, et al. 1985. Dexamethasone suppression test and mood following strokes. *Am J Psychiatry* 142:318–323.

Lipsey JR, Robinson RG, Pearlson GD, et al. 1984. Nortriptyline treatment for post-stroke depression: a double-blind trial. *Lancet* i:297–300.

Lipsey JR, Spencer WC, Rabins PV, et al. 1986. Phenomenological comparison of post-stroke depression and functional depression. *Am J Psychiatry* 143:527–529.

Malec JF, Richardson JW, Sinaki M, et al. 1990. Types of affective response to stroke. *Arch Phys Med Rehabil* 71:279–284.

Mayberg HS, Moran TH, Robinson RG. 1990. Remote lateralized changes in cortical [^{3}H] spiperone binding following focal frontal cortex lesions in the rat. *Brain Res* 516:127–132.

Mayberg HS, Robinson RG, Wong DF, et al. 1988. PET imaging of cortical S_2 serotonin receptors after stroke: lateralized changes and relationship to depression. *Am J Psychiatry* 145:937–943.

Millikan CK, McDowell F, Easton JD. 1987. *The Epidemiology of Stroke*. Philadelphia: Lea & Febiger.

Morris PLP, Robinson RG, Raphael B. 1990. Prevalence and course of post-stroke depression in hospitalized patients. *Int J Psychiatry Med* 20:327–342.

Murray GB, Shea V, Conn DK. 1987. Electroconvulsive therapy for post-stroke depression. *J Clin Psychiatry* 47:258–260.

Olsson T, Astrom M, Eriksson S, et al. 1989. Hypercorticolism revealed by the dexamethasone suppression test with acute ischemic stroke. *Stroke* 20:1685–1690.

Parikh RM, Robinson RG, Lipsey JR, et al. 1990. The impact of post-stroke depression on recovery in activities of daily living over a 2-year follow-up. *Arch Neurol* 47:785–789.

Reding MJ, Orto LA, Winter SW, et al. 1986. Antidepressant therapy after stroke: a double-blind trial. *Arch Neurol* 43:763–765.

Robinson RG, Bolduc PL, Price TR. 1987. Two-year longitudinal study of post-stroke mood disorders: diagnosis and outcome at one and two years. *Stroke* 18:837–843.

Robinson RG, Bolla-Wilson K, Kaplan E, et al. 1986. Depression influences intellectual impairment in stroke patients. *Br J Psychiatry* 148:541–547.

Robinson RG, Kubos KL, Starr LB, et al. 1984a. Mood disorders in stroke patients: importance of lesion location. *Brain* 107:81–93.

Robinson RG, Lipsey JR, Bolla-Wilson K, et al. 1985. Mood disorder in left-handed stroke patients. *Am J Psychiatry* 142:1424–1429.

Robinson RG, Price TR. 1982. Post-stroke depressive disorders: a follow-up study of 103 patients. *Stroke* 13:635–641.

Robinson RG, Starr LB, Lipsey JR, et al. 1984b. A two-year longitudinal study of post-stroke mood disorders: dynamic changes in associated variables over the first six months of follow-up. *Stroke* 15:510–516.

Schulz R, Tompkins CA, Rau MT. 1988. A longitudinal study of the psychosocial impact of stroke on primary support persons. *Psychol Aging* 3:131–141.

Sharpe M, Hawton K, House A, et al. 1990. Mood disorders in long-term survivors of stroke: associations with brain lesion location and volume. *Psychol Med* 20:815–828.

Sinyor D, Amato P, Kaloupek D, et al. 1986a. Post-stroke depression: relationship to functional impairment, coping strategies, and rehabilitation outcome. *Stroke* 17:1102–1107.

Sinyor D, Jacques P, Kaloupek DG, et al. 1986b. Post-stroke depression and lesion location: an attempted replication. *Brain* 109:537–546.

Starkstein SE, Bryer JB, Berthier ML, et al. 1991a. Depression after stroke: the importance of cerebral hemisphere asymmetries. *J Neuropsychiatry Clin Neurosci* 3:276–285.

Starkstein SE, Cohen BS, Fedoroff P, et al. 1990a. Relationship between anxiety disorders and depressive disorders in patients with cerebrovascular injury. *Arch Gen Psychiatry* 47:246–251.

Starkstein SE, Fedoroff P, Berthier ML, et al. 1991b. Manic-depressive and pure manic states after brain lesions. *Biol Psychiatry* 29:149–158.

Starkstein SE, Moran TH, Bowersox JA, et al. 1988a. Behavioral abnormalities induced by frontal cortical and nucleus accumbens lesions. *Brain Res* 473:74–80.

Starkstein SE, Pearlson GD, Boston JD, et al. 1987a. Mania after brain injury: a controlled study of causative factors. *Arch Neurol* 44:1069–1073.

Starkstein SE, Robinson RG. 1989a. Affective disorders and cerebral vascular disease. *Br J Psychiatry* 154:170–182.
Starkstein SE, Robinson RG, Berthier ML, et al. 1988b. Differential mood changes following basal ganglia vs thalamic lesions. *Arch Neurol* 45:725–730.
Starkstein SE, Robinson RG, Berthier ML, et al. 1988c. Depressive disorders following posterior circulation compared with middle cerebral artery infarcts. *Brain* 111:375–387.
Starkstein SE, Robinson RG, Honig MA, et al. 1989b. Mood changes after right-hemisphere lesions. *Br J Psychiatry* 155:79–85.
Starkstein SE, Robinson RG, Price TR. 1987b. Comparison of cortical and subcortical lesions in the production of post-stroke mood disorders. *Brain* 110:1045–1059.
Starkstein SE, Robinson RG, Price TR. 1988d. Comparison of patients with and without post-stroke major depression matched for size and location of lesions. *Arch Gen Psychiatry* 45:247–252.
Starkstein SE, Robinson RG, Price TR. 1988e. Comparison of spontaneously recovered versus nonrecovered patients with post-stroke depression. *Stroke* 19:1491–1496.
Wade DT, Legh-Smith JE, Hewer RA. 1987. Depressed mood after stroke: a community study of its frequency. *Br J Psychiatry* 141:200–205.

4

DEPRESSION IN ALZHEIMER DISEASE

David J. Loreck, M.D.
Marshal F. Folstein, M.D.

In 1907, Alzheimer described a 51-year-old woman suffering from multiple cognitive defects accompanied by delusions, hallucinations, and violent behavior (Alzheimer 1987). She died after 4.5 years of steady decline, and her brain showed what has come to be recognized as the characteristic features of Alzheimer disease: atrophy, neuronal loss, neurofibrillary tangles, and neuritic plaques. Although this patient cried and became fearful, depression of mood was not described. Despite recent studies indicating that depression often is an integral part of the psychiatric syndrome of Alzheimer disease, standardized methods for the assessment of depression in patients who are cognitively impaired are just emerging now. Depressed patients with Alzheimer disease appear to respond to standard antidepressant treatment, but depression remains an important predictor of a poor outcome. In this chapter, we report studies regarding the occurrence of depression in patients with Alzheimer disease and correlate the clinical features of depression with the neuropathologic and neurochemical changes found at autopsy.

CLINICAL DESCRIPTION OF THE SYNDROME

The clinical features of Alzheimer disease can be conceptualized as having two stages: an early stage, with symptoms and pathology related to the limbic system; and a late stage, related to the extension of the pathology into the parietal cortex. The earliest clinical manifestation typically is a memory disorder, and depression occurs during this early stage, when there is severe bilateral disease in the olfactory system and its connections in the amygdala, hippocampus, and hypothalamus. The ascending bioaminergic systems to the cortex, particularly the frontal lobe, pass through this area. As the dis-

Table 4.1. NINCDS-ADRDA Criteria for Clinical Diagnosis of Alzheimer Disease

I. The criteria for the clinical diagnosis of *probable* Alzheimer disease include:
   dementia established by clinical examination and documented by the Mini-Mental Test, Blessed Dementia Scale, or some similar examination, and confirmed by neuropsychological tests;
   deficits in two or more areas of cognitition;
   progressive worsening of memory and other cognitive functions;
   no disturbance of consciousness;
   onset between the ages of 40 and 90 years, most often after age 65; and
   absence of systemic disorders or other brain diseases that in and of themselves could account for the progressive deficits in memory and cognition.

II. The diagnosis of *probable* Alzheimer disease is supported by:
   progressive deterioration of specific cognitive functions, such as language (aphasia), motor skills (apraxia), and perception (agnosia);
   impaired activities of daily living and altered patterns of behavior;
   family history of similar disorders, particularly if confirmed neuropathologically; and laboratory results of:
      normal lumbar puncture as evaluated by standard techniques;
      normal pattern or nonspecific changes in EEG, such as increased slow-wave activity; and
      evidence of cerebral atrophy on CT with progression documented by serial observation.

III. Other clinical features consistent with the diagnosis of *probable* Alzheimer disease, after exclusion of causes of dementia other than Alzheimer disease, include:
   plateaus in the course of progression of the illness;
   associated symptoms of depression, insomnia, incontinence, delusions, illusions, hallucinations, catastrophic verbal, emotional, or physical outbursts, sexual disorders, and weight loss;
   other neurologic abnormalities in some patients, especially with more advanced disease and including motor signs such as increased muscle tone, myoclonus, or gait disorder;
   seizures in advanced disease; and
   CT normal for age.

IV. Clinical diagnosis of *possible* Alzheimer disease:
   may be made on the basis of the dementia syndrome, in the absence of other neurologic, psychiatric, or systemic disorders sufficient to cause dementia, and in the presence of variation in the onset, in the presentation, or in the clinical course;
   may be made in the presence of a second systemic or brain disorder sufficient to produce dementia, which is not considered to be *the* cause of the dementia; and
   should be used in research studies when a single, gradually progressive severe cognitive deficit is identified in the absence of other identifiable cause.

V. Criteria for diagnosis of *definite* Alzheimer disease are:
   the clinical criteria for probable Alzheimer disease, and
   histopathologic evidence obtained from a biopsy or autopsy.

VI. Classification of Alzheimer disease for research purposes should specify features that may differentiate subtypes of the disorder, such as:
   familial occurrence;
   onset before age 65;
   presence of trisomy 21; and
   coexistence of other relevant conditions such as Parkinson disease.

Source: McKhann et al. 1984.

ease advances to involve the parietal cortex, patients develop aphasia, apraxia, agnosia, delusions, and hallucinations.

The depression in Alzheimer disease often emerges gradually, with increased anxiety, crying, handwringing, pacing, hopelessness, sleep disturbance, and weight loss. Patients talk of death and suicide, but in our experience, suicide attempts rarely occur. This is perhaps because the patients lack the capacity to plan a suicide.

The diagnosis of depression in Alzheimer disease may be made in a patient who meets the requirements for probable Alzheimer disease set by National Institute for Neurological and Communicative Diseases and Stroke/Alzheimer's Disease and Related Disorders Association (Table 4.1), and who develops a depressive syndrome as defined in DSM-III-R (Table 4.2) criterion A. These criteria are more specific than those in the DSM-III, where a patient with depressed mood and disturbance of sleep as well as concentration impairment would meet the criteria for major depression. Because sleep and concentration disturbance occur in Alzheimer disease without depression, cases would be included that would not meet the DSM-III-R

Table 4.2. Diagnostic Criteria for Major Depressive Syndrome

At least five of the following symptoms have been present during the same 2-week period and represent a change from previous functioning, and at least one of the symptoms is either depressed mood or loss of interest or pleasure. (Do not include symptoms that are clearly due to a physical condition, mood-incongruent delusions or hallucinations, incoherence, or marked loosening of associations.)

1. Depressed mood (or can be irritable mood in children and adolescents) most of the day, nearly every day, as indicated either by subjective account or observation by others.
2. Markedly diminished interest or pleasure in all, or almost all, activities most of the day, nearly every day (as indicated either by subjective account or observation by others of apathy most of the time).
3. Significant weight loss or weight gain when not dieting (e.g., more than 5% of body weight in 1 month), or either decrease or increase in appetite nearly every day (in children, consider failure to make expected weight gains).
4. Insomnia or hypersomnia nearly every day.
5. Psychomotor agitation or retardation nearly every day (observable by others, not merely subjective feelings of restlessness or being slowed down).
6. Fatigue or loss of energy nearly every day.
7. Feelings of worthlessness or excessive or inappropriate guilt (which may be delusional) nearly every day (not merely self-reproach or guilt about being sick).
8. Diminished ability to think or concentrate, or indecisiveness, nearly every day (either by subjective account or as observed by others).
9. Recurrent thoughts of death (not just fear of dying), recurrent suicidal ideation without a specific plan, or a suicide attempt or a specific plan for committing suicide.

Source: American Psychiatric Association 1987.
Note: A "major depressive syndrome" is defined here as criterion A from the DSM-III-R.

criteria, which requires at least five criterion A symptoms; the DSM-III-R also includes a diagnosis of Alzheimer disease with depression that is less useful, as no specific criteria are provided.

Several investigators have questioned whether a depressive syndrome in Alzheimer disease can be distinguished from pseudodementia (also called *the dementia syndrome of depression*). In cases where the onset of dementia is recent and cognitive deterioration does not predate depressive symptoms, the diagnosis may be difficult, requiring time and treatment trials for clarification. However, in one study, no cases meeting the criteria for probable Alzheimer disease by NINCDS-ADRDA criteria and with depression emerged as reversible dementia on treatment or pathologic confirmation (Pearlson et al. 1990).

THE USE OF RATING SCALES FOR DEPRESSION IN ALZHEIMER DISEASE

There is limited research on the validity of standard depression scales when used with the demented patient. Gotlieb et al. (1988) evaluated the Brief Psychiatric Rating, Hamilton, and Zung scales in Alzheimer disease, and both the Brief Psychiatric Rating and Hamilton scales appeared to have good reliability and validity in mild cases, as well as fair reliability and validity in more severe cases. The Zung scale had only fair validity in mild cases and was not valid in severe cases. Sunderland et al. (1988) and Alexopoulos et al. (1988) attempted to address this issue by developing scales designed for the demented patient.

PREVALENCE

Estimates regarding the prevalence of depression in Alzheimer disease depend on the sampling and case-ascertainment methods. All estimates are from clinical samples, and these can be expected to be higher than true rates found in representative community samples.

Although reported prevalence estimates range from 0% to 86%, large studies using standard criteria for a major depressive syndrome in Alzheimer disease estimate the prevalence at from 10% to 20%. This is significantly higher than the reported rates of major depression in the general geriatric population (Blazer and Williams 1980) but similar to the rates of depression reported during other chronic medical conditions (Borson et al. 1986).

Reding et al. (1985) reported a prevalence of major depression (DSM-III criteria) of 19% in 99 patients with probable Alzheimer disease during the evaluation of 225 consecutive referrals to a dementia rehabilitation program. Reifler et al. (1982, 1986) reported the prevalence of major depression (DSM-III criteria) of 20% to 31% in patients with Alzheimer disease (DSM-III criteria) referred to a geriatric clinic, and Kral (1983) reported a prevalence of 15% in 40 patients with Alzheimer disease. Lopez et al. (1990) reported a 10% prevalence of major depression in patients with Alzheimer disease and a Mini-Mental Status score greater than 18.

Rovner et al. (1989) reported a prevalence of major depression (DSM-III criteria) of 17% in 144 patients with probable Alzheimer disease (NINCDS criteria). Pearlson et al. (1990) reported a 15% prevalence of DSM-III-R criteria major depression in 400 patients with Alzheimer disease (NINCDS criteria), which overlapped Rovner et al.'s sample of 144 referred to the Alzheimer Disease Research Center. Burns (1990) reported that 23.5% of 178 patients with probable Alzheimer disease who were evaluated at a British public health clinic by the Geriatric Mental State Schedule and Cambridge Diagnostic Examination for the Elderly schedules had "significant" depressive symptoms; 6% were on antidepressant medications even though no patients met the criteria for major depression.

Methods of sampling, case detection, and assessment account for the reports with extreme values, ranging from 0% to 86%. Knesevich et al. (1983) and Burke et al. (1988a) reported a prevalence of 0% but excluded all patients with a past or present history of major depression at the time of entry into the study. This exclusion criterion would powerfully affect the prevalence rate because most studies suggest both that a prior affective history is a risk factor for developing depression and that depression tends to occur early in the disease course. Similarly, Cummings et al. (1987) reported a 0% prevalence rate in a population of more advanced cases with a mean MMSE score of 10.8 and at a lower risk for depression.

The other extreme value (86% [Merriam et al. 1988]) was obtained by giving the Schedule for Affective Disorders and Schizophrenia–Change questionnaire to caregivers and not by examining the patients. This is consistent with studies that suggest caregivers rate patients as more depressed than the patients rate themselves. MacKenzie et al. (1989) evaluated 46 patients by DSM-III-R criteria and found the prevalence of depression by patient rating at 4.3% and by family rating at 30.6%. Teri and Wagner (1991) found that a mean Hamilton Depression Score in patients meeting the DSM-III-R criteria for major depression was 9.0% by patients and 15.2% by caregiver reports.

In summary, a review of studies suggests a prevalence of depression in Alzheimer disease of 10% to 20%. This value is affected by weighing informant versus patient data, selecting patients early versus late in the disease course, and using past or present psychiatric history as exclusion criteria for entry into studies. Higher rates also would be expected when drawing sample populations from psychiatric clinics or senior centers, which select for patients with impairments.

RISK FACTORS FOR DEPRESSION IN ALZHEIMER DISEASE

Pearlson et al. (1989) reported family history of depression to be a significant risk factor for developing depression in Alzheimer disease. They evaluated 400 consecutive patients referred to a dementia research clinic who met NINCDS-ADRDA criteria for probable Alzheimer disease by chart review. Fifteen percent had major depression (DSM-III criteria) at the initial or follow-up clinic visits. They excluded 18 of the patients who had a prior history of major depression before the onset of dementia, because they would be at high risk to have a family history of major affective illness. Of the 41 remaining patients with depression and Alzheimer disease, 46.3% had a first-degree relative with a major affective disorder compared with 11.3% of the nondepressed patients with Alzheimer disease. Family members with depression did not have an increased rate of dementia, thus suggesting that a genetic risk for depression, independent of Alzheimer disease, is associated with increased risk for depression during the course of Alzheimer disease.

Reifler et al. (1986a) and Lazarus et al. (1987) reported that depression occurs more frequently in women with Alzheimer disease than in men. Rovner et al. (1989a) reported a higher prevalence of depression in patients who were younger at the onset of Alzheimer disease. Rovner et al. also reported that past psychiatric history, particularly depression, is a risk factor; they found 33% of patients with Alzheimer disease and major depression had previous psychiatric treatment, most frequently for depression.

In summary, a prior history of depression, a family history of depression, younger age, and female gender have been reported as possible risk factors for depression in patients with Alzheimer disease.

DISEASE COURSE AND PROGNOSIS

Depression diminishes the patient's functional capacity, predicts early entry into nursing homes, and once in the nursing home, predicts greater morbidity and mortality. The majority of reports describe depression as occurring early in the disease course, and prevalence values above 20% are found in samples where Mini-Mental Status scores are 18 or higher. Lower prevalence values have been given in studies with Mini-Mental State scores below 15. Fisher et al. (1990) reported a correlation between depression and cognitive impairment of −0.5, indicating that patients with depression were less cognitively impaired than those without depression. Lazarus et al. (1987), however, reported one study that did not support this finding.

There have been no studies describing the duration, and few describing the severity, of depressive syndromes in Alzheimer disease. The existing studies report Hamilton scores for patients with depression and Alzheimer disease in the 12 to 18 range, compared with mean Hamilton scores above 20 for major depression in the general adult population. Lopez et al. (1990) reported that these patients did not differ significantly in their profile of neuropsychologic deficits or in the rate of cognitive deterioration compared with patients who are not depressed.

Recent studies suggest depression does affect the clinical course in Alzheimer disease. Pearson et al. (1989) evaluated 50 patients who met the criteria for probable Alzheimer disease; 20 of these 50 were diagnosed with a major depressive syndrome. Pearson et al. then proceeded to match the 20 patients with depression and the 20 patients without depression by age, physical mobility, and degree of cognitive impairment. Patients with depression were found to be much more impaired in activities of daily living.

These results are consistent with those of Steele et al. (1990), who evaluated the first 25 patients institutionalized from an Alzheimer's Disease Research Center patient cohort. These 25 patients were matched with 25 noninstitutionalized patients, and the Hamilton Depression score in the subsequently institutionalized patients was 7.9 compared with 3.0 for the noninstitutionalized patients. Also, Rovner et al. (1991) evaluated 454 consecutive admissions to local nursing homes and found that major depression independent of all other variables increased the 1-year mortality by 59 percent.

These studies indicate that depression has a profound effect on the prognosis of patients with Alzheimer disease. Depression is reported to diminish the patient's functional capacity, predict early entry into nursing homes, and once in the nursing home, predict greater morbidity and mortality.

PATHOGENESIS

The pathogenesis of depression in Alzheimer disease has not been established, but several probable mechanisms are emerging. The relatively high rate of autopsy in Alzheimer disease research populations allows clinicopathologic correlations seldom available in idiopathic depressive syndromes. These autopsies indicate extensive and disproportionate degeneration of the ascending aminergic systems in patients with depression and Alzheimer disease compared with nondepressed patients with Alzheimer disease.

Several studies report a consistent pattern of abnormalities in brainstem nuclei that produce biogenic amines. Specifically, there are relative decreases in the neurotransmitter levels in the locus ceruleus (norepinephrine), dorsal raphe nucleus (serotonin), and substantia nigra (dopamine) in patients with depression and Alzheimer disease. Zweig et al. (1988) reported a significantly more severe neuronal loss in both the locus ceruleus and the dorsal raphe nucleus in patients with depression and Alzheimer disease than in the nondepressed patients with Alzheimer disease. Zubenko et al. (1990) confirmed the extensive degeneration of locus ceruleus and also found neuronal loss in the substantia nigra, a major source for dopaminergic innervation; they found that the combination of locus ceruleus and substantia nigra pathology was a more powerful predictor for depression than pathology in either area alone. In a separate study, Zubenko and Moossy (1990) reported that patients with dementia and depression had a 10- to 20-fold decrease in cortical norepinephrine levels compared with patients suffering dementia who were not depressed. Serotonin levels also were decreased, but the decline was not statistically significant. D'Amato et al. (1987) reported similar findings as well, and Wolfe et al. (1990) reported low homovanillic acid (the primary dopamine breakdown metabolite) in the CSF of patients with Alzheimer disease who had extrapyramidal signs and depressive symptoms.

In contrast to studies indicating aminergic degeneration, Zubenko et al. (1990) reported relative preservation of the cholinergic system in patients with depression compared to those without depression. This is consistent with the study of Davis et al. (1987), where patients with Alzheimer disease became depressed after treatment with oxotremorine, a long-acting cholinergic agonist. Viewed together, these findings suggest that some level of cholinergic integrity is necessary for the expression of depressed mood, and they provide a pathologic basis for the observation that depression tends to occur early in the course of Alzheimer disease.

TREATMENT

Antidepressant treatments, including tricyclic antidepressants, monoamine oxidase inhibitors, and electroconvulsive therapy, have been reported to be effective in treating patients with Alzheimer disease who have a depressive syndrome. Most of these studies, however, have been limited to open trials and small sample sizes.

Reifler et al. (1989) reported a double-blind trial of imipramine in patients with Alzheimer disease and depression. Both the treatment and placebo groups experienced significant decrease in their Hamilton Depression score. Reifler (1986b) also gave 20 patients with depression and Alzheimer disease Doxepin or desipramine, with 85% improving in a 3-to-6-week period and the family reporting significant improvement in functional status, cheerfulness, and manageability; antidepressant treatment did not have a significant effect on cognitive status.

Reynolds et al. (1987) treated 16 patients with cognitive impairment and depression, eight of whom were diagnosed with Alzheimer disease. Of these eight patients, five were treated with nortriptyline at therapeutic levels and three with electroconvulsive therapy. Eighty-one percent had a positive clinical response, with the mean Hamilton score dropping from 17.0 to 9.0. There were no changes in Mini-Mental Status score either pre- or posttreatment. The concern that antidepressant medications might have negative effects on memory in Alzheimer disease was evaluated by Marcopoulos and Graves (1990), who found only a slight, but statistically significant, drop in memory performance.

There have been no controlled trials with monoamine oxidase inhibitors, although Ashford and Ford (1979) published a report of treating five patients having Alzheimer disease with notable improvement. Jenike (1985) also treated two patients who had failed tricyclic antidepressant medications using MAO inhibitors with a positive clinical response. Tariot et al. (1987) treated 17 patients with deprenyl (selegiline) and reported significant improvement in both anxiety and depressive symptoms.

There have been no placebo-controlled, double-blind studies with psychostimulants. Kaplitz (1975) treated 44 senile and apathetic patients with methylphenidate (10 to 30 mg) and reported significant improvement in energy, psychomotor retardation, and irritability. Branconnier and Cole (1980) reported treating patients with dementia using methylphenidate as well; the patients subsequently became less depressed and less confused.

Passeri et al. (1987) treated 63 patients with Alzheimer disease and 59 with multi-infarct dementia in a randomized, double-blind, placebo-controlled trial with minaprine (an aminopyridazine derivative) and reported improved mood in the treatment group compared with the placebo group. There also was cognitive improvement as well.

Several case reports indicate that patients with depression and Alzheimer disease respond to electroconvulsive treatment. Reynolds et al. (1987), Snow and Wells (1981), and Liang et al. (1988) all reported cases of electroconvulsive treatment improving affect in patients with depression and Alzheimer disease who have no cognitive complications.

CONCLUSIONS

Depression in Alzheimer disease constitutes a great burden for the individual patient and provides, through an experiment of nature, a model for idiopathic depression. For the patient with Alzheimer disease, depression must be detected early, because it is common, often predicts subsequent placement in a nursing home, increases mortality rates of institutionalized cases, and because effective treatment is available. As a model for affective disorders, Alzheimer disease invites further studies to illuminate the mechanism by which a genetically vulnerable aminergic system deteriorates. Depression is a syndrome, comparable to dementia or paralysis, and we can expect the etiology and pathogenesis to be heterogeneous. Further studies are likely to reveal pathology and etiology affecting several neurosystems and related in different cases to genetic, environmental, and possibly psychologic factors. Rational treatments will emerge from the comprehension of these mechanisms.

ACKNOWLEDGMENTS

This work was supported by the following grants: Alzheimer's Disease Research Center (NIA AG 05146), Columbia Predictors of Alzheimer's Disease (R01 AG07370-01A1), Genetic Linkage (NIHM 1 U01 MH46290), and Training Grant for Dementias of Aging (NIHM T32 AG00149).

REFERENCES

Alexopoulus GS, Abrams RC, Young RC, et al. 1988. Cornell Scale for depression in dementia. *Biol Psychiatry* 23:271–284.

Alzheimer A. 1987. About a peculiar disease of the cerebral cortex. *Alzheimer's Dis Assoc Disord* 1:7–8. (1907 article translated by Jarvik L).

American Psychiatric Association. 1987. *Diagnostic and Statistical Manual of Mental Disorders, 3rd Edition (Revised)*. Washington, D.C.: American Psychiatric Association Press.

Ashford JW, Ford CV. 1979. Use of MAO inhibitors in elderly patients. *Am J Psychiatry* 136:1466–1467.

Blazer D, Williams CD. 1980. Epidemiology of dysphoria and depression in an elderly population. *Am J Psychiatry* 137:439–443.

Borson S, Barnes RA, Kukull WA, et al. 1986. Symptomatic depression in elderly medical outpatients: I. Prevalence, demography, and health service utilization. *J Am Geriatr Soc* 34:341–347.

Branconnier RJ, Cole JO. 1980. The therapeutic role of methylphenidate in senile organic brain syndrome. In: Cole JO, Barrett JE, eds. *Psychopathology in the Aged*. New York: Raven Press.

Burke WJ, Rubin EH, Morris JC, et al. 1988a. Symptoms of depression in dementia of the Alzheimer type. *Alzheimer's Dis Assoc Disord* 2:356–362.

Burke WJ, Chung HD, Huang JS, et al. 1988b. Evidence of retrograde degeneration of epinephrine neurons in Alzheimer's disease. *Ann Neurol* 24:532–536.

Cummings J, Miller B, Hill MA, et al. 1987. Neuropsychiatric aspects of multi-infarct dementia and dementia of the Alzheimer type. *Arch Neurol* 44:389–393.

D'Amato RJ, Zweig RM, Whitehouse PJ, et al. 1987. Aminergic systems in Alzheimer's disease and Parkinson's disease. *Ann Neurol* 22:229–236.

Davis KL, Hollander E, Davidson M, et al. 1987. Induction of depression with oxotremorine in patients with Alzheimer's disease. *Am J Psychiatry* 144:468–471.

Fischer P, Simanyi M, Danielczyk W. 1990. Depression in dementia of the Alzheimer type and in multi-infarct dementia. *Am J Psychiatry* 147:1484–1487.

Gottlieb GL, Gur RE, Gur RC. 1988. Reliability of psychiatric scales in patients with dementia of the Alzheimer type. *Am J Psychiatry* 145:857–860.

Jenike MA. 1985. Monoamine oxidase inhibitors as treatment for depressed patients with primary degenerative dementia (Alzheimer's disease). *Am J Psychiatry* 142:763–764.

Kaplitz SE. 1975. Withdrawn, apathetic geriatric patients responsive to methylphenidate. *J Am Geriatr Soc* 23:271–276.

Knesevich JW, Martin RL, Berg L, et al. 1983. Preliminary report on affective symptoms in the early stages of senile dementia of the Alzheimer type. *Am J Psychiatry* 140:233–235.

Kral V. 1983. The relationship between senile dementia (Alzheimer type) and depression. *Can J Psych* 28:304–306.

Lazarus L, Newton N, Cohler B, et al. 1987. Frequency in presentation of depressive symptoms in patients with primary degenerate dementia. *Am J Psychiatry* 144:41–45.

Liang RA, Lam RW, Ancill RJ. 1988. ECT in the treatment of mixed depression. *Br J Psychiatry* 152:281–284.

Lopez OL, Boller F, Becker JT, et al. 1990. Alzheimer's disease and depression:neuropsychological impairment and progression of the illness. *Am J Psychiatry* 147:855–860.

Mackenzie TB, Robiner WN, Kropman DS. 1989. Differences between patient and family assessments of depression in Alzheimer's disease. *Am J Psychiatry* 146:1174–1178.

Marcopulos BA, Graves RE. 1990. Antidepressant effect on memory in depressed older persons. *J Clin Exp Neuropsychol* 12:655–663.

McKhann G, Drachman D, Folstein M, et al. Clinical diagnosis of Alzheimer's disease: report of the NINCDS-ADRDA Work Group under the auspices of the Department of Health and Human Services Task Force on Alzheimer's disease. *Neurology* 34:939–944.

Merriam AE, Aronson MK, Gaston P, et al. 1988. The psychiatric symptoms of Alzheimer's disease. *J Am Geriatr Soc* 36:7–12.

Passeri M, Cucinotta D, DeMello M, et al. 1987. Comparison of minaprine and placebo in the treatment of Alzheimer's disease and multi-infarct dementia. *Int J Geriatr Psychiatry* 2:97–104.

Pearlson GD, Ross CA, Lohr WD, et al. 1990. Association between family history of affective disorder and the depressive syndrome of Alzheimer's disease. *Am J Psychiatry* 147:452–456.

Pearlson GD, Rabins PV, Kim WS, et al. 1989. Structural brain CT changes and cognitive deficits in elderly depressives with and without reversible dementia ('pseudodementia'). *Psychol Med* 19:573–584.

Pearson JL, Teri L, Reifler BV, et al. 1989. Functional status and cognitive impairment in Alzheimer's patients with and without depression. *J Am Geriatr Soc* 37:1117–1121.

Reding M, Haycox J, Blass J. 1985. Depression in patients referred to a dementia clinic. *Arch Neurol* 42:894–896.

Reifler BV. 1986b. Mixed cognitive-affective disturbances in the elderly: a new classification. *J Clin Psychiatry* 47:354–356.

Reifler B, Larson E, Harley R. 1982. Coexistence of cognitive impairment and depression in geriatric outpatients. *Am J Psychiatry* 139:623–626.

Reifler BV, Larson E, Teri L, et al. 1986a. Dementia of the Alzheimer's type and depression. *J Am Geriatr Soc* 34:855–859.

Reifler BV, Teri L, Raskind M, et al. 1989. Double-blind trial of imipramine in Alzheimer's disease patients with and without depression. *Am J Psychiatry* 146:45–49.

Reynolds CF III, Perel JM, Kupfer DJ, et al. 1987. Open-trial response to antidepressant treatment in elderly patients with mixed depression and cognitive impairment. *Psychiatr Res* 21:111–122.

Rovner BW, Broadhead J, Spencer M, et al. 1989a. Depression and Alzheimer's disease. *Am J Psychiatry* 146:350–353.

Rovner BW, German PS, Brant LJ, et al. 1991. Depression and mortality in nursing homes. *JAMA* 265:993–996.

Rovner BW, Morriss RK. 1989b. Depression and Alzheimer's disease. In: Robinson RG, Rabins PV, eds. *Depression in Coexisting Disease.* New York: Ihaku-Shoin Medical Publishers, Inc., 14:202–211.

Snow SS, Wells CE. 1981. Case studies in neuropsychiatry: diagnosis and treatment of coexistent dementia and depression. *J Clin Psychiatry* 42:439–441.

Steele C, Rovner B, Chase GA, et al. 1990. Psychiatric symptoms and nursing home placement of patients with Alzheimer's disease. *Am J Psychiatry* 147:1049–1051.

Sunderland T, Alterman IS, Yount D, et al. 1988. A new scale for the assessment of depressed mood in demented patients. *Am J Psychiatry* 145:955–959.

Tariot PN, Sunderland T, Weingartner H, et al. 1987. L-Deprenyl in Alzheimer's disease. *Arch Gen Psychiatry* 44:427–433.

Teri L, Wagner AW. 1991. Assessment of depression in patients with Alzheimer's disease: concordance among informants. *Psychol Aging* 6:280–285.

Wolfe N, Katz D, Albert ML, et al. 1990. Neuropsychological profile linked to low dopamine: in Alzheimer's disease, major depression, and Parkinson's disease. *J Neurol Neurosurg Psychiatry* 53:915–917.

Zubenko GS, Moossy J. 1988. Major depression in primary dementia. *Arch Neurol* 45:1182–1186.
Zubenko GS, Moossy J, Kopp U. 1990. Neurochemical correlates of major depression in primary dementia. *Arch Neurol* 47:209–214.
Zweig RM, Ross CA, Hedreen JC, et al. 1988. The neuropathology of aminergic nuclei in Alzheimer's disease. *Ann Neurol* 24:233–242.

5

DEPRESSION IN EPILEPSY

Howard A. Ring, M.D.
Michael R. Trimble, M.D.

Depression is a clinically important concomitant of epilepsy. Hippocrates described a link between the two states: "Melancholics ordinarily become epileptics, and epileptics melancholics: of these two states what determines the preference is the direction the malady takes; if it bears upon the body, epilepsy, if upon the intelligence, melancholy" (Lewis 1934). This association has continued to intrigue observers (Temkin 1971). In his textbook on epilepsy, written at the beginning of the scientific approach to its treatment, Reynolds (1861) discussed the variety of interactions between mental state and seizures; he noted emotional disturbance as a cause of epilepsy, "depression of spirits" as an immediate prodroma of epileptic paroxysms, and depression and timidity as common interparoxysmal symptoms (particularly in men). More recently, a number of reviews have documented the nature of the association between depression and epilepsy (Barraclough 1981, Dodrill and Batzel 1986, Robertson 1988, Robertson 1989, Blumer 1991, Devinsky and Bear 1991). This chapter describes the nature of the affective disturbances reported in patients with epilepsy, summarizes the clinical and physiologic associations between the conditions, and explores potential biologic links that may underlie them as well as treatments suggested by these observations.

PREVALENCE

Most authors accept that depression is seen more often in epilepsy while bipolar affective disturbance is rare. The significance of the association, however, depends on the population studied.

Very few studies have investigated the absolute prevalence of psychiatric morbidity in epilepsy in the community, but two studies in

England assessed all patients with epilepsy who were registered with a number of primary health-care family physicians. In a sample of 218 patients, Pond and Bidwell (1959) recorded psychologic difficulties in 29%; in half of these, the difficulties were "neurotic" in nature. Fifteen years later, in a similar community-based survey of 88 patients, Edeh and Toone (1985) recorded neurotic depression in 22% of the sample. Hence, psychiatric disturbances often are seen in epilepsy, but in the absence of a similarly assessed, community control population, the significance of this frequency is difficult to interpret. Rutter et al. (1976), in their community-based Isle of Wight survey, found psychiatric disturbance in 58% of 8- to 10-year-old children with epilepsy. Considering a sample of patients with a single type of epilepsy, Currie et al. (1971) described clinically apparent anxiety in 19% and depression in 11% in their survey of 666 patients with temporal lobe epilepsy attending a London hospital for any reason over an 18-year period.

Studies investigating the prevalence of depression in epilepsy compared with control populations have recruited subjects from various sources, so a consensus result is unavailable. Kogeorgos et al. (1982) compared 66 outpatients with epilepsy and a matched group of chronic neurologic outpatients without epilepsy. These 66 outpatients also were compared with data from the general population using two self-rated questionnaire measures of psychopathology: the General Health Questionnaire and the Crown-Crisp Experiential Index. Kogeorgos et al. concluded that nearly half the patients with epilepsy had probable psychiatric disorders, and that more males than females were affected in comparison with their two other groups. Psychiatric morbidity was more prevalent in the group with epilepsy, but not significantly so when compared with the neurologic group. However, on measures of "free-floating anxiety," "depression," and "hysteria," the patients with epilepsy who were defined as having psychiatric disorders obtained significantly higher scores than the neurologic patients who were similarly defined, thus suggesting these problems were more severe in the epileptic group. Mendez et al. (1986) also investigated the prevalence of depression in 175 outpatients with epilepsy and 70 nonepileptic controls who attended similar vocational services for disabled people, and the authors describe their two populations as comparably disabled. Assessment was by means of a self-rated questionnaire, however, which only 35% of the patients with epilepsy and 38% of control subjects returned. Of these, 55% of the patients with epilepsy reported depression, compared with 30% of the matched controls.

The importance of understanding depression in epilepsy is highlighted when the frequency of suicide and parasuicide in this population is reviewed. Barraclough (1981), reviewing 11 previous studies, reported a suicide rate five times that of the general population. Mathews and Barabas (1981) reviewed eight studies and noted a suicide rate among patients with epilepsy of 5%, compared with 1.4% in control populations.

Mania is rarely associated with epilepsy; Williams (1956) described elation in just three of 2000 patients. The few cases reported in the literature are anecdotal accounts of individual cases (Barczak et al. 1988, Hurwitz et al. 1985).

There is clear evidence that depression is more common in people with epilepsy than in the population at large. The suggestion that it also is more common in these patients than in comparably disabled nonepileptic subjects supports a specific link between depression, but not mania, and epilepsy. To increase our understanding of this link between these conditions, we can examine the nature of affective disturbances in epilepsy.

DIAGNOSIS

Because an epileptic seizure is an event defined in time, many authors have used temporal definitions to characterize different associations between epilepsy and affective disturbance. This approach also may be of mechanistic interest because of the different cerebral processes operating both during and between seizures. The most common temporal separation is into prodromal, peri-ictal and interictal periods. The peri-ictal period includes the aura, the ictus itself, and the immediately postictal period. The affective disturbance associated with each of these stages initially is described separately, before the interaction between these is considered.

PRODROMAL PHENOMENA

The prodroma, occurring hours to days before a seizure, was investigated by Blanchet and Frommer (1986), who reported a prospective study in which 27 patients with epilepsy self-rated their moods using Personal Feelings Scales and recorded life events on a daily basis for at least 56 days. During this time, 13 patients had at least one seizure; the authors observed that in these patients, the mean ratings of mood on eight of the 10 scales showed a decline on the day or days preceding and an increase after the seizure. In four of these patients, the mean Depression Scale rating on the day preceding the seizure also was significantly lower than the mean rating on normal days. An increase in negative life events was reported by patients whose mood fell before seizures, but this correlation was not significant.

There are several possible explanations for the association between lowered mood ratings and the subsequent occurrence of seizures. Lower mood may be a symptom of the prodromal phase of seizure activity, initiated by the same biologic processes that bring about the seizure. Alternatively, it may be that the mood change itself precipitates a seizure. Blanchet and Frommer discussed these possibilities but concluded the question remains without a definitive answer, because in their study, the relationship of life events and mood to seizures apparently were independent.

PERI-ICTAL PHENOMENA

The aura is the earliest stage of the subjective awareness of seizure activity, and many different sensations have been recorded (Lennox and Cobb, 1933). The study of auras may be of value in locating lesions within the brain and the understanding of the neurophysiologic and psychopathologic mechanisms underlying the epileptic event itself as well as broader areas of cerebral functioning (Taylor and Lochery, 1987). Taylor and Lochery explored these issues by investigating 215 aura experiences of 88 patients with temporal lobe epilepsy. They recorded details of auras of various complexities and types, but it is noteworthy that even though there were 24 experiences of "epigastric fear," there were no reports of any other affective states.

Williams (1956) investigated emotional phenomena in 2000 patients with epilepsy and found that 100 reported an emotion as part of the "epileptic experience." As in the study by Taylor and Lochery (1987), the most commonly reported emotion was fear, occurring in 61% of the 100 patients with emotional phenomena in Williams' sample. On some occasions, this fear was quite pervasive, with psychic and somatic features; in contrast, depression was reported less often, in just 21% (i.e., 1% of the entire group). Williams observed, however, that when depression did occur, it tended to last for longer than the other peri-ictal phenomena, persisting for up to several days after the ictus. This was interpreted as being akin to naturally occurring depression, which tends to be self-sustaining. It may be severe in intensity and associated with suicidal behavior (Betts 1982).

Thus, peri-ictal depression, though it does occur, is not common but is characterized by a greater persistence than other emotional phenomena. It is interesting to note that depressive auras appear to be particularly rare, whereas fear is more common.

Peri-ictal mania is rare as well. Barczak et al. (1988) published a series of three patients with postictal hypomania, and all three cases were middle-aged men with right-sided temporal lobe epilepsy who became hypomanic following a series of seizures. Each displayed affect-laden hallucinations as well as delusions with a religious theme. These symptoms dispersed over 1 to 2 weeks.

INTERICTAL PHENOMENA

Several studies have investigated the phenomenology of interictal depression. Mendez et al. (1986) compared 20 depressed epileptic inpatients with 20 nonepileptic depressed subjects. Both groups met DSM-III criteria for major depression, and there were no differences between the groups with respect to the overall depression-scale scores and number of previous suicide attempts. The depressed control group, however, were significantly older and, interestingly, had a significantly more common family history of depression than the epilepsy group (11 versus 3 cases, respectively). Behavior and psychiatric symptoms were investigated in both groups using clinical interviews and medical records as well as the Hamilton Depression Scale and the Brief Psychiatric Rating Scale. All patients had endogenous features of depression (anergia, anhedonia, appetite and sleep disturbance), but the authors concluded that the major distinguishing characteristics of the patients with depression and epilepsy in respect to the nonepileptic group were a chronic dysthymic background, relative lack of neurotic traits such as somatization or self-pity, and a history of periods of agitated psychotic behavior. These psychotic episodes were described as having been peri-ictal.

Robertson et al. (1987) described the depressive phenomenology of a larger group of patients with epilepsy meeting Research Diagnostic Criteria for major depressive disorder. They assessed 66 patients using clinical examination and a number of standardized rating scales. In common with the findings of Mendez et al. (1986), the type of depression often was endogenous, on this occasion in approximately 40% as measured by the Newcastle Scale. The average severity of depression measured with the Beck Depression Inventory was 24.9, corresponding to a moderately severe depressive state. Patients in this study obtained very high state and trait anxiety scores using the Spielberger Inventory. The authors suggest that the high level of state anxiety may have been caused by the depression, because it decreased significantly during a 6-week, double-blind, placebo-controlled antidepressant trial (Robertson and Trimble 1985). Only 3% of the subjects had a history of bipolar illness.

ISSUES IN THE DIAGNOSIS OF DEPRESSION IN EPILEPSY

The research studies this chapter reviews generally have utilized various combinations of diagnostic criteria as well as self- and observer-rated questionnaires to make the diagnosis of depression. In routine clinical practice, the diagnosis most often will rely on the history and mental state examination, and in this context, it is important to consider the differential diagnosis of depression in epilepsy. In the first instance, this will depend on whether the patient already is known to have epilepsy. Betts (1982) described several instances in which affective disturbances were the presenting features of epilepsy and that in some cases led to initial misdiagnoses, for instance, hysteria or primary depression. In a further case history, Betts illustrated the situation in which an anxiety disorder may present with hyperventilation attacks that are misdiagnosed as epilepsy. All these examples serve to emphasize the importance of careful observation of the clinical phenomena manifested by the patient. In those known to have epilepsy, it is important to distinguish the development of depression requiring specific antidepressant treatment from toxicity associated with excessive anticonvulsant medication and peri-ictal affective disturbances associated with an increase in seizure frequency and the loss of affective responsiveness that may be seen in those patients developing a schizophreniform psychosis (Slater and Beard 1963).

ASSOCIATIONS OF DEPRESSION IN EPILEPSY

To seek some insight into the possible mechanisms of depression in epilepsy, it is important to examine the psychiatric and seizure characteristics that have been associated with depression in the various published studies including such data. Unfortunately, even though a number of studies have examined affective disturbance in epilepsy, data from these investigations are not strictly comparable. Patients were selected by various, differing entry criteria; affective disturbance was rated using different measures; and populations sampled have been drawn from the community (Edeh and Toone 1985), neuropsychiatric (Robertson et al. 1987) and neurologic (Kogeorgos et al. 1982) hospital outpatient clinics, psychiatric (Mendez et al. 1986) and general (Altshuler et al. 1990) inpatient units, and from patients awaiting temporal lobe surgery (Hermann and Wyler 1989). Table 5.1 lists some of the seizure- and treatment-related as well as other variables described in association with epilepsy and has been culled largely from the studies discussed here. It is far from exhaustive, but it does include conclusions drawn by various authors about the nature of some of the associations of depression in epilepsy. Consideration of these observations may suggest possible mechanisms that underlie the association of these two conditions.

Examination of the data suggests that some general observations may be made. It appears that neither seizure type (complex partial with or without secondary generalization or primary generalized seizures), frequency, nor duration of epilepsy are often associated with depression. The situation is more equivocal regarding the co-occurrence of a left-sided focus and interictal depression, and it appears

Table 5.1. The Associations of Depression in Epilepsy

Association	Studies Finding an Association	No Association
Seizure characteristics		
Type	8	5,9,14,18
Temporal focus	8,11	14
Left focus	1,8,11	3,7,9,14,18
Frequency	10	1,6,8,14
Duration	14	1,5,7,11
Treatment-related		
Polypharmacy	14,15,16	1,7,8
Phenobarbitone	2,14	
Low serum folate	4,12,13,17	
Personal factors		
Male preponderance	5	3,14
Loss of control	7	8
Family depression history	14	8

Note: Studies providing data: 1 = Altshuler et al. 1990; 2 = Brent et al. 1987; 3 = Currie et al. 1971; 4 = Edeh and Toone 1985; 5 = Kogeorgos et al. 1982; 6 = Kramer et al. 1987; 7 = Hermann and Wyler 1989; 8 = Mendez et al. 1986; 9 = Mendez et al. 1989; 10 = Moller and Froscher 1990; 11 = Perini and Mendius 1984; 12 = Reynolds et al. 1966; 13 = Robertson 1985; 14 = Robertson et al. 1987; 15 = Shorvon and Reynolds 1979; 16 = Thompson and Trimble 1982; 17 = Trimble et al. 1980; 18 = Williams 1956.

that a temporal focus is associated more often with depression than not. It should be noted that many of the studies in the literature did not contribute to these latter observations, because their entrance requirements included the diagnosis of temporal lobe epilepsy.

TREATMENT ASSOCIATIONS

Polypharmacy has been associated with depression by some authors, but others have failed to confirm this. Thompson and Trimble (1982) observed improvements in psychologic test performances, particularly those involving concentration and motor ability, in 20 patients who underwent a reduction in the number of different anticonvulsants prescribed from a mean of 2.8 to 1.6 drugs. In addition, this group also achieved significant reductions in anxiety and depression scores on the Middlesex Hospital Questionnaire when they were seen 6 months after the medication changes (Fig. 5.1). In this same study, a further group of 15 patients were prescribed carbamazepine after complete (in 7 patients) or partial withdrawal of other anticonvulsants. In the subgroup of these patients who had initially high depression scores on the Middlesex Hospital Questionnaire, there were significant reductions in the mean depression scores at both 3 and 6 months following the medication change (Fig. 5.2).

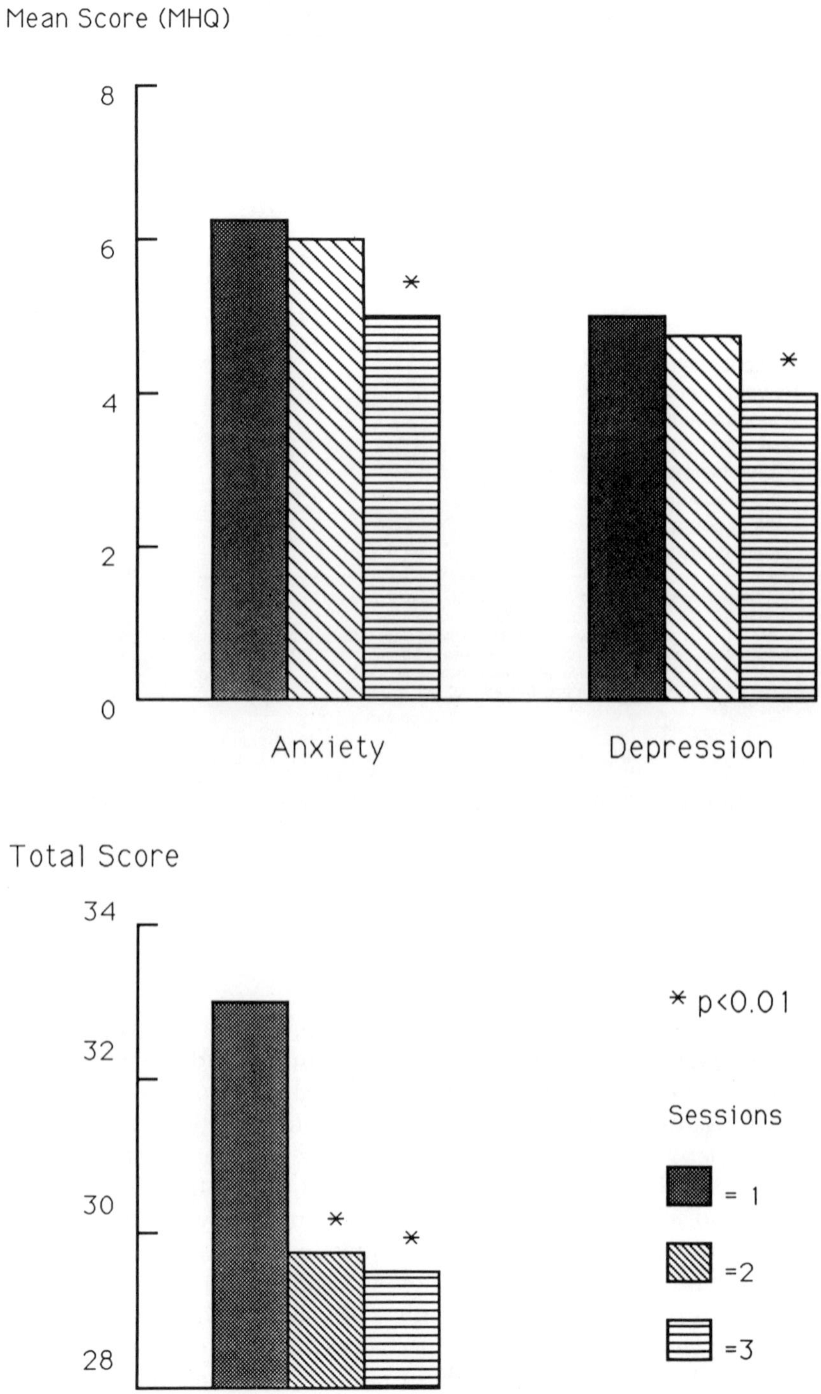

Figure 5.1. Middlesex Hospital Questionnaire (*MHQ*) anxiety and depression scores at baseline (*session 1*), 3 months (*session 2*), and 6 months (*session 3*) after the reduction of anticonvulsant polypharmacy.

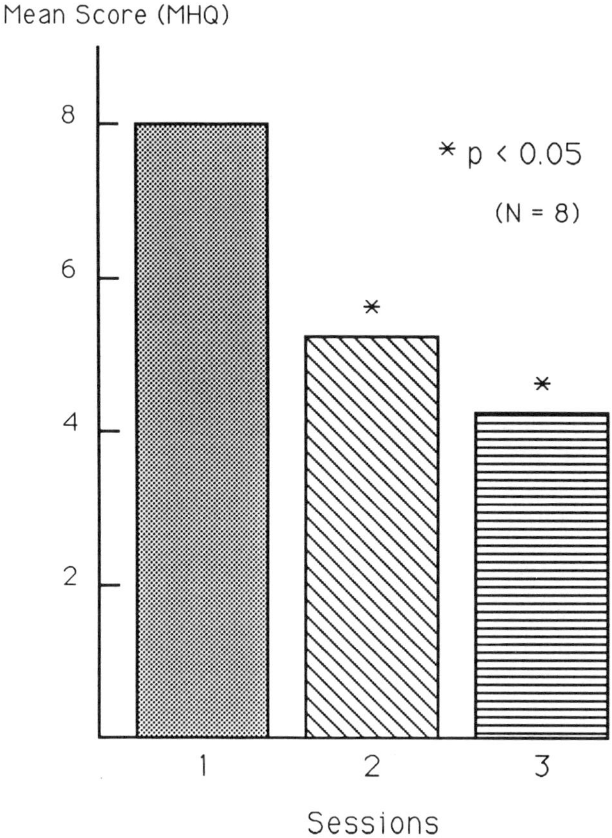

Figure 5.2. Middlesex Hospital Questionnaire (*MHQ*) depression scores in those with initially high values at baseline (*session 1*), 3 months (*session 2*), and 6 months (*session 3*) after the introduction of carbamazepine.

There is support for the observation that the use of phenobarbital is linked to the development of depression. This association has been reported in both adults (Robertson et al. 1987) and adolescents. Regarding adolescents, Brent et al. (1987) showed a much higher prevalence of major depressive disorder (40% versus 4%) and suicidal ideation (47% versus 4%) in those treated with phenobarbital who had a family history of depression.

Although only investigated in a limited number of studies, there also is some evidence that low folate may be associated with depression. Red blood cell folate is a more reliable guide to folate status than serum folate (Reynolds 1991), and the two studies contributing data to Table 5.1 both found that red blood cell folate was significantly lower in their subgroups having both epilepsy and depression than in the comparison groups (Reynolds et al. 1966, Edeh & Toone 1985).

Depression is more common in women in the population at large, but this gender difference does not appear to be maintained with interictal depression. Other recognized associations of depression in the general literature have not yet clearly been demonstrated or refuted in patients with epilepsy. In particular, associations with a family history of depression and a psychologic sense of loss of control in life remain equivocal.

POTENTIAL MECHANISMS FOR THE PATHOGENESIS OF DEPRESSION IN EPILEPSY

There is no currently established mechanism by which epilepsy may bring about clinical depression. However, based in part on some of the associations described in the preceding section, several hypotheses may be explored.

PSYCHOSOCIAL FACTORS

The social sequelae of having epilepsy were present more than 2000 years ago, when Hippocrates referred to the condition as the "sacred disease." Since that time, much has been written on the social stigmatization of those with epilepsy; even in our own, more enlightened times, there is evidence that this stigmatization persists (Betts 1982). The most powerful means for reducing this prejudice is educating the public to the realities of epilepsy. Such education for the families of those with epilepsy will reduce the stresses within some of those families; these stresses may contribute to the development of depression. Herman and Wyler (1989) investigated the adverse effects of stigma, discrimination, and the vocational difficulties and attendant strains of often unpredictable losses of consciousness using the psychologic construct of locus of control. Regarding a population of patients awaiting temporal lobe surgery for epilepsy, they concluded there was a significant association between an external locus of control (indicating a feeling of loss of personal control over life) and depression. In the following review of the potential biologic mechanisms of depression, it will be seen that the contribution of psychosocial factors may be the critical element in determining which of those individuals with a particular biologic state will develop depression.

SEIZURE-RELATED FACTORS

The frequency of temporal lobe foci in patients with depression is of interest in the light of animal studies regarding kindling. Experimental kindling is a phenomenon in which repeated subthreshold electrical stimulation leads to the subsequent development of seizure activity; it is produced most readily in limbic structures, particularly the amygdala and hippocampus (Trimble 1988, Adamec 1990). Although kindling in the strictest sense is not ethically demonstrable in humans, it has been demonstrated in every other vertebrate tested (Racine et al. 1989), and in humans, the kindling model has been applied to a number of clinical states, including initial seizure development, the progression of clinical epilepsy, and several behavioral disturbances (Bolwig and Trimble 1989).

Adamec (1990) reviewed the relevance of kindling models for understanding human neurologic and psychiatric disorders. In particular, he reported that patients with epilepsy who were also classified as having a psychiatric condition were more likely to report auras involving formed images, humming or buzzing, and irritability. These experiences, experimentally, are associated with the stimulation of limbic structures in humans. Adamec argues that if the intensity of subjective experience is related to the intensity of limbic activation, then the kindling analogy is viable, and repeated seizure involvement of limbic tissue (regardless of the seizure type) may lead to kindling-like processes that alter limbic function interictally. It is thus suggested that limbic activation during seizures is associated with interictal psychopathology. However, recalling that only a minority of patients with limbic involvement in their epilepsy develop significant psychopathology, Adamec concluded that the proposed change in limbic functioning does not cause depression directly but rather increases the individual's vulnerability to both psychologic and social stresses.

The role of the temporal lobe in the generation of affective states also may be investigated by considering the effects of temporal lobe surgery performed for the control of epilepsy. Jensen and Larsen (1979), after following up 74 patients treated with an anterior temporal lobectomy, concluded that improvement in psychiatric status correlated with relief from seizures. This was most true for behavioral disturbances, including those associated with attempted suicide, but was not the case for schizophrenia-like psychoses.

It is difficult to establish the relative contributions to an improved mood from the understandable relief and change in life circumstances that are associated with a dramatic reduction in seizures and from a possible biologic role of decreased limbic seizure activity, but the findings of Hermann & Wyler (1989) may shed some light on this relationship. They reported that of 24 patients rendered seizure-free following surgery, 18 showed a subsequent decrease in measures of depression (using the CES-D Scale), while only four increased their depression scores. However, of the 13 subjects who continued to have occasional seizures (but with at least a 75% reduction in frequency), there was no overall change in depression scores. The authors observed there was no concomitant shift in locus of control in the group with lower depression scores, while preoperatively, an external locus of control correlated positively with depression. Interpretations of these results include the possibility that the preoperative correlation was not meaningful or that, if it was, the psychiatric improvement postoperatively may have been from biologic effects of decreased seizures rather than a psychologic reaction to the change in state.

There also is some suggestion that in a minority of patients with chronic epilepsy, depression has worsened or developed de novo after temporal lobectomy (Devinsky and Bear 1991). If this should occur, then there is some evidence that it will do so acutely. Of 72 patients followed postoperatively for 1 to 2 years, six made suicide attempts; in every case, these attempts were in the first month after the operation (Jensen and Larsen 1979). An increase in depression following anterior temporal lobectomy also was described by Bruton (1988) in an analysis of the Falconer series of patients from the Maudsley Hospital. In this group of 249 patients, only one was considered depressed at the time of surgery, but during postoperative follow-up, the incidence of depression rose to 10% and six patients committed suicide. The mechanism of this effect is unknown, but the postoperative increase in depression may be in part an artifact of comparing rates at a single point in time preoperatively with those obtained over a prolonged postoperative follow-up period, extending from at least 1 year to more than 20 in several patients.

The studies contributing to Table 5.1 report conflicting results regarding laterality of the seizure focus in the genesis of depression. There are a number of studies in the neurologic literature, however, that demonstrated major depression is more often associated with left as opposed to right hemisphere cerebrovascular lesions whereas the rare development of post-stroke mania is strongly associated with a right hemisphere lesion in a limbic-connected area (Starkstein and Robinson 1989). With respect to epilepsy, the debate over the association of lateralization and psychopathology was initiated by Flor-Henry (1969), who suggested that a nondominant hemisphere abnormality was related to manic-depressive psychoses. There is little evidence to support this view, however, and those studies that demonstrated an association between the side of the lesion and depression have concluded (as with the findings concerning stroke) that a left hemisphere focus is more likely (Altshuler et al. 1990, Mendez et al, 1986, Perini and Mendius 1984).

Hurwitz et al. (1985) reported a woman with independent left- and right-sided temporal lobe discharges. After a left temporal discharge, she developed agitation, insomnia, and suicidal ideation; right-sided discharges evoked laughing and sexually disinhibited behavior. The authors suggested these changes resulted from release of the contralateral hemisphere after ipsilateral seizure inactivation. Also, although not providing an explanation of the association of hemisphere and psychopathology, Cutting (1990) reviewed suggestions that the right hemisphere has a lower "emotional baseline" than the left and is more sensitive to negative information. These observations, like those of Adamec (1990) described earlier, suggest that depression in epilepsy represents a combination of an increased biologic vulnerability and the action of psychosocial factors.

The reason that disagreement exists between studies concerning the existence of a left hemisphere–depression association (Table 5.1) is unclear. It is possible that it may relate to the observation by Starkstein and Robinson (1989) that this relationship only appears to hold for major and not minor depression; however, while it is difficult to test this hypothesis because of the different depression measures used in the various studies, this does not appear to be the solution. The mean Beck Depression Inventory scores described for their depressed subjects by Altshuler et al. (1990) of 12.2 and by Perini and Mendius (1984) of 9.5 correspond to relatively mild depression, while in the study by Robertson et al. (1987), who failed to find any lateralizing difference, one of the entry criteria was that subjects meet the Research Diagnostic Criteria for major depressive disorder. A relationship between depression and the side of epileptic focus, together with the implications of such a relationship, remains to be proven.

TREATMENT-RELATED FACTORS

Relationships between epilepsy, anticonvulsant medications, and mood have been reported (Robertson 1989, Robertson et al. 1987), and these authors noted that patients receiving phenobarbital were more depressed whereas those taking carbamazepine were both less depressed and less anxious. Phenobarbital is thought to enhance γ-aminobutyric acid (GABA) mediated postsynaptic inhibition as part of its anticonvulsant activity both experimentally and in patients (Engel 1989). A new anticonvulsant drug, vigabatrin, also increases activity in GABAergic pathways, and a small minority of patients who take vigabatrin become depressed in association with this treatment (Ring et al. 1990). In the study cited, this proportion was approximately 10%, but the prevalence of depressive symptoms is considerably lower in many other published studies investigating this drug (Ring and Reynolds 1992).

The development of depression following treatment with a substance that increases brain GABA concentrations is of particular interest considering the discussion over recent years as to whether GABA agonists have a role as antidepressants (Bartholini et al. 1986). As yet, evidence for such an effect is weak and, at times, even contradictory (Lloyd et al. 1987). Hence, the possibility that a treatment which increases GABA may be associated with the development of depression is worthy of examination. The involvement of GABAergic mechanisms in depression have been discussed widely (Bartholini et al. 1986), and a number of studies have measured CSF GABA concentrations in patients with psychiatric disorders. A common finding in several of these studies is significantly decreased GABA concentrations in patients with depression (Petty and Schlesser 1981, Petty and Sherman 1984, Gerner and Hare 1981, Gold et al. 1980, Kasa et al. 1982) and euthymic, medication-free, unipolar and bipolar patients (Berrettini et al. 1982, Berrettini et al. 1983).

The situation, however, is far from clear. Two studies (Post et al. 1980, Joffe et al. 1986) failed to find lower CSF GABA concentrations in patients with depression compared to normal individuals. In addition, it has been demonstrated (Gale 1989) that equivalent changes in GABAergic activity have different effects in different brain regions, such that experimentally, GABA elevation in most brain regions was not anticonvulsant, this effect being seen only following GABA augmentation in the substantia nigra. Thus, CSF GABA levels that reflect whole-brain GABA activity are unlikely to shed light on GABA concentrations in particular brain regions associated with specific functions. If increased GABA activity were antidepressant, then it might be expected that a clinically effective treatment such as electroconvulsive shock therapy would increase GABA concentrations; however, there is evidence to suggest that repeated electroconvulsive shock leads to a reduction in GABA release in the nucleus accumbens and striatum (Willner 1985). Thus, by implication, it may be that increased GABA release in these areas could be depressant.

Direct evidence that increased GABA activity may be depressant is limited. A small study (Nurnberger et al. 1986) in which GABA was administered intravenously to normal volunteers found an anxiogenic effect. It has been reported in a series using high-dose alprazolam in the study of panic disorder (Lydiard et al. 1987) that a major depressive disorder emerged in 33%, despite remission of their panic symptoms. The presumed mechanism of action of benzodiazepines is to augment the physiologic effects of GABA by acting at a site coupled to a postsynaptic GABA receptor to increase GABA binding (McGeer and McGeer 1989).

Thus, treatment-related depression in epilepsy may be mediated through increases in GABAergic activity. There is no evidence, however, that similar processes operate in those patients with epilepsy who become depressed in the absence of drug effects.

Another biochemical and treatment-related mechanism that has been suggested as contributing to depression in epilepsy is folate depletion (Reynolds 1991); a relationship between mental illness and folate deficiency was reported by Carney (1967). Phenytoin and barbiturates both may lead to falls in serum, red blood cell, and CSF folate. Edeh and Toone (1985) examined serum and red blood cell folate levels in a community sample of patients with epilepsy who were on mono- or polytherapy. They found significantly lower folate concentrations in those receiving polytherapy and in those achieving psychiatric "caseness" using the Clinical Interview Schedule. This was true for the depressive neurosis subgroup but not the anxiety subgroup; however, the authors emphasize that association does not imply causality and that the links between folate deficiency and mood change are unclear. There have been no successful therapeutic trials of folate in patients with depression and epilepsy, but a recent double-blind, placebo-controlled study of methylfolate in patients with DSM-III major depression (without epilepsy) demonstrated significantly improved clinical and social recovery associated with methylfolate administration (Godfrey et al. 1990). Regarding a possible mechanism of action, it has been pointed out that the folate cycle is involved in synthesizing methyl groups that in turn become involved in the action of S-adenosylmethionine, a methyl donor involved in the methylation of (among other things) neurotransmitters (Reynolds 1991).

TREATMENT

Because several factors may contribute to the development of depression in epilepsy, any treatment approach should address all of these areas. First, a clinical assessment of the severity of depression should be made because of the increased risk of suicide in those with epilepsy; subsequent actions will be determined by the result of this assessment. In addition, epilepsy, anticonvulsant, and psychosocial variables also should be examined.

SEIZURE STATUS

Seizure control should be optimized in treatment, and any change in the nature of the seizures should be considered. For instance, a recent increase in frequency or the development of secondarily generalized seizures in a patient with a focal epilepsy may be associated with the development of depression, both by virtue of the cerebral effects of the seizures and because of the increased disruption in the daily life of the patient. Both the development of depression and increase in seizure frequency may reduce patient compliance with anticonvulsant medication, thus leading to a vicious circle of worsening epilepsy and greater mood disturbance. It also may be the case that worsening epilepsy and changes in mental state indicate a progressive intracerebral pathology.

ANTICONVULSANT STATUS

The contributions of polytherapy and specific anticonvulsants (e.g., barbiturates, vigabatrin) to the development of depression have been discussed. Reduction in polytherapy has been reported to reduce depression, and the introduction of carbamazepine may be antidepressant (Thompson and Trimble 1982). Dalby (1975) drew together evidence that carbamazepine was associated with an improvement in affective state; this effect has been described in patients with epilepsy in whom carbamazepine was introduced and who were then observed to obtain lower depression scores on the Middlesex Hospital Questionnaire over the next 6 months (Thompson and Trimble 1982). Carbamazepine also has been demonstrated to be antidepressant in some patients with depression but not epilepsy in a double-blind, placebo-controlled trial (Post et al. 1986) as well as having a role as a prophylactic agent in the control of manic-depressive illness. Current evidence suggests that carbamazepine monotherapy is the optimum treatment for patients with seizures and affective disturbance.

SPECIFIC ANTIDEPRESSANT TREATMENTS

There appears to be little evidence that the use of monoamine oxidase inhibitors is associated with the occurrence of seizures (Robertson 1988). Seizures have been reported occasionally in depressed patients who are taking therapeutic doses of tricyclic antidepressants (Trimble 1978); however, a causal relationship is difficult to establish, in part because a small proportion of any large sample studied over time is likely to have a seizure caused by the onset of epilepsy during this time (Edwards 1985). A prospective study of the incidence of antidepressant-induced seizures found that those requiring treatment with an anticonvulsant medication occurred in less than one case in 1000 (Jick et al. 1983). All of these observations were made in patients without epilepsy, and the implications for those who have the condition are unclear. Edwards (1985) suggested that a family history of epilepsy is relevant, but Blumer (1991) concluded that lowering of the seizure threshold with modest doses of a tricyclic antidepressant is very rarely of clinical significance. Our experience, however, is less encouraging. The combined use of antidepressant and anticonvulsant medications has been associated with the development of drug interactions that require blood-level monitoring and dose adjustments of both classes of agents to maintain optimal therapeutic benefits (Richens et al. 1983). Thus, antidepressants that inhibit hepatic drug metabolism may increase serum anticonvulsant concentrations (Shader et al. 1978), and anticonvulsants may lower blood antidepressant concentrations.

Clinical practice varies, but successful treatment of depression in patients with epilepsy using antidepressant medications has been reported by several authors (Blumer 1991, Robertson and Trimble 1985). Regarding the choice of antidepressant, there is no clear answer. Monoamine oxidase inhibitors appear to be among the least likely to provoke seizures, but these have other difficulties associated with their use, such as the need for a special diet. Doxepin was investigated by Ojemann et al. (1983), who performed a retrospective analysis of its effect on seizure frequency in 19 patients with depression and epilepsy; depression improved to some extent in all patients. In addition, 15 patients experienced a reduction in seizure frequency during treatment. The mechanism of this latter effect is unknown, but the observation indicates doxepin was not associated with an exacerbation of seizures in this population. Fluvoxamine, protriptyline, and nortriptyline also have been suggested as being safer than other antidepressants (Robertson 1988), but their use has been associated with seizures.

Limited experience exists concerning the use of electroconvulsive therapy in epilepsy. Betts (1981) reported that it is not contraindicated in severe, treatment-resistant depression. With the attendant risk of suicide, it may be life-saving.

In view of the interplay of psychosocial and biologic factors in the genesis of depression, several authors also have pointed out the value of including the appropriate type of psychotherapy within the overall management plan (Devinsky and Bear 1991; Robertson 1988).

CONCLUSIONS

Good evidence exists that epilepsy and depression are associated in some way. There clearly is an increased suicide rate in those who have epilepsy; however, despite the large number of studies that have investigated the relationship between affective disturbance and seizures, the nature of this relationship remains obscure. Studies have reported both for and against various specific associations between affective state and psychosocial, seizure, and biochemical variables. In the absence of any clear consensus, it is impossible to define the mechanisms underlying an association. The many discrepancies between research methodologies utilized also make it difficult to meaningfully compare results across different studies. It is possible, however, to remain optimistic that as more comparable results are obtained, valuable insights will be gained into the relationship between a defined electrophysiologic disorder and the more ephemeral characteristics of depression. We then will have gained both a better understanding of how the brain works and a means to further reduce the suffering of those living with epilepsy.

ACKNOWLEDGMENTS

The authors are grateful for the support of the Raymond Way Memorial Fund.

REFERENCES

Adamec RE. 1990. Does kindling model anything clinically relevant? *Biol Psychiatry* 27:249–279.

Altshuler LL, Devinsky O, Post RM, et al. 1990. Depression, anxiety, and temporal lobe epilepsy: laterality of focus and symptoms. *Arch Neurol* 47:284–288.

Barczak P, Edmunds E, Betts T. 1988. Hypomania following complex partial seizures: a report of three cases. *Br J Psychiatry* 152:137–139.

Barraclough B. 1981. Suicide and epilepsy. In: Reynolds EH, Trimble MR, eds. *Epilepsy and Psychiatry*. Edinburgh: Churchill Livingstone, pp. 72–76.

Bartholini G, Lloyd KG, Morselli PI. 1986. *GABA and Mood Disorders: Experimental and Clinical Research*. New York: Raven Press.

Berrettini WH, Nurnberger JI, Hare T, et al. 1982. Plasma and CSF GABA in affective illness. *Br J Psychiatry* 141:483–487.

Berrettini WH, Nurnberger JI, Hare TA, et al. 1983. Reduced plasma and CSF gamma-aminobutyric acid in affective illness: effect of lithium carbonate. *Biol Psychiatry* 18:185–194.

Betts TA. 1981. Depression, anxiety and epilepsy. In: Reynolds EH, Trimble MR, eds. *Epilepsy and Psychiatry*. Edinburgh: Churchill Livingstone, pp. 60–71.

Betts TA. 1982. Psychiatry and epilepsy. In: Laidlaw J, Richens A, eds. *A Textbook of Epilepsy*. Edinburgh: Churchill Livingstone, pp. 227–270.

Blanchet P, Frommer GP. 1986. Mood change preceding epileptic seizures. *J Nerve Ment Dis* 174:471–476.

Blumer D. 1991. Epilepsy and disorders of mood. In: Smith D, Treiman D, Trimble M, eds. *Advances in Neurology, Vol. 55*. New York: Raven Press, pp. 185–195.

Bolwig TG, Trimble MR. 1989. *The Clinical Relevance of Kindling*. Chichester: John Wiley & Sons, 1989.

Brent DA, Crumrine PK, Varma RR, et al. 1987. Phenobarbital treatment and major depressive disorder in children with epilepsy. *Pediatrics* 80:909–917.

Bruton CJ. 1988. The neuropathology of temporal lobe epilepsy. Maudsley Monographs. Oxford: Oxford University Press.

Carney MWP. 1967. Serum folate values in 423 psychiatric patients. *BMJ* 4:512–516.

Currie S, Heathfield KWG, Henson RA, et al. 1971. Clinical course and prognosis of temporal lobe epilepsy: a survey of 666 patients. *Brain* 94:173–190.

Cutting J. 1990. *The Right Cerebral Hemisphere and Psychiatric Disorders.* Oxford: Oxford University Press.

Dalby MA. 1975. Behavioural effects of carbamazepine. In: Penry JK, Daly DD, eds. *Complex Partial Seizures and Their Treatment.* New York: Raven Press, pp. 331–344.

Devinsky O, Bear DM. 1991. Varieties of depression in epilepsy. *Neuropsychiatry Neuropsychol Behav Neurol* 4:49–61.

Dodrill CB, Batzel LW. 1986. Interictal behavioural features of patients with epilepsy. *Epilepsia* 27(Suppl 2):S64–S76.

Edeh J, Toone BK. 1985. Antiepileptic therapy, folate deficiency, and psychiatric morbidity: a general practice survey. *Epilepsia* 26:434–440.

Edwards JG. 1985. Antidepressants and seizures: epidemiological and clinical aspects. In: Trimble MR, eds. *The Psychopharmacology of Epilepsy.* Chichester: John Wiley & Sons, pp. 119–139.

Engel J Jr. 1989. *Seizures and Epilepsy.* Philadelphia: F.A. Davis.

Flor-Henry P. 1969. Psychosis and temporal lobe epilepsy: a controlled investigation. *Epilepsia* 10:363–395.

Gale K. 1989. GABA in epilepsy: the pharmacologic basis. *Epilepsia* 30 (Suppl 3):S1–S11.

Gerner RH, Hare TA. 1981. CSF GABA in normal subjects and patients with depression, schizophrenia, mania, and anorexia nervosa. *Am J Psychiatry* 138:1098–1101.

Godfrey PSA, Toone BK, Carney MWP, et al. 1990. Enhancement of recovery from psychiatric illness by methyfolate. *Lancet* 336:392–395.

Gold BI, Bowers MB, Roth RH, et al. 1980. GABA levels in CSF of patients with psychiatric disorders. *Am J Psychiatry* 137:362–364.

Hermann BP, Wyler AR. 1989. Depression, locus of control, and the effects of epilepsy surgery. *Epilepsia* 30:332–338.

Hurwitz TA, Wada JA, Kosaka BD, et al. 1985. Cerebral organization of affect suggested by temporal lobe seizures. *Neurology* 35:1335–1337.

Jensen I, Larsen JK. 1979. Mental aspects of temporal lobe epilepsy: follow-up of 74 patients after resection of a temporal lobe. *J Neurol Neurosurg Psychiatry* 42:256–265.

Jick H, Dinan BJ, Hunter JR, et al. 1983. Tricyclic antidepressants and convulsions. *J Clin Psychopharmacol* 3:182–185.

Joffe RT, Post RM, Rubinow DR, et al. 1986. Cerebrospinal fluid GABA in manic-depressive illness. In: Bartholini G, Lloyd KG, Morselli PL, eds. *GABA and Mood Disorders. Experimental and Clinical Research.* New York: Raven Press, pp. 187–199.

Kasa K, Otsuki S, Yamamoto M, et al. 1982. Cerebrospinal fluid gamma-aminobutyric acid and homovanillic acid in depressive disorders. *Biol Psychiatry* 17:877–883.

Kogeorgos J, Fonagy P, Scott DF. 1982. Psychiatric symptom patterns of chronic epileptics attending a neurological clinic: a controlled investigation. *Br J Psychiatry* 140:236–243.

Kramer LD, Fralin C, Berman NG, et al. 1987. Relationship of seizure frequency and interictal depression. *Epilepsia* 28:629.

Lennox WG, Cobb S. 1933. Epilepsy. XIII. Aura in epilepsy: a statistical review of 1359 cases. *Arch Neurol Psychiatry* 30:374–387.

Lewis AJ. 1934. Melancholia: a historical review. *J Ment Sci* 80:1–42.

Lloyd KG, Morselli PL, Bartholini G. 1987. GABA and affective disorders. *Med Biology* 65:159–165.

Lydiard RB, Laraia MT, Ballenger JC, et al. 1987. Emergence of depressive symptoms in patients receiving alprazolam for panic disorder. *Am J Psychiatry* 144:664–665.

Mathews WS, Barabas G. 1981. Suicide and epilepsy: a review of the literature. *Psychosomatics* 22:515–524.

McGeer PL, McGeer EG. 1989. Amino acid neurotransmitters. In: Siegel G, Agranoff B, Ablers RW, et al., eds. *Basic Neurochemistry*. New York: Raven Press, pp. 311–332.

Mendez MF, Cummings JL, Benson F. 1986. Depression in epilepsy: significance and phenomenology. *Arch Neurol* 43:766–770.

Mendez MF, Lanska DJ, Manon-Espaillat R, et al. 1989. Causative factors for suicide attempts by overdose in epileptics. *Arch Neurol* 46:1065–1068.

Moller AA, Froscher W. 1990. Depressive disorder of the epilepsy patient—symptoms and factors of influence. *Schweiz Arch Neurol Psychiatry* 141: 139–148.

Nurnberger JI, Berrettini WH, Simmons-Alling S, et al. 1986. Intravenous GABA administration is anxiogenic in man. *Psychiatr Res* 19:113–117.

Ojemann LM, Friel PN, Trejo WJ, et al. 1983. Effect of doxepin on seizure frequency in depressed epileptic patients. *Neurology* 33:646–648.

Perini G, Mendius R. 1984. Depression and anxiety in complex partial seizures. *J Nerve Ment Dis* 172:287–290.

Petty F, Schlesser MA. 1981. Plasma GABA in affective illness. A preliminary investigation. *J Affect Disord* 3:339–343.

Petty F, Sherman AD. 1984. Plasma GABA levels in psychiatric illness. *J. Affect Disord* 6:131–138.

Pond DA, Bidwell BH. 1959. A survey of epilepsy in fourteen general practices. II. Social and psychological aspects. *Epilepsia* 1:285–299.

Post RM, Ballenger JC, Hare TA, et al. 1980. CSF GABA in normals and patients with affective disorder. *Brain Res Bull* 5(suppl 2):755–759.

Post RM, Uhde TW, Roy-Byrne PP, et al. 1986. Antidepressant effects of carbamazepine. *Am J Psychiatry* 143:29–34.

Racine RJ, Ivy GO, Milgram NW. 1989. Kindling: clinical relevance and anatomical substrate. In: Bolwig TG, Trimble MR, eds. *The Clinical Relevance of Kindling*. Chichester: John Wiley & Sons, pp. 15–34.

Reynolds EH, Chanarin I, Milner G, et al. 1966. Anticonvulsant therapy, folic acid and vitamin B12 metabolism and mental symptoms. *Epilepsia* 7: 261–270.

Reynolds EH. 1991. Interictal psychiatric disorders. Neurochemical aspects. In: Smith D, Treiman D, Trimble M, eds. *Advances in Neurology, Vol. 55*. New York: Raven Press, pp. 47–58.

Reynolds JR. 1861. Epilepsy: Its Symptoms, Treatment and Relation to Other Chronic Convulsive Diseases. London: John Churchill.

Richens A, Nawishy S, Trimble M. 1983. Antidepressant drugs, convulsions and epilepsy. *Br J Clin Pharmacol* 15:295–298.

Ring HA, Heller AJ, Farr IN, et al. 1990. Vigabatrin: rational treatment for chronic epilepsy. *J Neurol Neurosurg Psychiatry* 53:1051–1055.
Ring HA, Reynolds EH. 1992. Vigabatrin. In: Pedley T, Meldrum BS, eds. *Recent Advances in Epilepsy* 5. London: Churchill Livingstone, pp. 177–195.
Robertson MM. 1988. Depression in patients with epilepsy reconsidered. In: Pedley TA, Meldrum BS, eds. *Recent Advances in Epilepsy, Vol. 4*. Edinburgh: Churchill Livingstone, pp. 205–240.
Robertson MM. 1989. The organic contribution to depressive illness in patients with epilepsy. *J Epilepsy* 2:189–230.
Robertson MM. 1985. Depression in patients with epilepsy: an overview and clinical study. In: Trimble MR, ed. *The Psychopharmacology of Epilepsy*. Chichester: John Wiley & Sons, pp. 65–82.
Robertson MM, Trimble MR. 1985. The treatment of depression in patients with epilepsy. A double-blind trial. *J Affect Disord* 9:127–136.
Robertson MM, Trimble MR, Townsend HRA. 1987. Phenomenology of depression in epilepsy. *Epilepsia* 28:364–372.
Rutter M, Tizard J, Yule W, et al. 1976. Isle of Wight studies, 1964–1974. *Psychol Med* 6:313–332.
Shader RI, Weinberger DR, Greenblatt DJ. 1978. Problems with drug interactions in treating brain disorders. *Psychiatr Clin North Am* 1:51–69.
Shorvon SD, Reynolds EH. 1979. Reduction in polypharmacy for epilepsy. *BMJ* 2:1023–1025.
Slater E, Beard AW. 1963. The schizophrenia-like psychoses of epilepsy. *Br J Psychiatry* 109:95–150.
Starkstein SE, Robinson RG. 1989. Affective disorders and cerebral vascular disease. *Br J Psychiatry* 154:170–182.
Taylor DC, Lochery M. 1987. Temporal lobe epilepsy: origin and significance of simple and complex auras. *J Neurol Neurosurg Psychiatry* 50:673–681.
Temkin O. 1971. *The Falling Sickness*. Baltimore: Johns Hopkins University Press.
Thompson PJ, Trimble MR. 1982. Anticonvulsant drugs and cognitive functions. *Epilepsia* 23:531–544.
Trimble M. 1978. Non-monoamine oxidase inhibitor antidepressants and epilepsy: a review. *Epilepsia* 19:241–250.
Trimble MR, Corbett JA, Donaldson D. 1980. Folic acid and mental symptoms in children with epilepsy. *J Neurol Neurosurg Psychiatry* 43:1030–1034.
Trimble MR. 1988. *Biological Psychiatry*. Chichester: John Wiley & Sons.
Williams D. 1956. The structure of emotions reflected in epileptic experiences. *Brain* 79:29–67.
Willner P. 1985. *Depression. A Psychological Synthesis*. New YorK: John Wiley & Sons.

6

DEPRESSION IN MULTIPLE SCLEROSIS*

Steven J. Huber, Ph.D.
Stephen M. Rao, Ph.D.

Multiple sclerosis (MS) is a common neurologic disease with a prevalence rate of approximately 60 per 100,000 individuals (Baum and Rothschild 1981, Kurtzke 1984). MS primarily is a disease of early to middle adulthood, the average age at onset of symptoms being approximately 30 years (Matthews et al. 1985). Pathologic changes primarily involve the central nervous system white matter; there are multiple patchy lesions that result from destruction of the myelin sheath and subsequent formation of demyelinated plaques (Matthews et al. 1985). The areas surrounding the ventricles are the most common sites of lesions (Brownwell and Hughes 1962).

The principal physical symptoms include motor weakness, incoordination, fatigue, spasticity, visual disturbances (e.g., reduced acuity, double vision), paresthesia, and bladder disturbance (Sibly 1990). The course of MS is highly variable; some patients experience frequent clinical exacerbations, with accumulating neurologic deficit, while others experience chronic progressive physical deterioration. A minority of patients experience a benign course that is characterized by few exacerbations followed by nearly complete remission of symptoms.

In addition to the physical symptoms, significant cognitive and emotional disturbances are common in patients with MS. Charcot (1877) first described the emotional changes and suggested that "the dominant feeling in the patients appears to be a sort of almost stupid indifference in reference to all things. It is not rare to see them give way to foolish laughter for no cause, and sometimes, on the contrary, melt into tears without reason." Cottrell and Wilson (1926) provided

*Portions of this chapter were adapted from Rao SM, Huber SJ, Borenstein RA. Emotional changes with multiple sclerosis and Parkinson's disease. *J Consult Clin Psychol* 1992; 60:369–378.

the first systematic description of the psychiatric symptoms, which they considered to be a common and integral aspect of MS.

Despite the early recognition of neurobehavioral symptoms in MS, this aspect did not receive serious and consistent attention until approximately 15 years ago (Rao 1990). This research coincided with the development of objective neuropsychologic procedures that allowed the researchers to examine behavioral symptoms in a quantifiable manner. It now is well recognized that neurobehavioral symptoms not only are common but also can represent a major source of disability for patients with MS. Proper clinical management includes careful examination of these symptoms.

Several emotional disturbances have been described in patients with MS, and these include bipolar disorders (Schiffer et al. 1986, Kellner et al. 1984), euphoria (Pratt 1951, Rabins et al. 1986), mania (Peselow et al. 1981, Kellner et al. 1984), and pathologic crying and laughing where there is dissociation between the expression of emotion and the internal mood state (Schiffer et al. 1985). Depression is the most common emotional change in MS (Ron and Logsdail 1989, Schiffer and Babigian 1984, Whitlock and Siskind 1980) and will be the focus of this chapter.

PREVALENCE

Depression in MS most often is characterized by anger, worry about the future, irritability, and discouragement (Minden et al. 1987, Whitlock and Siskind 1980). It also is important to consider that even in patients without major depression, a high proportion experience milder symptoms, including sadness or feeling blue, difficulty concentrating, social withdrawal, or lack of interest in usual activities (Minden et al. 1989).

The common occurrence of depression in MS is well established, but little is known regarding its prevalence, severity, and natural history. For example, prevalence estimates of depression in MS range from 27% to 54% (Minden and Schiffer 1990). Variation in patient populations and methods used to define depression probably accounts for these differences.

PATIENT SELECTION

Studies concerning prevalence require careful selection of the patient sample. The vast majority of studies relating to depression in MS are based on relatively small patient populations, which can differ in terms of several potentially important clinical variables. MS is a heterogeneous disorder in respect to the severity, nature and course of the symptoms, and the demographic characteristics. In addition to variability among patients, there may be considerable within-subject variability as well; for example, patients with MS are more likely to report emotional disorders when evaluated during an exacerbation than during periods of remission (Cleeland et al. 1970, Dalos et al. 1983). Because of this variability, prevalence studies need to document pertinent disease-related characteristics.

Recruitment bias represents another methodologic consideration in these studies. Most have examined patients from university settings, and such selection bias yields prevalence estimates that may not be applicable to the general population. In most cases, such patients tend to be affected more by the disease than is the case in the general-illness population (Nelson et al. 1988).

DIAGNOSIS AND ASSESSMENT

Early studies of depression in MS utilized subjective, and often unspecified, criteria to make the diagnosis. This lack of standardized criteria and objective evaluations made comparing the results of these studies difficult if not impossible. Thus, little progress was achieved in terms of defining the prevalence or characteristic features of depression in MS.

More recent studies have employed two methods to examine depression in MS. Some have focused on the symptoms of depression by using rating scales, whereas others used a syndrome approach by examining the proportion of patients who meet accepted diagnostic criteria for depressive disorders. There are advantages and disadvantages associated with each approach (Ron 1986).

Studies employing the syndrome model have been facilitated greatly by the development of formal diagnostic criteria, such as those defined in the DSM-III-R (American Psychiatric Association 1987). Application of these criteria permits the reliable identification of patient groups that can be compared with other studies using similar diagnostic criteria. The syndrome approach has a statistical disadvantage, however, because it provides only dichotomous data pertaining to depression.

The symptom approach has utilized several rating scales, including the Beck Depression Inventory (Beck et al. 1961), the Hamilton Depression Scale (Hamilton 1960), the Zung Depression Scale (Zung 1965), and the Minnesota Multiphasic Personality Inventory. The primary advantage of these procedures is that they provide continuous data, which allows examination of the relationship between the severity of depressive symptoms and the disease or demographic variables of interest.

The major disadvantage of both approaches when used to examine patients with MS concerns the overlap between depressive and neurologic symptoms (e.g., fatigue, sleep disturbances, psychomotor retardation); thus, total scores derived from depression scales may be difficult to interpret because of overlapping somatic features of depression and those related to MS. This confounding factor may distort attempts to examine the relationship between the severity of depressive symptoms and the disease-related factors, including severity or duration. In addition, this overlap would tend to inflate prevalence estimates of depression in MS. This problem may be most evident when examining patients with advanced disease.

Some studies using rating scales have attempted to avoid this problem by excluding those items with an apparent content overlap (Marsh et al. 1982). This approach is based on the assumption that specific features of depression in MS vary as a function of the disease severity (e.g., somatic features) while others (e.g., mood) may not. Thus, the relationship between depressive and motor changes might be evident for only some aspects of depression.

We examined the relationship between disease severity and specific features of depression as measured by the Beck Depression Inventory (Huber et al. 1992). Disease severity was rated according to the Expanded Disability Status Scale (Kurtzke 1965), and patients with a score of 0 to 2 were classified as mild and those with a score of 3 to 9 were classified as moderate to severe. Items from the Beck Depression Inventory were divided into those related to mood, self-reproach, vegetative, and somatic features of depression. Our results suggested there was no systematic relationship between the disease severity and any of the specific features of depression (Table 6.1). Symptoms related to mood, self-reproach, and somatic features were significantly higher in the patients having MS when compared with an age- and education-matched control group, but the magnitude of these elevated symptoms did not vary as a function of disease sever-

Table 6.1. Mean Beck Depression Inventory Scores

			Multiple Sclerosis Group			
Feature	Control Group[*]		Mild[†]		Moderate to Severe[‡]	ANOVA
Total	5.2	<	11.5	=	12.1	$P < 0.01$
Mood	1.7	<	3.2	=	3.5	$P < 0.01$
Self-reproach	0.9	<	2.6	=	3.0	$P < 0.01$
Vegetative	1.2	=	2.0	=	2.2	$P < 0.03$
Somatic	1.3	<	3.4	=	3.7	$P < 0.01$

Note: The pattern of post-hoc comparisons are indicated (=, <).
[*]$n = 47$.
[†]$n = 27$.
[‡]$n = 62$.

ity. This suggests that disease severity is not a confounding factor when examining depressive symptoms in MS.

CAUSES OF DEPRESSION IN MULTIPLE SCLEROSIS

The factors responsible for the high prevalence of depression in MS are unclear. Some have suggested that depression is an integral symptom of MS and is directly related to the alterations in brain function caused by demyelinated lesions (Schiffer et al. 1983, Schiffer and Babigian 1984, Whitlock and Siskind 1980). Others have suggested that the emotional changes result from a psychologic reaction to a progressively disabling and unpredictable disease (Surridge 1969, Baretz and Stevenson 1981, McIvor et al. 1984).

There is evidence to support both positions, suggesting that depression in MS results from a variety of causes. Variability exists even among the results of studies that used the same technique to evaluate this question. For example, the relationship between the severity of motor and depressive symptoms has been assumed to provide information related to the reactive versus endogenous distinction; some have found a modest correlation (McIvor et al. 1984), while others have found no relationship (Huber et al. 1992, Maybury and Brewin 1984, Schiffer and Wineman 1990, Rabins et al. 1986). This suggests that depression in MS is more complicated than the simple endogenous–reactive dichotomy would imply and is more likely to result from a multidimensional process. The following discussions review evidence supporting both the role of direct brain dysfunction and indirect reactive factors in depression during MS.

DIRECT MANIFESTATIONS OF BRAIN DYSFUNCTION

This section reviews evidence suggesting that depression in MS results directly from brain dysfunction. The four approaches discussed include comparison with other disabling conditions, clinical subgroups of patients, the relationship between depression and cognitive dysfunction, and the correlations with brain involvement using recently developed neuroimaging techniques.

Comparison with Other Disabling Conditions. Few areas of investigation pertaining to depression in MS have provided consistent results. One exception is the comparison of patients with MS to patients with other chronic physical disabilities; comparison groups include patients who suffer similar degrees of physical disability from diseases that do not primarily involve the central nervous system. Controlled studies on selected samples of patients with MS found that emotional disorders are more common in MS than in rheumatoid arthritis (Ron and Logsdail 1989), spinal cord injury

(Dalos et al. 1983, Rabins et al. 1986), muscular dystrophy (Surridge 1969), and amyotrophic lateral sclerosis (Schiffer and Babigian 1984). This suggests that the emotional changes associated with MS extend beyond those expected from a simple reaction to physical disability.

Clinical Subgroups. The identification of specific patient subgroups has been taken to support the hypothesis that the presence of brain lesions partly determines depressive symptoms. Two types of evidence have been proposed. Some studies have found that up to 20% of patients with MS and depression experience this emotional change before the onset of physical symptoms (Schiffer et al. 1983, Whitlock and Siskind 1980). In addition, two studies (Schiffer and Babigian 1984, Rabins et al. 1986) divided patients with MS into those with predominantly cerebral involvement and those with spinal cord lesions on the basis of clinical, EEG, and CT scan information; patients with cerebral involvement were more depressed in both studies. Thus, evidence derived from clinical subgroup studies suggests that direct brain involvement influences depressive symptoms.

Relationship Between Depression and Cognitive Impairment. Some degree of cognitive dysfunction is common in MS, occurring in 40% to 60% of patients (Peyser et al. 1990, Rao et al. 1991a). Two studies (Peyser et al. 1980, Rao et al. 1984) examined the relationship between cognitive impairment and Minnesota Multiphasic Personality Inventory profiles, and results suggested that patients with cognitive impairment and/or severe memory disturbance had elevations on scale 8 (schizophrenia) and those with normal cognitive status or mild memory disturbances were more likely to have elevations on scales 1 (hypochondriasis), 2 (depression), and 3 (hysteria). This suggests that patients having moderate to severe cognitive impairment are less likely to endorse items on scales that comprise the "neurotic triad" and more likely to endorse the unusual mental experiences that comprise scale 8. In contrast, patients with normal or mild cognitive disturbance are more likely to report concerns with physical functioning.

A more recent study (Rao et al. 1991b) examined this issue using two methods. Patients with MS completed the Zung Depression Scale (Zung 1965) and the State-Trait Anxiety Inventory (Spielberger et al. 1970), and their relatives or close friends completed the Katz Adjustment Scale (Katz and Lyerly 1963). There was no difference on the self-report scales between patients with and without cognitive impairment; however, patients with cognitive impairment were rated (Katz Adjustment Scale) as significantly more confused, apathetic, disinterested, helpless, and socially withdrawn than patients who were cognitively intact.

Neuroimaging Studies. Magnetic resonance imaging is the most sensitive imaging technique to detect brain lesions in MS (Gebarski et al. 1985, Stewart et al. 1987); the location of lesions visualized using MRI are similar to those of autopsy findings (Stewart et al. 1986). Attempts to correlate MRI findings with physical disability have provided inconsistent results (Huber et al. 1988, Stewart et al. 1987). In contrast, a more systematic relationship exists between MRI findings and neurobehavioral symptoms in MS. Total lesion area and atrophy of the corpus callosum consistently have been found to correlate with the severity of overall cognitive dysfunction as well as with several discrete cognitive functions, including memory, conceptual reasoning, speed of information processing, and interhemispheric transfer of information (Franklin et al. 1988, Huber et al. 1987, Rao et al. 1989).

Attempts to establish a relationship between MRI findings and emotional disturbances in MS also have met with some success. Ron and Logsdail (1989) did not find a significant relationship between total lesion area and the overall severity of psychiatric morbidity; further, they found no relationship with ratings of anxiety, depression, flattened affect, delusions, or thought disorder. There also was no relationship with the extent of cerebral demyelination, but significant relationships were established with the distribution of lesions. Ron and Logsdail found significant correlations between lesions in the temporoparietal regions and flattened affect, delusions, and thought disorder.

In a related study, Honer et al. (1987) compared the MRI findings in patients with MS and clinically significant affective disorders (e.g., bipolar affective disturbance, major depression, organic personality disorder) and those in patients with MS but no signs of affective disturbance. Consistent with Ron and Logsdail (1989), no group difference in respect to total lesion area was found, but the affectively disturbed MS group had significantly greater temporal lobe involvement than did the control group.

INDIRECT OR REACTIVE MECHANISMS

Multiple sclerosis is an unpredictable disease, with fluctuating symptoms that frequently mimic psychophysiologic disorders. It is not uncommon during the period between symptom onset and diagnosis, that patients are referred to psychotherapists for treatment of "conversion disorders." Thus, one could expect that these factors alone would play a major role in causing emotional distress, and to address these issues, investigators have examined the emotional change of patients in relation to both disease (e.g., clinical exacerbations, physical disability) and psychologic traits (e.g., locus of control, coping skills).

In general, emotional distress appears to increase with changes in physical symptoms. Two studies demonstrated that patients with MS display more psychopathology during periods of exacerbation (Cleeland et al. 1970, Dalos et al. 1983), and reported a modest relationship between depression and severity of the disease. The majority of studies have not found a significant relationship, but all have found that this relationship is positive. These associations suggest that changes in physical well-being have some effect on emotional status.

Some research also has been directed toward identification of the psychologic constructs that mediate emotional response to physical disability. It has been suggested that an internal locus of control correlates with better emotional adjustment (Brooks and Matson 1982, Halligan and Reznikoff 1985), that is, realistic recognition of greater dependency on others represents an important factor in the emotional adjustment to physical disability associated with MS. Further, patients who maintain social contact with able-bodied individuals appear to achieve better emotional adjustment to MS than patients who do not (Maybury and Brewin 1984).

THE TREATMENT OF DEPRESSION IN MULTIPLE SCLEROSIS

Only a small percentage of patients with MS receive treatment for psychiatric disturbances (Minden et al. 1987). In addition, there are relatively few studies related to the treatment of affective disturbances in MS; additional research in this area is necessary to improve the clinical management of MS.

Tricyclic antidepressant medications are used widely in clinical practice for a variety of illnesses, and they have been shown to be effective in neurologic disorders including stroke (Lipsey et al. 1984) and Parkinson disease (Anderson et al. 1980). To our knowledge, only one study has examined their effectiveness in treating depression associated with MS; Schiffer and Wineman (1990) performed a double-blind trial of desipramine in patients with MS and a major depressive disorder. Results indicated that a significantly greater proportion of treated patients had improved depressive symptoms compared with untreated controls, and this effect was unrelated to disability status. There were, however, side effects, including postural hypotension, dry mouth, and constipation, in approximately half the treated patients. The authors concluded that desipramine provides modest benefit for patients with MS and serious depression, but side effects from this medication may be more common in patients with MS than in other patient groups.

Psychotherapy has been shown to be effective in the treatment of depression in MS, and Larcombe and Wilson (1984) evaluated the effectiveness of cognitive-behavioral psychotherapy. The rationale for this approach was based on the assumption that part of the depression in MS represents a stress reaction to having a chronic debilitating disorder. The physical disability reduces engagement in previously rewarding and pleasurable activities, and adjustment is required to deal appropriately with these new constraints. There may be a negative self-image related to the loss of ability to engage in previous activities and to dealing with new problems associated with physical disability. Larcombe and Wilson found a significant reduction in posttreatment compared with pretreatment depressive symptoms, as measured by the Beck Depression Inventory and Hamilton Depression Rating Scale, in the treatment group only. In fact, the mean posttreatment score was similar to that observed in a group of patients without depression, which suggests the improvement was significant clinically. In addition, this level of improvement was sustained at the 1-month follow-up and was not considered to be a transient effect.

Rabins et al. (1986) reported that corticosteroids had no effect on depression or euphoria in MS; however, another study (Minden et al. 1988) found that approximately 20% of patients with MS become hypomanic or manic when treated with corticotropin or prednisone. This reaction was significantly more common with corticotropin compared with prednisone, and these symptoms subsided with discontinuation of drug. The occurrence of these episodes was unrelated to the severity or duration of the disease, type of MS, age, or gender. The primary risk factor for this complication was a history of major depression before the onset of MS; a family history of depression or alcoholism were more weakly related. These findings suggest that treating high-risk patients with corticotropin requires either the careful monitoring of side effects or the use of lower dosages (Cass et al. 1966).

CONCLUSIONS

The exact cause of depression in MS remains uncertain. Existing research suggests that depression does not have a single cause but rather is caused by an interaction of biologic and psychologic factors.

A better understanding of depression in MS is of both theoretic and practical significance. Theoretically, MS represents an excellent model to study the relationship between changes in emotion and subcortical structures and their related neurotransmitter systems; this disorder also provides an opportunity to examine the interaction between biologic and psychologic changes in relation to mood. From a practical perspective, improved diagnostic and monitoring procedures will allow both systematic and objective evaluation of rational treatment strategies.

All studies to date that are related to both clinical and demographic correlates of depression in MS have used cross-sectional designs. Longitudinal studies are required to adequately examine the natural history of depression in MS.

Changes in the immune system are related to physical symptoms, but no studies have attempted to examine the relationship between immunologic changes and depression in MS. Further, results of studies examining the relationship between structural changes (using MRI) and depression are preliminary but promising. Given the high correspondence between MRI and autopsy findings in MS, this area of research deserves further attention.

Few studies have examined the treatment of depression in MS. A related issue concerns the development of rating scales to monitor changes in depressive symptoms that are not confounded by changes in physical symptoms.

The practical significance of depression in MS is not understood well. Few studies have attempted to examine systematically the impact of depression on daily activities, social function, or employment, and studies that examine the impact of depression on work-related status may be an especially important disability consideration in this patient population.

REFERENCES

American Psychiatric Association. 1987. *Diagnostic and Statistical Manual of Mental Disorders, 3rd Ed. Revised.* Washington, D.C.: American Psychiatric Association.

Anderson J, Aabro E, Gulman N, et al. 1980. Antidepressive treatment of Parkinson's disease. *Acta Neurol Scand* 6:210–219.

Baretz RM, Stephenson GR. 1981. Emotional responses to multiple sclerosis. *Psychosomatics* 22:117–127.

Baum HM, Rothschild BB. 1981. The incidence and prevalence of reported multiple sclerosis. *Ann Neurol* 10:420–428.

Beck AT, Ward CH, Mendelson M, et al. 1961. An inventory for measuring depression. *Arch Gen Psychiatry* 1:561–571.

Brooks NA, Matson RR. 1982. Social-psychological adjustment to multiple sclerosis: a longitudinal study. *Soc Sci Med* 16:2129–2135.

Brownell B, Hughes JF. 1962. The distribution of plaques in the cerebrum in multiple sclerosis. *J Neurol Neurosurg Psychiatry* 25:315–320.

Cass LJ, Alexander L, Enders M. 1966. Complications of corticotropin therapy in multiple sclerosis. *JAMA* 197:105–111.

Charcot JM. 1877. *Lectures on the Disease of the Nervous System*. London: New Sydenham Society.

Cleeland CS, Matthews CG, Hopper CL. 1970. MMPI profiles in exacerbation and remission of multiple sclerosis. *Psychol Rep* 27:373–374.

Cottrell SS, Wilson SAK. 1926. The affective symptomatology of disseminated sclerosis: a study of 100 cases. *J Neurol Psychopathol* 7:1–30.

Dalos NP, Rabins PV, Brooks BR, et al. 1983. Disease activity and emotional state in multiple sclerosis. *Ann Neurol* 13:573–583.

Devins GM, Seland TP. 1987. Emotional impact of multiple sclerosis: recent findings and suggestions for future research. *Psychol Bull* 101:363–375.

Franklin GM, Heaton RK, Nelson LM, et al. 1988. Correlation of neuropsychological and MRI findings in chronic/progressive multiple sclerosis. *Neurology* 38:1826–1829.

Gebarski SS, Gabrielson TO, Gilman S. 1985. The initial diagnosis of multiple sclerosis: clinical impact of MRI. *Ann Neurol* 17:469–474.

Halligan FR, Reznikoff M. 1985. Personality factors and change with multiple sclerosis. *J Consult Clin Psychol* 53:547–548.

Hamilton M. 1960. A rating scale for depression. *J Neurol Neurosurg Psychiatry* 23:56–62.

Honer WG, Hurwitz T, Li DKB, et al. 1987. Temporal lobe involvement in multiple sclerosis patients with psychiatric disorders. *Arch Neurol* 44: 187–190.

Huber SJ, Paulson GW, Shuttleworth EC, et al. 1987. Magnetic resonance imaging correlate of dementia in multiple sclerosis. *Arch Neurol* 44:732–736.

Huber SJ, Paulson GW, Shuttleworth EC. 1988. Depression in Parkinson's disease. *Neuropsychiatry Neuropsychol Behav Neurol* 1:47–51.

Huber SJ, Rammahon KW, Christy JA, et al. The pattern of depressive symptoms with progression of multiple sclerosis. *Neuropsychiatry Neuropsychol Behav Neurol* (in press).

Katz MM, Lyerly SB. 1963. Methods of measuring adjustment and behavior in the community: I. Rationale, description, discriminative validity, and scale development. *Psychol Rep* 13:503–535.

Kellner CH, Davenport Y, Post RM, et al. 1984. Rapidly cycling bipolar disorder and multiple sclerosis. *Am J Psychiatry* 114:112–113.

Kurtzke JF. 1965. Further notes on disability evaluation in multiple sclerosis with scale modification. *Neurology* 15:654–661.

Kurtzke JF. 1984. Neuroepidemiology. *Ann Neurol* 16:265–277.

Larcombe NA, Wilson PH. 1984. An evaluation of cognitive-behavior therapy for depression in patients with multiple sclerosis. *Br J Psychiatry* 145:366–371.

Lipsey JR, Robinson RG, Pearlson GD, et al. 1984. Nortriptyline treatment of post-stroke depression: a double-blind study. *Lancet* i:297–300.

Marsh GG, Hirsch SH, Leung G. 1982. Use and misuse of the MMPI in multiple sclerosis. *Psychol Rep* 51:1127–1134.

Matthews WB, Acheson ED, Batchelor JR, et al. 1985. *McAlpine's Multiple Sclerosis*. New York: Churchill Livingstone.

Maybury CP, Brewin CR. 1984. Social relationships, knowledge and adjustment to multiple sclerosis. *J Neurol Neurosurg Psychiatry* 47:372–376.

McIvor GP, Riklan M, Reznikoff M. 1984. Depression in multiple sclerosis as a function of length and severity of illness, age, remissions, and perceived social support. *J Clin Psychol* 40:1028–1033.
Minden SL, Schiffer RB. 1990. Affective disorders in multiple sclerosis: review and recommendations for clinical research. *Arch Neurol* 47:98–104.
Minden SL, Orav J, Reich P. 1987. Depression in multiple sclerosis. *Gen Hosp Psychiatry* 9:426–434.
Minden SL, Orav J, Reich P. 1989. Characteristics and predictors of depression in multiple sclerosis. In: Jensen K, Knudsen L, Stenager E, et al. *Mental Disorders and Cognitive Deficits in Multiple Sclerosis.* London: John Libbey, pp. 129–139.
Minden SL, Orav J, Schildkraut JJ. 1988. Hypomanic reactions to ACTH and prednisone treatment for multiple sclerosis. *Neurology* 38:1631–1634.
Nelson LM, Franklin GM, Hamman RF, et al. 1988. Referral bias in multiple sclerosis research. *J Clin Epidemiol* 41:187–192.
Peselow ED, Fieve RR, Deutsch SI, et al. 1981. Coexistent manic symptoms and multiple sclerosis. *Psychosomatics* 22:824–825.
Peyser JM, Edwards KR, Poser CM. 1980. Psychological profiles in patients with multiple sclerosis: a preliminary investigation. *Arch Neurol* 37:437–440.
Peyser JM, Edwards KR, Poser CM, et al. 1980. Cognitive function in patients with multiple sclerosis. *Arch Neurol* 37:577–579.
Peyser JM, Rao SM, LaRocca NG, et al. 1990. Guidelines for neuropsychological research in multiple sclerosis. *Arch Neurol* 47:94–97.
Pratt RTC. 1951. An investigation of the psychiatric aspects of disseminated sclerosis. *J Neurol Neurosurg Psychiatry* 14:326–335.
Rabins PV, Brooks BR, O'Donnell P, et al. 1986. Structural brain correlates of emotional disorder in multiple sclerosis. *Brain* 109:585–597.
Rao SM. 1990. *Neurobehavioral Aspects of Multiple Sclerosis.* New York: Oxford University Press.
Rao SM, Hammeke TA, McQuillen MP, et al. 1984. Memory disturbance in chronic progressive multiple sclerosis. *Arch Neurol* 41:625–631.
Rao SM, Leo GJ, Bernadin L, et al. 1991a. Cognitive dysfunction in multiple sclerosis: I. Frequency, patterns, and prediction. *Neurology* 41:685–691.
Rao SM, Leo GJ, Ellington L, et al. 1991b. Cognitive dysfunction in multiple sclerosis: II. Impact on social functioning. *Neurology* 41:692–696.
Rao SM, Leo GJ, Haughton VM, et al. 1989. Correlation of magnetic resonance imaging with neuropsychological testing in multiple sclerosis. *Neurology* 39:161–166.
Ron MA. 1986. Multiple sclerosis: psychiatric and psychometric abnormalities. *J Psychosomat Res* 30:3–11.
Ron MA, Logsdail SJ. 1989. Psychiatric morbidity in multiple sclerosis: a clinical and MRI study. *Psychol Med* 19:887–895.
Schiffer RB, Babigian HM. 1984. Behavioral disorders in multiple sclerosis, temporal lobe epilepsy, and amyotrophic lateral sclerosis: an epidemiologic study. *Arch Neurol* 41:1067–1069.
Schiffer RB, Caine ED, Bamford KA, et al. 1983. Depressive episodes in patients with multiple sclerosis. *Am J Psychiatry* 140:1498–1500.
Schiffer RB, Herndon RM, Rudick RA. 1985. Treatment of pathologic laughing and weeping with amitriptyline. *N Engl J Med* 312:1480–1482.
Schiffer RB, Wineman NM. 1990. Antidepressant pharmacotherapy of depression associated with multiple sclerosis. *Am J Psychiatry* 147:1493–1497.

Schiffer RB, Wineman NM, Weitkamp LR. 1986. Association between bipolar affective disorder and multiple sclerosis. *Am J Psychiatry* 143:94–95.

Sibley WA. 1990. Diagnosis and course of multiple sclerosis. In: Rao SM, ed. *Neurobehavioral Aspects of Multiple Sclerosis*. New York: Oxford University Press, pp. 5–14.

Spielberger CD, Gorsuch RL, Lushene RE. 1970. *STAI Manual for the State-Trait Anxiety Inventory*. Palo Alto, CA: Consulting Psychologists Press, Inc.

Stewart WA, Hall LD, Berry K, et al. 1986. Magnetic resonance imaging in multiple sclerosis: pathological correlation studies in eight cases. *Neurology* 36(suppl 1):320.

Stewart JM, Houser OW, Baker HC, et al. 1987. Magnetic resonance imaging and clinical relationships in multiple sclerosis. *Mayo Clin Proc* 62:174–184.

Surridge D. 1969. An investigation into some psychiatric aspects of multiple sclerosis. *Br J Psychiatry* 115:749–764.

Whitlock FA, Siskind MM. 1980. Depression as a major symptom of multiple sclerosis. *J Neurol Neurosurg Psychiatry* 48:361–365.

Zung WK. 1965. A self-rating depression scale. *Arch Gen Psychiatry* 12:63–70.

7

DEPRESSION IN PARKINSON DISEASE

Sergio E. Starkstein, M.D., Ph.D.
Helen S. Mayberg, M.D.

Parkinson disease (PD) is a disorder of middle or late life, with a gradual and chronic progression. The main symptoms are stiffness and slowness of movement (rigidity and bradykinesia), a 3 to 5 cycles/second resting tremor, and postural instability. Taken together, these symptoms may produce the well-known phenomenology of PD, which is characterized by fatigue, diminution in automatic movements, a soft and monotonous voice, masked facial expression, constipation, decreased libido, and impairments of both perceptual motor and visual spatial functions; some of these also may be found among patients with "functional" (i.e., no known brain injury) depression as well.

In his description of PD, Parkinson (1817) described a group of patients who were so demoralized by the disease that they refused treatment. From then on, the association between PD and depression was well recognized. PD was explained in early studies as resulting from psychologic trauma or losses, and the motor symptoms were considered to be physical manifestations of an unconscious behavior (Janet 1924). Moreover, PD was described as an "illness of the ambitious, moralistic man" and the result of "suppressed hostility" (Dakof and Mendelsohn 1986). After the biologic basis of the disease was discovered, these explanations of PD as a somatic manifestation of psychiatric conflicts faded, but it became quite clear that psychiatric problems (and mainly depression) were quite prevalent among patients with PD.

Several theories have been advanced to explain the high frequency of depression in PD. It was suggested that depression is an understandable consequence of the progressive physical impairment, thus giving rise to the "psychologic hypothesis" of depression in PD (Mindham 1970). Some investigators suggested that depression may result from biochemical abnormalities (the "biologic" hypothesis) Van Praag et al. (1975), while others have supported the role of social factors underlying these mood changes (the "psychosocial" hypothesis) (McCarthy and Brown 1989). Studies on depression in PD began more than 50 years ago, but structured psychiatric interviews and diagnostic criteria for the assessment of depression only recently have been used in this research.

THE FREQUENCY OF DEPRESSION IN PARKINSON DISEASE

Several prospective studies have examined the frequency of depression in PD. Patrick and Levy (1922) found a "depressive reaction" in 34% of 140 patients with PD, and while others have reported a higher frequency of depression, methodologic problems may have biased those reports toward the higher values. For instance, Mindham (1970) reported a frequency of depression at 90% of patients with PD; however, patients in this study were selected from admissions to a psychiatric unit.

One of the main problems in research concerning depression in this disease is that depression has been diagnosed either on a clinical basis or based on a cutoff score of a depression scale in most studies; standardized questionnaires have not been used. Only two studies have used a standardized interview (such as the PSE) (Wing et al. 1974) as well as defined criteria for depression (such as in the DSM-III) (APA, 1980). In one, we assessed the frequency of depression in a consecutive series of patients examined in a general neurology clinic on regular follow-up visits (Starkstein et al. 1990a). We explicitly avoided the inclusion of patients with PD who were attending a specialized Movement Disorders Unit and who may have had a more severe form of the disease. The most important finding was that 41% of our sample was depressed; half of these patients met DSM-III criteria for major depression, while the other half met DSM-III criteria for minor (dysthymic) depression. Moreover, 20% of the 64 patients with PD who were not depressed at the psychiatric evaluation acknowledged a previous history of depression.

In the other study that used adequate psychiatric instruments, Brown and MacCarthy (1990) examined 40 patients with PD using the PSE. They found a high frequency of simple depression, tension, irritability, worrying, and loss of interest and concentration. Seventy percent of patients had at least one of these symptoms, and 55% had two or more.

These findings demonstrate a high frequency of depression in PD, but an important question is whether the frequency of this depression is higher than in other diseases with comparable physical impairments. Several studies have examined the frequency of depression in patients with PD and in those with other chronic health problems such as hemiplegia, rheumatoid arthritis, and so on (Warburton 1967, Marsh & Markham 1973, Horn 1974, Robins 1976). These studies consistently have shown a significantly higher frequency of depression in patients with PD compared with those having other diseases. The study by Gotham et al. (1986), however, where no significant differences in the prevalence of depression between patients with PD and those with rheumatoid arthritis were found, is an exception, but in this study, patients were mailed self-report questionnaires. Also, no standardized diagnostic criteria for depression were used. Whether these methodologic limitations explain the lack of significant between-group differences remains unknown, and the subject will require further prospective studies.

In conclusion, depression is a frequent finding in patients with PD. Cross-sectional studies have demonstrated that approximately 20% of patients have major and another 20% minor depression. Longitudinal studies may show that more than 50% of patients with PD will develop depression at some point in the evolution of the disease, and several studies suggest that the frequency of depression is higher in PD compared with that in other diseases producing important physical limitations. Other studies, however, could not find significant differences.

THE PHENOMENOLOGY OF DEPRESSION IN PARKINSON DISEASE

One of the most important issues in the study of depression in PD is the reliability with which depression can be diagnosed. Slowness, difficulties in concentration, and loss of energy may be frequent features of both PD and depression; thus, to examine the specificity of affective and autonomic symptoms of depression in PD, we measured the frequency of these symptoms in patients having PD both with and without a depressive mood (Starkstein et al. 1990b). We selected a consecutive series of patients who reported depressive feelings (depressed group) and who denied a depressive mood (nondepressed group). The groups were matched for important variables that might influence the frequency of depressive or depressivelike symptoms, such as age, Hoehn and Yahr stage of illness, and duration of the disease. The most important finding was that patients with a depressive mood had a significantly higher frequency of every single affective and autonomic symptoms of depression, except for early morning awakening, anergia, and motor retardation. Based on these empiric findings, we suggested specific modifications to the DSM-III criteria for both major and minor depression (dysthymia) to be used in patients with PD (Table 7.1). Moreover, we found that the presence of at least three affective and three autonomic symptoms of

Table 7.1. Criteria for Major and Minor Depression

Major Depression	Minor Depression (Dysthymia)
Dysphoric mood	Dysphoric mood
Presence of at least four of the following symptoms:	Presence of at least three of the following symptoms:
Poor appetite or significant weight loss	Insomnia
Insomnia	Feelings of inadequacy, loss of self-esteem, or self-depreciation
Loss of interest or pleasure in usual activities, or decrease in sexual drive	Decreased effectiveness or productivity
Feelings of worthlessness, self-reproach, or excessive or inappropriate guilt	Decreased attention, concentration, or ability to think clearly
Complaints or evidence of diminished ability to think or concentrate, such as slowed thinking, or indecisiveness	Social withdrawal
Recurrent thoughts of death, suicidal tendencies, wishes to be dead, or suicide attempt	Loss of interest in or enjoyment of pleasurable activities
	Inability to respond with apparent pleasure to praise or rewards
	Pessimistic attitude toward the future, brooding about past events, or feeling sorry for self
	Tearfulness or crying
	Recurrent thoughts of death or suicide

Source: Modified from American Psychiatric Association 1980.

depression had a sensitivity of 96% and specificity of 100% for the diagnosis of major depression, as well as a sensitivity of 88% and specificity of 97% for the presence of either minor or major depression.

Studies by Gotham et al. (1986) and Huber et al. (1990) found both affective and autonomic symptoms to be common features of depression in PD. Also, Levin et al. (1988) demonstrated that autonomic symptoms of depression can be measured reliably in patients with PD and do not constitute a somatic artifact. It should be mentioned, however, that the pattern of depressive features may change with progression of the disease; Huber et al. (1990) reported that affective symptoms of depression were similarly frequent along the different stages of the illness but that autonomic symptoms mainly were observed in the late stages of the disease.

Symptoms of anxiety frequently may be found among patients with PD and depression, and Schiffer et al. (1988) found that 75% of these patients met the criteria for past or present generalized anxiety disorder. Also, Stein et al. (1990) reported that while 34% of 24 patients with PD had a current anxiety disorder, 29% also had clinically significant, social phobic symptoms.

In conclusion, several studies have demonstrated that both affective and autonomic symptoms of depression in patients with PD truly reflect the presence of a mood disorder, and except for early morning awakening, anergia, and motor retardation, these symptoms are not related to the severity of the illness. Thus, the use of a standardized psychiatric interview as well as diagnostic criteria may diagnose reliably the presence of both major and minor (dysthymic) depression in patients with PD.

THE COURSE OF DEPRESSION IN PARKINSON DISEASE

When does depression start in patients with PD? This question is not only relevant in terms of a better treatment of depression in PD but also may shed light on the mechanism of such depression. If depression is significantly more frequent during the late stages of the illness, it may be explained as a reaction to the severe physical impairments. However, if depression starts in the early stages of the disease, or even before the onset of motor symptoms, a "biologic" mechanism would seem more appealing.

In a study that included 34 patients with a recent onset of PD, Santamaría et al. (1986) found that in 10 of 11 patients with symptoms of depression, this depression began before the onset of the motor symptoms. Also, Todes and Lees (1985) reported that a high proportion of patients with PD exhibit characteristic personality traits, such as emotional and attitudinal inflexibility, a lack of affect, and a predisposition to depressive illness; these introspective, overcontrolled, and anhedonic personality traits may precede the development of motor symptoms by several decades.

In our cross-sectional study of depression in PD, we found that 29% of 21 patients with major depression were depressed before the onset of motor symptoms (Starkstein et al. 1990a). However, only 5% of patients with minor depression and 2% of 64 patients without depression had a prior history of depressive mood ($X^2 = 16.6$, $P < 0.001$), thus suggesting that patients with PD and a history of depression before the onset of motor symptoms may have a high risk of developing major depression after the onset of the illness.

In a prospective, 1-year follow-up study of this population, we found that 56% of patients with major depression at the initial evaluation still had a major depression at follow-up, 33% a minor depression, and 11% were not depressed (Starkstein et al. 1992). Among patients with an initial diagnosis of minor depression, 26% still had a minor depression at the 1-year follow-up, 11% a major depression, and 63% no depression. The hypothesis of unequal frequency of depression (major or minor) among patients with an initial diagnosis of major or minor depression was substantiated statistically ($X^2 = 11.5$, df $= 1$, $P < 0.001$). Also, among patients with an initial diagnosis of no depression, 82% were not depressed at the 1-year follow-up, and the remaining 18% had a minor depression (Fig. 7.1). These findings suggest that in the majority of patients with PD and major depression, this depression may last for at least 1 year, while most patients with minor depression may recover in a shorter time. This finding of a significantly different duration of depression among patients with PD and major or minor depression gives partial validation to this diagnostic scheme, and the fact that 18% of patients without depression were depressed at the 1-year evaluation suggests most patients with PD may show depression at some point during the longitudinal evolution of the illness.

In conclusion, depression in PD may start before the onset of motor symptoms, mainly in patients who later develop a major depression. The duration of depression is longer than 1 year in the majority of patients with major depression but shorter in those with minor depression.

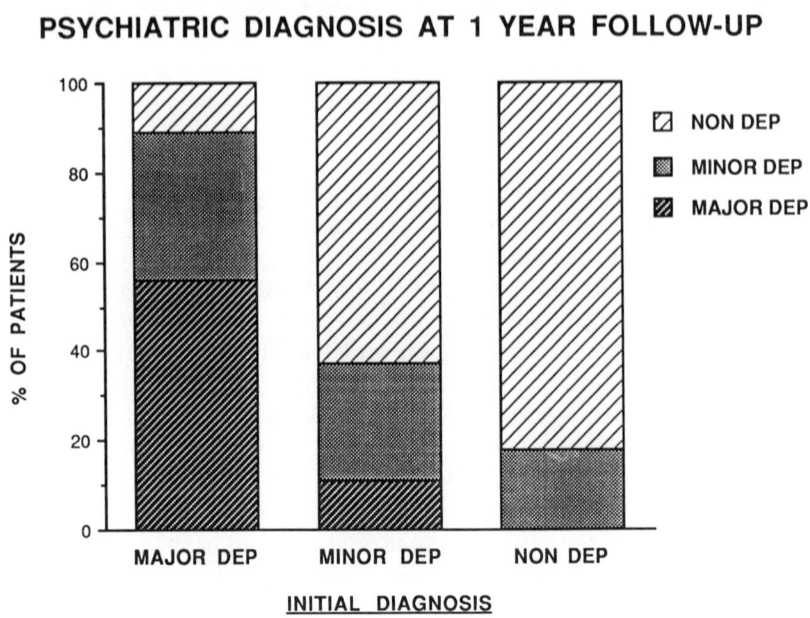

Figure 7.1. Patients with an initial diagnosis of major depression (*DEP*) showed a significantly higher frequency of depression at 1 year compared with patients having an initial diagnosis of minor or no depression.

DEPRESSION AND ASSOCIATED VARIABLES

Patients with PD may show important limitations in their ADLs. The presence of rigidity and akinesia may impair daily activities such as dressing oneself, toilette activities, and eating. Voice pitch and speech articulation also may be impaired, thus making communication difficult, and postural disequilibrium may affect locomotion. Finally, in the late stages of the illness, patients may no longer be able to work and may give up their previous physical activities and hobbies; in this context, the presence of depression would not be surprising. If depression in PD is significantly related to the greater impairments of the ADLs, then the prevalence of depression should be significantly higher in the late stages than the early stages of the illness. However, in our cross-sectional study, we found that the prevalence of depression in early versus late stages was similar (Starkstein et al. 1990a) (Fig. 7.2).

While several studies have found a significant correlation between impairment in activities of daily living (ADLs) and depression

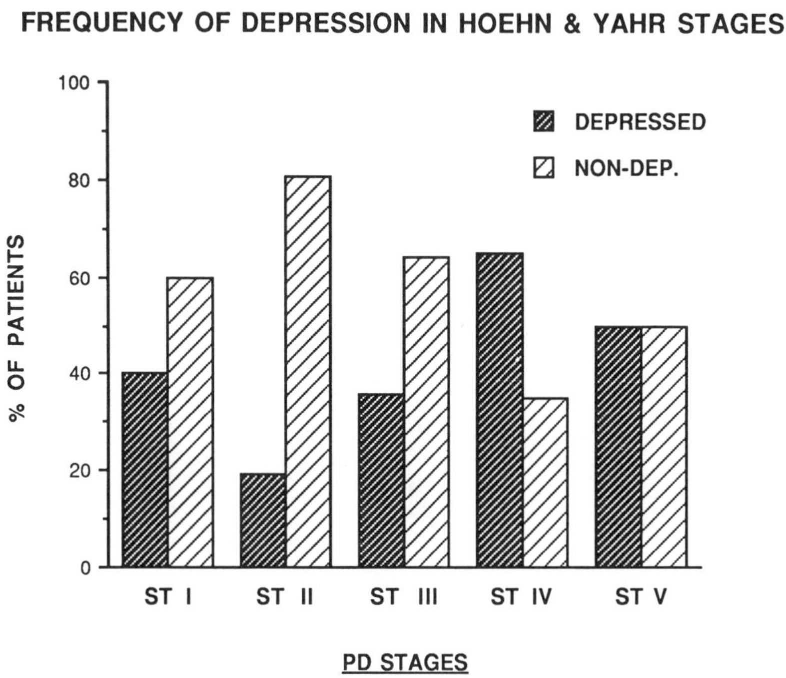

Figure 7.2. Patients in stage (*ST*) I of their disease showed a similar frequency of depression (*DEP*) as patients in the late stages of the illness (i.e., stages IV and V).

scores (Gotham et al, 1986), this association was not equally strong among different stages of the illness. In our cross-sectional study, we carried out a stepwise regression analysis to examine the association between depression and important variables such as age, duration of the disease, levodopa dosage, Mini-Mental State Examination, and ADL scores for each of the five Hoehn and Yahr stages of illness (Starkstein et al. 1990a). For stage I, both duration of illness and levodopa dosage independently accounted for a significant part of the variance ($R^2 = 0.52$, $P < 0.01$), while impairments in ADL scores accounted for most of the variance with depression scores in stage IV ($R^2 = 0.19$, $P < 0.05$). These findings have two important implications. First, they demonstrate that different correlates of depression exist in early versus late stages of PD, thus suggesting that the mechanisms of depression may be different. Second, they demonstrate that the association between depression scores and impairments in ADLs is significant only during the late stages of the illness.

The significant correlation between ADL and depression scores also may be interpreted as depression producing further impairments in ADLs. In a recent follow-up study, we examined twice (with a 1-year interval) a consecutive series of patients with PD and

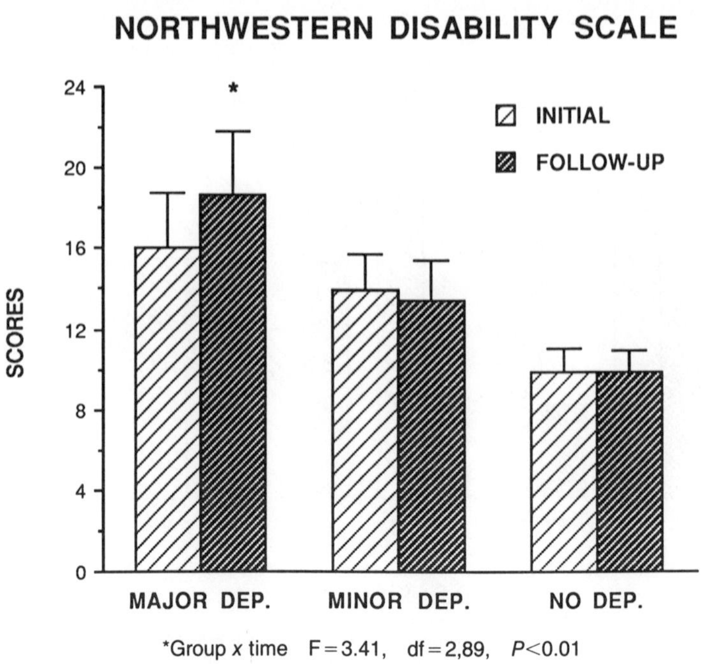

Figure 7.3. Patients with major depression (*DEP*) showed a significantly faster decline in activities of daily living.

either major, minor, or no depression (Starkstein et al. 1992). We analyzed impairments in ADLs using a two-way ANOVA with repeated measures, where factor 1 was group (major versus minor versus no depression), factor 2 was time (initial examination versus 1-year follow-up), and the repeated measure were ADL scores. A significant group by time interaction (F = 3,41; df = 2,89; $P < 0.05$) showed that the decline in ADL scores was significantly greater in patients with major depression (Fig. 7.3). Moreover, a significant group by time interaction in Hohen and Yahr stages existed (F = 5,13; df = 2,89; $P < 0.01$), showing a faster progression along the stages of the illness in patients with major depression (Fig. 7.4). By the 1-year follow-up, 10 of the 15 patients (67%) in the major-depression group had progressed to the next Hoehn and Yahr stage, compared with seven of 17 patients (41%) with minor depression and 10 of 49 patients (20%) with no depression ($X^2 = 11.6$, df = 2, $P < 0.01$). Similar findings were reported by Brown et al. (1988) in a study where self-report questionnaires (the Beck Depression Inventory and an ADL scale) were mailed to 152 patients with PD 1 year after they had returned similar questionnaires; approximately two thirds of the

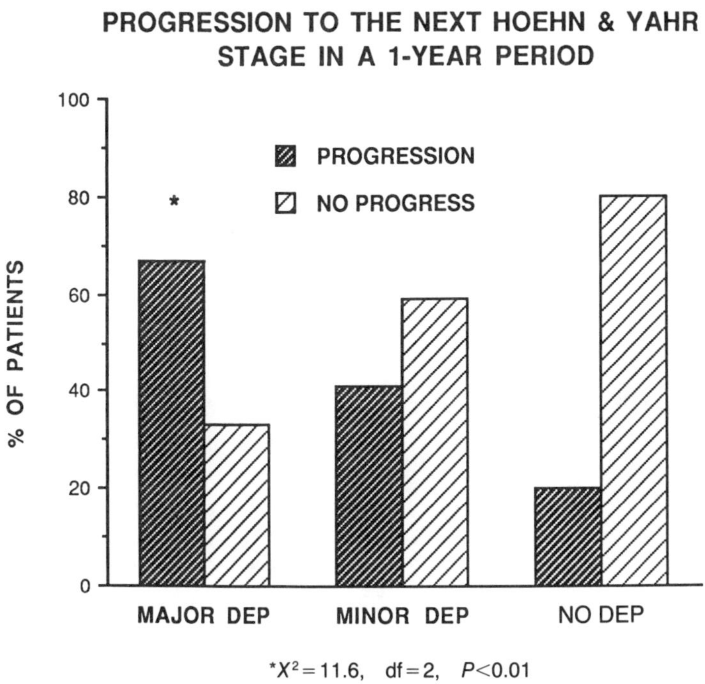

Figure 7.4. Patients with major depression (*DEP*) showed a significantly faster progression along the stages of the illness.

original cohort returned the follow-up questionnaires, with the greatest decline in ADL scores found in patients who became depressed during the follow-up period.

DEPRESSION IN EARLY VERSUS LATE ONSET OF PARKINSON DISEASE

In a cross-sectional study, Santamaría et al. (1986) reported that patients with PD who were depressed at the time of the evaluation were significantly younger at the onset of PD than patients without depression. In a recent study, we compared a group of patients with PD who had the onset of motor symptoms before the age of 55 years (early onset) and patients with PD who had the onset of motor symptoms after age 55 (late onset) (Starkstein et al. 1989a). Figure 7.5 shows the frequences of major, minor, and no depression in these groups. Patients with an early onset showed a significantly higher frequency of major depression ($X^2 = 9.92$, df $= 1$, $P < 0.001$) than did patients with a late onset; this difference remained significant even after the early and late onset groups were matched for duration of illness. Thus, while patients with an early onset of PD may show

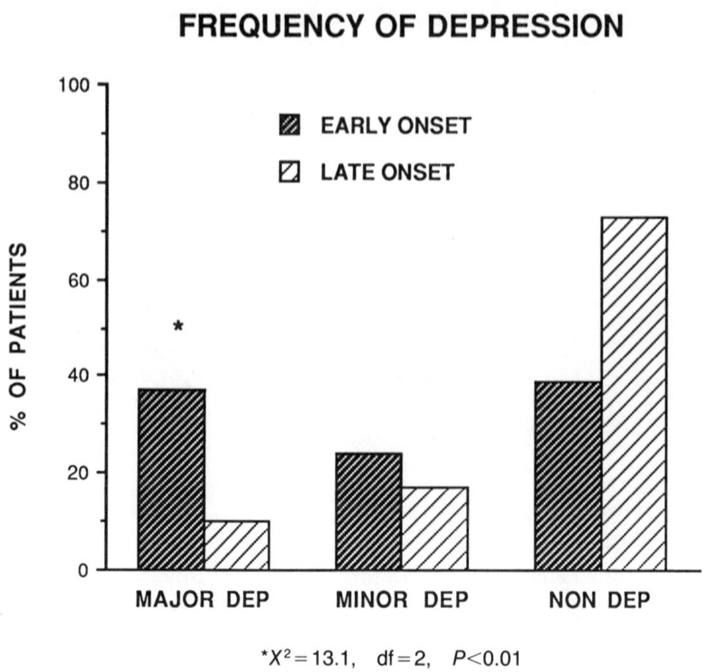

Figure 7.5. Patients with an early onset of PD showed a significantly higher frequency of depression (*DEP*) than patients with a late onset.

a slow progression of motor symptoms, high frequency of depression, and a significant association between depression and cognitive impairments, those patients with a late onset of PD may have a faster progression of motor symptoms, significantly lower frequency of depression, and a significant association between depression and impairments in ADLs.

We also found different correlates of depression in early versus late onset groups. We carried out a stepwise regression analysis, where depression scores were the dependent variable and age, duration of illness, levodopa dosage, tremor, rigidity, akinesia, and ADL and Mini-Mental State Examination scores were independent variables. Within the early onset group, duration of the illness and Mini-Mental State Examination scores accounted for a significant part of the variance ($R^2 = 0.27$, $P < 0.05$), but in the late-onset group, ADL scores accounted for a significant part of the variance ($R^2 = 0.22$, $P < 0.01$).

In conclusion, a significant association between depression and impairment in ADLs was present only during the late stages of the illness and mainly in patients who had late onset of motor symptoms. Recent findings suggest that depression is not a reaction to physical impairments, but the presence of major depression may produce further impairments in ADLs. Other findings further support the hypothesis that impairments in ADLs cannot account for depression in PD. First, depression may precede the onset of motor symptoms in at least 25% of patients with major depression, and the frequency of depression during the early stages of the illness (when physical impairments are mild) is similar to the frequency of depression in late stages (when physical impairments are severe).

DEPRESSION AND COGNITIVE IMPAIRMENTS

Cognitive impairments are a frequent finding in patients with PD, and recent studies suggest that the presence of major depression may account for at least part of this intellectual decline. We empirically examined whether the presence of either major or minor depression was associated with cognitive deficits in patients with PD; we found that patients with major depression had significantly lower Mini-Mental State Examination scores than patients with minor or no depression (Starkstein et al. 1990a). In another study, we also found that patients with PD and major depression had significantly more impairments on tasks that assess frontal-lobe functions than patients without depression who were matched for age, duration, and stage of illness (Starkstein et al. 1989b). In conclusion, data suggests that patients with PD and major depression may show the phenomenon of depression-related cognitive impairments.

DEPRESSION AND LATERALIZATION OF PARKINSON DISEASE SYMPTOMS

The initial stage of PD (stage I of Hoehn and Yahr) is characterized by unilateral (left or right) motor symptoms. Positron-emission tomography studies have demonstrated that patients with unilateral PD have both abnormal metabolic activity and levodopa uptake in the basal ganglia contralateral to the side of motor symptoms (Eidelberg et al. 1990, Nahmics et al. 1985).

We examined whether the presence of exclusive or predominantly unilateral symptoms of PD were associated with a different frequency of depression; our study included 19 patients with left sided PD and 19 patients with right sided PD (Starkstein et al. 1990a). Inclusion criteria were the presence of unilateral PD symptoms or ratio between extremities in symptom-severity ratings using a scale for tremor, rigidity, and akinesia of at least 2:1. No significant differences were found on demographic variables, but patients with right sided PD showed a significantly higher frequency of both major and minor depression (53% versus 21%, $X^2 = 4.07$, df = 1, $P < 0.05$)

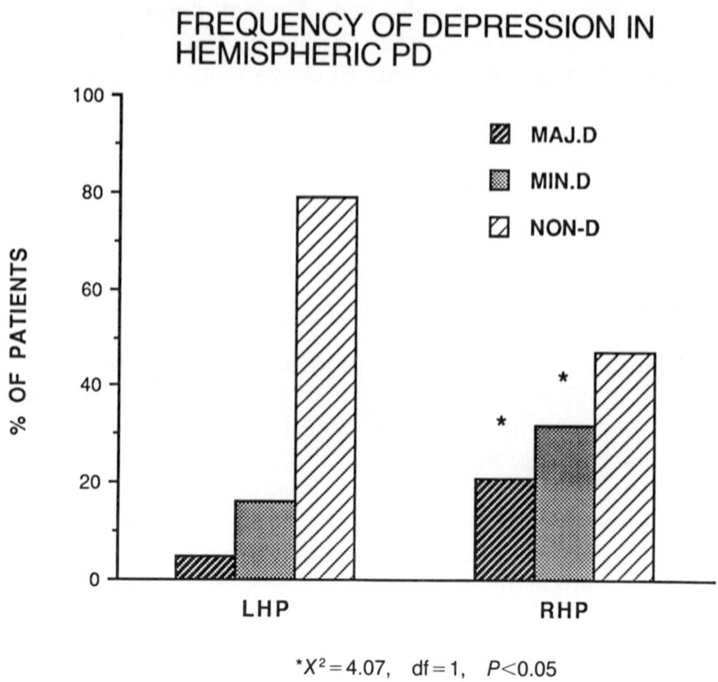

Figure 7.6. Patients with right sided PD (*RHP*) showed a significantly higher frequency of major (*MAJ. D*) and minor depression (*MIN. D*) than patients with a left sided PD (*LHP*).

and significantly higher depression scores than patients with left hemisphere PD (Fig. 7.6).

In conclusion, patients with right sided PD (left hemisphere dysfunction) showed a significantly higher frequency of depression than patients with left hemisphere PD (right hemisphere dysfunction). These findings are similar to the significantly higher frequency of depression reported in patients with left basal ganglia infarctions (Starkstein et al. 1988), and they suggest that biologic factors may be related to the production of depression in the early stages of PD.

THE BIOLOGIC MARKERS OF DEPRESSION IN PARKINSON DISEASE

The dexamethasone suppression test has been used as a biologic marker of depression in patients with "functional" (i.e., no known brain injury) depression. Although the sensitivity and specificity of DST may vary between studies, most patients with major depression will not suppress the secretion of cortisol after the dexamethasone injection (Carroll et al. 1989).

Two studies examined the usefulness of DST as a biologic marker of depression among patients with PD. Kostic et al. (1990) found a nonsuppressor response in 75% of patients with PD and depression and in 28% of patients with PD and no depression. No significant association was found between nonsuppression and gender, age, duration of illness, or severity of depression. The second study (Frochtengarten et al. 1987) reported very different results; only five of 35 (14%) of patients with PD and depression were nonsuppressors, and none of the 21 patients with PD and no depression were nonsuppressors. When the 4:00 pm values of plasmatic cortisol are considered, the specificity and sensitivity in Kostic et al.'s study was 83% and 69%, respectively, while in Frochtengarten et al.'s study, the specificity was 100% and sensitivity only 14%.

In conclusion, DST does not seem to be a very useful marker of depression in PD, because the sensitivity of this test is very low. Future studies may examine the sensitivity and specificity of other biologic markers of depression in these patients with depression.

THE MECHANISM OF DEPRESSION IN PARKINSON DISEASE

Psychologic, biologic, and psychosocial factors have been proposed to explain the high prevalence of depression in PD. We already have discussed evidence against a psychologic explanation of depression in PD (depression may start before the onset of motor symptoms, impairments in ADLs only explain a small part of the variance in the correlation with depression scores, and it is the depression that accelerates progression of illness).

Among biologic factors explaining the presence of depression in PD, a genetic vulnerability for mood disorders should be considered. In our cross-sectional study of mood disorders in PD, we found a positive family history of psychiatric disorders in 23% of patients with major depression, 33% of patients with minor depression, and 24% of patients without depression (Starkstein et al. 1990a). These findings demonstrate that a genetic predisposition for mood disorders may not play an important role in the production of depression in PD.

Which other biologic factors may produce depression in PD? In another study, we found that patients with PD and depression had significantly lower metabolic activity in the head of the caudate and the orbitofrontal cortex compared with patients having PD without depression; Mayberg et al. (1990) this is similar to our findings in stroke patients, where stroke lesions involving the head of the caudate and the frontal cortex produced the highest frequency of depression (Starkstein et al. 1988). Because these areas of the brain are important afferents of biogenic amine pathways, it is possible that dysfunction of specific dopaminergic and/or catecholaminergic pathways may play an important role in the production of depression in PD, and several observations support this hypothesis. Studies have reported significant changes in mood and anxiety in parallel with fluctuations in motor symptoms. In most of these studies, patients with severe parkinsonism ("off" state) reported significantly more depression and anxiety than during the state of relatively normal motor function ("on" state), thus suggesting that the "on-off" mood changes may be related to swings in central dopaminergic function (Nizenbaum et al. 1987, Menza et al. 1990, Cantello et al. 1986, Friedenberg & Cummings 1989).

Cantello et al. (1989) examined the euphoric response to intravenous methylphenidate in patients having PD both with and without depression using a double-blind, placebo-controlled study. They found that the depressed group had a significant lack of response to the euphoriant effects of methylphenidate compared with the nondepressed PD group. Because euphoria produced by central stimulants is related to the activity of dopaminergic synapses in limbic terminals, the authors suggest that degeneration of the mesolimbic dopaminergic system may play an important role in the production of depression in PD.

If dopamine deficits are either necessary or sufficient to produce depression in PD, then why does levodopa therapy fail to improve mood in patients with PD and depression? Moreover, why are homovanillic acid concentrations (a dopamine metabolite) in the CSF of patients with and without depression not significantly different (i.e., significantly lower in patients with PD and depression) (Mayeux et al. 1986)? First, CSF homovanillic acid values may not truly reflect brain dopamine metabolism (Hildebrand et al. 1990). Second, if depression in PD is primarily related to dopamine mesolimbic, but not dopamine nigrostriatal, dysfunction, then levodopa replacement acting primarily on striatal dopamine receptors may not influence mesolimbic dopamine terminals. In laboratory research, Kelly et al. (1975) demonstrated that at high levels of stimulation, the behavioral output of the nigrostriatal system may suppress the output of the mesolimbic system; they suggested this shift in balance between the nigrostriatal and mesolimbic systems may result in mood changes. Dopamine depletion in both systems may explain the depression observed during the "off" periods of PD, but the overstimulation of the nigrostriatal system (by producing an inhibitory effect on the mesolimbic system) may explain the depression found during dyskinesias.

Other neurotransmitters also may be involved in the production of depression in PD. Mayeux et al. (1986) showed significantly lower levels of the serotonin metabolite 5-hydroxyindoleacetic acid in the CSF of patients with PD and depression than in those without depression. Whether serotonergic changes are necessary or important to produce depression, or whether depression results from an abnormal interaction between serotonergic, dopamine, or noradrenergic systems, remains to be examined.

In conclusion, patients with PD and depression show significantly lower metabolic activity in the inferior frontal cortex and head of the caudate than do patients with PD without depression. These regions are richly innervated by dopaminergic axons originating in the ventral tegmental area and constituting the mesocorticolimbic circuit. The degeneration of these mesocorticolimbic dopamine fibers in patients with PD may lead to a metabolic dysfunction of the inferior frontal lobes, which may affect secondarily the serotonergic cell bodies originating in the dorsal raphe nucleus. This combination of dopaminergic and serotonergic dysfunction may underlie the clinical aspects of the depression in patients with PD.

THE TREATMENT OF DEPRESSION IN PARKINSON DISEASE

Tricyclic antidepressant medications have efficacy in the treatment of depression in PD. The usefulness of imipramine, desipramine, and nortriptyline has been demonstrated in double-blind, randomized, and placebo-controlled studies (Denmark et al. 1961, Laitinen 1969, Strang 1965, Andersen et al. 1980). Among these diverse tricyclic drugs, nortriptyline may constitute one of the best choices, because it has a lower frequency of orthostatic hypotension, sedation, and anticholinergic side effects than other tricyclic drugs. Patients usually are started on small dosages (10 to 25 mg/day) of nortriptyline and the dosage gradually increased by 10 to 25 mg every 3 to 4 days until a 70- to 75-mg dose is reached (Andersen et al. 1980). The medication may be taken as a single dose at bedtime or may be given in divided doses. With nortryptyline, there is both a lower limit (50 ng/ml) and an upper limit (150 ng/ml) for serum concentration (the therapeutic "window"); the other tricyclic drugs have a lower limit but not an upper limit established.

The most common, serious side effect in patients with PD is orthostatic hypotension. Because levodopa medications may produce orthostatic hypotension by themselves, the addition of a tricyclic antidepressant may potentiate this side effect. In the only controlled trial of nortriptyline in PD, these side effects seemed to be quite mild (Andersen et al. 1980). The mean systolic blood pressure in the standing position was only slightly lower with active treatment, and none of the patients on active treatment had arrythmias or electrocardiograph changes. Other side effects of tricyclic antidepressants include sedation, dry mouth, increased intraocular pressure in patients with narrow-angle glaucoma, urinary retention, delirium, and visual blurring. Of major concern, however, are the cardiovascular side effects; in addition to orthostatic changes, the tricyclic antidepressants reduce cardiac conduction and are contraindicated in patients with heart blocks or conduction abnormalities, severe arrhythmias, or a recent myocardial infarction.

Monoamine oxidase inhibitors have not been used regularly in patients with PD because of concerns about causing a hypertensive crisis when using levodopa with a nonselective monoamine oxidase inhibitor. However, one patient with PD recently was treated with the monoamine oxidase inhibitor phenelzine combined with amantadine (a drug that stimulates the release of dopamine from presynaptic dopaminergic nerve terminals) (Greenberg and Meyers 1985). The patient, who developed important side effects such as confusion and cardiac slowing with nortryptyline, was very much improved on a regimen of 45 mg/day of phenelzine. Another monoamine oxidase inhibitor that may constitute a good therapeutic choice for depression in PD is selegiline; this drug has been demonstrated to diminish the rate of progression of PD. A recent double-blind, placebo-controlled trial also demonstrated that selegiline is a good antidepressant drug when used in dosages of 15 mg/day in two doses. The advantage of selegiline over other monoamine oxidase inhibitors is that, being a selective monoamine oxidase inhibitor β-blocker, it is devoided of the "cheese and wine" reactions of the others when used in low doses. The efficacy of this drug in PD as well as its safety in this population will be demonstrated in future randomized, double-blind, placebo-controlled studies.

In patients with PD and a severe affective disorder, electroconvulsive therapy constitutes an important therapeutic modality. Several studies have reported the usefulness of electroconvulsive therapy in treating major depression in patients with PD who are either unable to tolerate or unresponsive to antidepressant medications (Burke et al. 1988; Asnis 1977; Holcomb et al. 1983; Young et al. 1985; Douyon et al. 1989). Improvement after electroconvulsive therapy correlated positively with age at treatment and with duration of levodopa therapy. The depression of some patients not only improves, but the motor symptoms of these patients may improve as well. Parkinsonian symptoms may improve in the absence of mood improvement, or at a different rate, and electroconvulsive therapy also may reduce the "on-off" phenomena in subjects with longstanding PD. Parkinsonian symptoms may return over a period of days, stay in remission for several months, or become more responsive to pharmacotherapy. Moreover, some patients who respond to electroconvulsive therapy may develop dyskinesias, which improve after the dopaminergic agonist doses are reduced. In most studies, no correlation exists between the improvement of parkinsonian symptoms and mood changes after electroconvulsive therapy. The ultimate mechanism for the beneficial influence of electroconvulsive therapy in PD is unknown, but electroconvulsive therapy may decrease the sensitivity of dopaminergic autoreceptors, which may lead to enhanced dopaminergic release.

CONCLUSIONS

Depression is a frequent finding among patients with PD. In cross-sectional studies, 20% of patients show major depression and another 20% minor depression. In longitudinal studies, most patients with PD show depression at some point in their disease. The diagnosis of depression may be made reliably by using slightly modified DSM-III criteria, and patients with major depression show a faster decline in ADLs and cognitive functions as well as a faster progression along the stages of the illness compared with patients having PD and minor or no depression. While the mechanism of depression in PD is unknown, several studies suggest that depression may be related to frontal lobe and/or biogenic amine dysfunction. Depression in PD is amenable to treatment with the usual tricyclic antidepressant medications, but the possibility of side effects such as orthostatic hypotension should be monitored closely. Electroconvulsive therapy is another valid treatment modality in cases of major depression refractory to drug treatment.

ACKNOWLEDGMENTS

This work was supported in part by a Young Investigator Award from the National Alliance for Research in Schizophrenia and Depression, a grant from the Raúl Carrea Institute of Neurological Research, and a grant from the Sandoz Foundation for Gerontological Research.

REFERENCES

Andersen J, Aabro E, Gulmann N, et al. 1980. Anti-depressive treatment in Parkinson's disease. *Acta Neurol Scand* 62:210–219.

American Psychiatric Association. 1980. *Diagnostic and Statistical Manual of Mental Disorders, 3rd Ed.* Washington, D.C.: American Psychiatric Press.

Asnis G. 1977. Parkinson's disease, depression, and ECT: a review and case study. *Am J Psychiatry* 134:191–195.

Brown RG, MacCarthy B. 1990. Psychiatric morbidity in patients with Parkinson's disease. *Psychol Med* 20:77–87.

Brown RG, MacCarthy B, Gotham AM, et al. 1988. Depression and disability in Parkinson's disease: a follow-up of 132 cases. *Psychol Med* 18:49–55.

Burke WJ, Peterson J, Rubin EH. 1988. Electroconvulsive therapy in the treatment of combined depression and Parkinson's disease. *Psychosomatics* 29:341–346.

Cantello R, Gilli M, Riccio A, et al. 1986. Mood changes associated with "end-of-dose deterioration" in Parkinson's disease: a controlled study. *J Neurol Neurosurg Psychiatry* 49:1182–1190.

Cantello R, Maguggia M, Gilli M, et al. 1989. Major depression in Parkinson's disease and the mood response to intravenous methylphenidate: possible role of the "hedonic" dopamine synapse. *J Neurol Neurosurg Psychiatry* 52:724–731.

Carroll BJ, Feinberg M, Gredent JF. 1981. A specific laboratory test for the diagnosis of melancholia: standardization, validation and clinical utility. *Arch Gen Psychiatry* 38:15–22.

Dakof GA, Mendelsohn GA. 1986. Parkinson's disease: the psychological aspects of a chronic illness. *Psychol Bull* 99:375–387.

Denmark JC, Powell JD, McComb SG. 1961. Imipramine hydrochloride (Tofranil) in parkinsonism. *Br J Clin Prac* 15:523–524.

Douyon R, Serby M, Klutchko B, et al. 1989. ECT and Parkinson's disease revisited: a "naturalistic" study. *Am J Psychiatry* 146:1451–1455.

Eidelberg D, Moeller JR, Dhawan V, et al. 1990. The metabolic anatomy of Parkinson's disease: complementary (18F) fluorodeoxyglucose and (18F) fluorodopa positron emission tomographic studies. *Movement Disord* 5:203–213.

Friedenberg DL, Cummings JL. 1989. Parkinson's disease, depression, and the on-off phenomenon. *Psychosomatics* 30:94–99.

Frochtengarten ML, Villares JCB, Maluf E, et al. 1987. Depressive symptoms and the dexamethasone suppression test in Parkinsonian patients. *Biol Psychiatry* 22:386–389.

Gotham AM, Brown RG, Marsden CD. 1986. Depression in Parkinson's disease: a quantitative and qualitative analysis. *J Neurol Neurosurg Psychiatry* 49:381–389.

Greenberg R, Meyers BS. 1985. Treatment of major depression and Parkinson's disease with combined phenelzine and amantadine. *Am J Psychiatry* 142:273–274.

Hildebrand J, Bourgeois F, Buyse M, et al. 1990. Reproducibility of monoamine metabolite measurements in human cerebrospinal fluid. *Acta Neurol Scand* 81:427–430.

Holcomb HH, Sternberg DE, Heninger GR. 1983. Effects of electroconvulsive therapy on mood, parkinsonism, and tardive dyskinesia in a depressed patient: ECT and dopamine systems. *Biol Psychiatry* 18:865–873.

Horn S. 1974. Some psychological factors in Parkinsonism. *J Neurol Neurosurg Psychiatry* 37:27–31.

Huber SJ, Freidenberg DL, Paulson GW, et al. 1990. The pattern of depressive symptoms varies with progression of Parkinson's disease. *J Neurol Neurosurg Psychiatry* 53:275–278.

Janet P. 1924. *Leçons sur les Maladies du Système Nerveux (2nd ed.).* Paris: Delahaye.

Kelly PH, Seviour PW, Iversen SD. 1975. Amphetamine and apomorphine responses in the rat following 6-OHDA lesions of the nucleus accumbens septi and corpus striatum. *Brain Res* 94:507–522.

Kostic VS, Sternic NC, Bumbasirevic LB, et al. 1990. Dexamethasone suppression test in patients with Parkinson's disease. *Movement Disord* 5:23–26.

Laitinen L. 1969. Desipramine in treatment of Parkinson's disease. *Acta Neurol Scand* 45:109–113.

Levin BE, Llabre MM, Weiner WJ. 1988. Parkinson's disease and depression: psychometric properties of the Beck Depression Inventory. *J Neurol Neurosurg Psychiatry* 51:1401–1404.

MacCarthy B, Brown R. 1989. Psychosocial factors in Parkinson's disease. *Br J Clin Psychol* 28:41–52.

Marsh GG, Markham CH. 1973. Does levodopa alter depression and psychopathology in Parkinsonism patients? *J Neurol Neurosurg Psychiatry* 36:925–935.

Mayberg HS, Starkstein SE, Sadzot B, et al. 1990. Selective hypometabolism in the inferior frontal lobe in depressed patients with Parkinson's disease. *Ann Neurol* 28:57–64.

Mayeux R, Stern Y, Williams JBW, et al. 1986. Clinical and biochemical features of depression in Parkinson's disease. *Am J Psychiatry* 143:756–759.

Menza A, Sage J, Marshall E, et al. 1990. Mood changes and "on-off" phenomena in Parkinson's disease. *Movement Disord* 5:148–151.

Mindham RHS. 1970. Psychiatric symptoms in parkinsonism. *J Neurol Neurosurg Psychiatry* 33:188–191.

Nahmias C, Garnett ES, Firnau G, et al. 1985. Striatal dopamine distribution in parkinsonian patients during life. *J Neurol Sci* 69:223–230.

Nissenbaum H, Quinn NP, Brown RG, et al. 1987. Mood swings associated with the "on-off" phenomenon in Parkinson's disease. *Psychol Med* 17:899–904.

Parkinson J. 1817. *An Essay on the Shaking Palsy.* London: Sherwood, Neely & Jones.

Patrick HT, Levy DM. 1922. Parkinson's disease: a clinical study of 146 cases. *Arch Neurol Psychiatry* 7:711–720.

Robins AH. 1976. Depression in patients with Parkinsonism. *Br J Psychiatry* 128:141–145.

Santamaría J, Tolosa E, Valles A. 1986. Parkinson's disease with depression: a possible subgroup of idiopathic parkinsonism. *Neurology* 36:1130–1133.

Schiffer RB, Kurian R, Rubin A, et al. 1988. Evidence for atypical depression in Parkinson's disease. *Am J Psychiatry* 145:1020–1022.

Starkstein SE, Berthier ML, Bolduc PL, et al. 1989a. Depression in patients with early versus late onset of Parkinson's disease. *Neurology* 39:1441–1445.

Starkstein SE, Mayberg HS, Preziosi TJ, et al. 1992. A prospective longitudinal study of depression, cognitive decline, and physical impairments in patients with Parkinson's disease. 1982. *J Neurol Neurosurg Psychiatry* 55:377–382.

Starkstein SE, Preziosi TJ, Berthier ML, et al. 1989b. Depression and cognitive impairment in Parkinson's disease. *Brain* 112:1141–1153.

Starkstein SE, Preziosi TJ, Bolduc PL, et al. 1990a. Depression in Parkinson's disease. *J Nervous Mental Dis* 178:27–31.

Starkstein SE, Preziosi TJ, Forrester AW, et al. 1990b. Specificity of affective and autonomic symptoms of depression in Parkinson's disease. *J Neurol Neurosurg Psychiatry* 53:869–873.

Starkstein SE, Robinson RG, Berthier ML, et al. 1988. Differential mood changes following basal ganglia vs thalamic lesions. *Arch Neurol* 45:725–730.

Stein MB, Heuser IJ, Juncos JL, et al. 1990. Anxiety disorders in patients with Parkinson's disease. *Am J Psychiatry* 147:217–220.

Strang RR. 1965. Imipramine in the treatment of parkinsonism: a double-blind placebo study. *BMJ* 2:33–34.

Todes CJ, Lees AJ. 1985. The pre-morbid personality of patients with Parkinson's disease. *J Neurol Neurosurg Psychiatry* 48:97–100.

Van Praag HM, Korf J, Lakke JPWF, et al. 1975. Dopamine metabolism in depressions, psychoses, and Parkinson's disease: the problem of the specificity of biological variables in behaviour disorders. *Psychol Med* 5:138–146.

Warburton JW. 1967. Depressive symptoms in parkinsonian patients referred for thalamotomy. *J Neurol Neurosurg Psychiatry* 30:368–370.

Wing JK, Cooper E, Sartorius N. 1974. *Measurements and Classification of Psychiatric Symptoms.* Cambridge: Cambridge University Press.

Young RC, Alexopoulos GS, Shamoian CA. 1985. Dissociation of motor response from mood and cognition in a parkinsonian patient treated with ECT. *Biol Psychiatry* 20:566–569.

8

DEPRESSION IN HUNTINGTON DISEASE

Carol E. Peyser, M.D.
Susan E. Folstein, M.D.

In 1872, Huntington described the three clinical features of the hereditary brain disorder that now bears his name. In addition to chorea, he described the patients as having a dementia and "that form of insanity which leads to suicide." Huntington disease (HD) is an autosomal dominant genetic disease, but the onset of clinical disease usually is delayed until the middle of adult life. Symptoms worsen for approximately 16 years and end in death, usually from aspiration or general debilitation.

Many authors have described depressive symptoms in HD, and there were two early reports of bipolar disorder in this disease. Kraepelin (1915) noted that the patients with HD in his clinic often had manic-depressive illness, and in their early survey of HD on the eastern seaboard of the United States, Davenport and Muncey (1916) noted that manic-depressive illness was frequent both in patients with HD and their at-risk children. In the early 1970s, when psychopathology in HD was interpreted as being largely a psychologic reaction to fatal illness, McHugh and Folstein (1975) reemphasized the frequent occurrence of this syndrome of major affective disorder in HD; they also suggested that with its clear neuropathology, HD might provide clues to the pathophysiology of idiopathic affective disorder.

Several compelling reasons exist for concluding that the mood disorder in patients with HD cannot be explained simply as an understandable psychologic reaction to adversity. Ten percent of all patients with HD have episodes of mania or hypomania (Table 8.1), which is certainly not an easily understandable response to a fatal and debilitating illness. Some patients have delusions or hallucinations when manic or depressed; and again, this is not within the realm of an adjustment reaction. Also, the phenomenology of major depression in HD is strikingly similar to the phenomenology of id-

Table 8.1. Lifetime Prevalence of Affective Disorders and Schizophrenia in Huntington Disease

	Subjects with Diagnosis, *n (%)*		
DSM-III Diagnosis	Blacks*	Whites†	Total‡
All Affective Disorders	10(20)	60(44)	70(38)§
Unipolar	3(6)	38(28)	41(22)
Bipolar	2(4)	16(12)	18(10)
Cyclothymia	0(0)	2(1)	2(1)
Dysthymia	5(10)	4(3)	9(5)
Schizophrenia	1(2)	7(5)	8(4)

*$n = 50$.
†$n = 136$.
‡$n = 186$.
§$P < 0.05$.

iopathic major depression. The episodes of both depression and mania come and go without respect to life events and, if untreated, have a duration similar to that in idiopathic affective disorder. Mood disorders are not distributed randomly in the HD population; they are more common in certain families (Folstein et al. 1983), in caucasian patients (Table 8.1), and in persons with an older age at the onset of HD (Folstein et al. 1987). Affective disorder often precedes other symptoms of HD as well, on average by 5 years (Minski and Guttmann 1938, Folstein et al. 1983); in some kindreds, affected persons have intermittent depression for as long as 20 years before any motor or cognitive signs appear. That this often occurs in patients who do not know they are at risk for HD makes it unlikely these depressive episodes are psychologic reactions to the fear of developing HD. Depressed and manic patients with HD also respond to appropriate pharmacologic treatments used in idiopathic affective disorders unrelated to HD. These epidemiologic and clinical characteristics suggest that biologic factors are involved in the genesis of the mood disorder in patients with HD.

PREVALENCE

Reports concerning the rates of depression in selected populations of patients with HD (Rosenbaum 1941, Heathfield 1967, Dewhurst et al. 1970, Bolt 1970, Mattson 1974, Folstein et al. 1983, Caine and Shoulson 1983, Pflanz et al. 1991) vary from 4% (Oliver 1970) to 44% (Mindham et al. 1985). The discrepancies between these studies are not surprising, because different methods were used and differing definitions of depression employed. Some samples were small, and others reported on only patients in psychiatric hospitals. In most of the studies with larger, more representative samples, diagnoses were based on a review of case notes alone without interviews (Pflanz et al. 1991).

To study the prevalence of psychiatric illness in patients with HD among a representative sample, unbiased by referral to a psychiatric clinic or hospital, a survey in Maryland attempted to locate every patient with HD in that state who was alive and symptomatic on April 1, 1980 (Folstein et al. 1987). Multiple case-finding methods were used, including record searches of short- and long-term hospitals, psychiatric hospitals, and nursing homes; letters to individual physicians, home- and foster-care agencies, and social workers; and inquiries at neurology and genetics clinics as well as voluntary organizations for families with HD. Of the 217 living patients found with a clear diagnosis, 186 could be examined psychiatrically or adequate psychiatric information otherwise could be obtained to make a psychiatric diagnosis according to DSM-III criteria (American Psychiatric Association 1980). For major depression, the modifications to these criteria were: the requirement that an "organic basis" for mood disorder be excluded was ignored; and an episode of depression was called *major depression* only if it lasted 1 month or longer and was not associated temporally with the diagnosis of HD, divorce, job loss, or death of a family member (Folstein et al. 1983, Folstein and Folstein 1983). Some patients could not be interviewed because of death or advanced disease, and the diagnostic criteria just described also were used for patients about whom information was obtained only through review of case notes. If information was available from family members alone, then the diagnostic criteria were required, such as depressed mood, weight loss, loss of time from work, and medical treatment. Thompson et al. (1982) showed this method results in less sensitivity, but not less specificity, of diagnosis of affective disorder. The effects of these modifications to DSM-III criteria would be expected to make the diagnostic criteria for major depression more stringent. Therefore, elicit symptoms systematically, a structured psychiatric interview (the National Institute of Mental Health Diagnostic Interview Schedule) (Robins et al. 1981) was conducted with the patient by an experienced clinician, using the spouse as an additional informant; the Diagnostic Interview Schedule was never the sole source of information. Diagnosis was based on all available information, often including many years of longitudinal follow-up, and on this basis, the cumulative lifetime prevalence of psychiatric disorder up to the patient's last examination was calculated.

Table 8.1 shows the lifetime prevalence of both affective disorder and schizophrenia in the Maryland survey population, and it shows the differing prevalence of these disorders in black and the white populations. Thirty-eight percent of all patients with HD met criteria for affective disorder at some time in life. However, 40% of caucasians but only 10% of blacks met criteria for major affective disorder (major depression or mania) at some time during their illness; 28% of caucasian patients with HD had unipolar depression and 12% episodes of mania or hypomania. It should be noted that cases classified as bipolar included many subjects who had recurrent depression with brief periods of hypomania (falling into the "Bipolar II" category or Bipolar Not Otherwise Specified according to the DSM-III-R classification system).

In a controlled study that also employed the Diagnostic Interview Schedule, Mindham et al. (1985) personally interviewed 27 randomly selected patients with HD and 27 randomly selected patients with Alzheimer disease who were attending the Johns Hopkins Alzheimer disease and HD clinics. A lifetime psychiatric history was taken, and information from relatives was invariably obtained. For the patients with HD, 44% had a history of major affective disorder before the onset of dementia; among patients with Alzheimer disease, this was true for 22% of cases. This study provides further documentation of the high incidence of mood disorder in the HD population and also indicates that affective disorder cannot be regarded simply as an early, nonspecific sign of any dementing process.

THE CLUSTERING OF AFFECTIVE DISORDER IN A SUBSET OF FAMILIES WITH HUNTINGTON DISEASE

Davenport and Muncy (1916) observed that mood disorders in HD tended toward a subset of families with HD. In 1938, Minski and Guttmann reported that many of the suicides in patients with HD clustered among a few families who had evidence of severe mood disorders. The Folstein survey in Maryland confirmed these earlier clinical observations that affective disorder in HD seemed to be restricted to a (large) subset of families with HD (Folstein et al. 1983). From this case series, five probands with both HD and major affective disorder and five with HD and no other psychiatric disorder (except dementia) were selected; these comprised probands from 10 different, unrelated families. Of the five probands with affective disorder, four had bipolar disorder, and one had recurrent major depressions.

In these 10 families, attempts were made to contact and interview the probands' siblings; parents; parents' siblings; and available, biologically unrelated family members (e.g., spouses or "in-laws"). One hundred forty-three of the 160 designated relatives and 76 of the in-laws were contacted and interviewed. For those patients with HD and their at-risk relatives, the interview methods followed those described previously; family informants and case notes were used if patients were deceased or too advanced in their disease to interview. For relatives not at risk for HD, an experienced nurse clinician conducted telephone interviews. The format for these psychiatric interviews was an unstructured, but lengthy, interview that was designed to elicit enough information to determine whether the subject had ever had an episode, lasting at least 2 weeks, meeting DSM-III-R criteria for major depression. When any suggestion at all emerged for an episode of depression, all DSM-III-R criteria were covered in the questioning, and all subjects were asked if they had ever received or sought counselling or psychiatric treatment as part of the interview. In some cases, the spouse or parent of a patient with HD served as an informant about other members of their own sibship, and in some cases, siblings of the caregiver of the HD patient were contacted.

For the five HD probands with affective disorder, 20 of the 23 relatives who also had HD had affective disorder and 3 did not. For the 5 HD probands with no history of mood disorder, five of their 23 relatives with HD had affective disorder and 18 did not. The chi-squared distribution for this comparison is 19.7 ($P < 0.001$).

None of the probands' "non-HD" parents or the non-HD parents' 42 siblings met criteria for major affective disorder. Several had minor depressive symptoms, however, and five were alcoholic. The lifetime prevalence of major affective disorder in the sample of subjects not at risk for HD was found to be 2%, and this provides evidence that the mood disorder in these 10 families likely was inherited through the "HD side" of these families and not from chance intermarriage with families afflicted by affective disorder.

This conclusion is strengthened by the very high prevalence of mood disorder in patients with HD. If the mood disorder was inherited from the "non-HD" side of the family, then one would expect a prevalence similar to that in the general population. Weissman et al. (1989) reviewed epidemiologic studies concerning the lifetime prevalence of idiopathic affective disorder, which have found lifetime risk rates of from 2% to 18%. In the epidemiologic catchment-area study in Baltimore during the early 1980s (Robins et al. 1984), the lifetime prevalence of major affective disorder was 4.3% (3.7% for major depression, and 0.6% for mania).

Assortative mating is common for patients with idiopathic affective disorder, that is, patients with mood disorders tend to select spouses with mood disorders at a higher rate than would occur by chance (Dunner et al. 1976, Merikangas and Spiker 1982). Our data are insufficient to exclude assortative mating of patients with HD and persons with mood disorders (and we certainly have seen occasional examples of mood disorders in the "non-HD" parents of patients with HD and mood disorders), but this is not a likely explanation of the very high rate of mood disorder among patients with HD in our sample. We conclude this based on the low rate of affective disorder found in the "non-HD" spouses and parents described previously and from clinical impressions based on years of experience with the spouses of patients with HD.

In conclusion, the inheritance pattern of affective disorder in families with HD appears to have a distinct pattern, with a higher prevalence of mood disorder in some families, patients with late onset of illness, and caucasians. This pattern differs from that in Alzheimer disease, for example; in Alzheimer disease, Pearlson et al. (1990) showed that affective disorder relates to family history of idiopathic affective disorder in unaffected relatives. We have shown clearly this is not the case in HD. The distinct inheritance pattern of affective disorder in HD described here remains to be confirmed by other investigators.

PHENOMENOLOGY OF MAJOR DEPRESSION IN HUNTINGTON DISEASE

The phenomenology of major depression early in HD, as well as during the time when those bearing the *HD* gene have no neurologic signs, is strikingly similar to the phenomenology of idiopathic affective disorder. Patients generally feel sad, dysphoric, or empty. Anhedonia is common, and patients can lose all hope for the future. There is often (but not invariably) a change in self-attitude, with unrealistic guilt and self-blame. There generally is a change in vital sense, with increased fatigue and a deterioration of ability to concentrate, and depressed patients can become suicidal. More commonly, however, they wish for death or see no point to living. Loss of appetite and insomnia are often seen, but in some cases, patients become hypersomnolent and withdraw to bed. Anxiety is common but not universal in patients with HD and depression, and some patients with anxious depressions have increased chorea when depressed. Prominent obsessions and compulsions are seen that subside in intensity or disappear when the patient becomes euthymic. Major depression in HD can be accompanied by psychotic phenomena, that is, delusions and in some cases hallucinations; the delusions or hallucinations often are mood-congruent. A wide variety of depressive delusions can be seen, for example, hypochondriac delusions (such as the belief that one is dying of cancer), delusions of guilt (such as believing that the individual deserves to be punished for having committed some horrible crime), the delusional belief that the HD victim's family is about to desert the patient, or delusions of persecution or catastrophe. Mood-congruent hallucinations also can occur, delusions are more common than hallucinations in our experience. When hallucinations do occur, most commonly these are auditory.

The duration of episodes of major depression in HD is similar to that in idiopathic major depression, generally lasting 6 months or less if untreated. In 21 cases from the Maryland survey (Folstein et al. 1983) with untreated affective disorder, 13 had an episode with a duration of less than 7 months, four had an episode lasting from 7 to 12 months, and four had an episode with a duration of over 1 year.

Affective disorder often precedes other symptoms of HD by 5 years on average (Folstein et al. 1983, Minski and Guttmann 1938). In 44 patients with affective disorder from the Maryland survey, mood disorder preceded chorea in 23. In six of the 44 cases, the onset of affective disorder was concurrent with chorea, and in 5 of the 44, mood disorder developed after chorea was first noted. We have observed some kindreds in which most affected persons suffer intermittent depression for many years before any motor or cognitive signs appear; in some cases, mood disorder can precede motor signs of HD by as long as 20 years. Episodes of depression commonly are most frequent during the first few years after the onset of chorea. Late in the course of HD, patients with affective disorder often cease having episodes of depression, or have less frequent episodes.

DEPRESSION IN ADVANCED HUNTINGTON DISEASE

During the middle stages of HD, the phenomenology of depression often is as previously described, but variations are common. Psychomotor retardation can be juxtaposed on the bradykinesia of HD, the bradykinesia improving somewhat with resolution of the depression. Sometimes patients seem to be alexithymic; they appear to be experiencing intense emotional pain yet are unable to identify the emotion. Such patients are unable to put their feelings into words but will acknowledge them when expressed by others and clearly act on them. For example, one patient with moderate HD jumped off a bridge, nearly ending his life. He was unable to describe spontaneously his feelings but looked miserable, and when the feelings that patients with depression often experience were described to him, he immediately identified with them.

A second phenomena in some patients with depression during the middle stages of HD is a presentation most notable for withdrawal and anhedonia with sleep disturbance and weight loss. Such patients can express quite profound feelings of sadness and worthlessness when probed, but they do so in such a flat and monotonous way that others may not take these complaints seriously. These patients with HD and depression often have masked facies and look blunted rather than sad. Masked facies also are present in patients who are not depressed (and deny any depression) but rather are apathetic; this apathetic, disconnected quality of some patients with HD, both when depressed and when euthymic, probably is the major reason they have been thought by some observers to resemble patients with schizophrenia.

Late in the course of HD, patients with affective disorder often have fewer episodes of mood disturbance, or the affective disorder subsides entirely. However, some patients have episodes of depression even in endstage disease. It becomes more difficult to identify episodes very late in HD because in advanced HD speech can be monosyllabic and sparse. Also, many patients are totally mute even when not depressed; when such patients become depressed, behavior changes. Patients become more irritable and hard to please, develop insomnia, and withdraw socially, becoming unresponsive to attention and affection, and they can become agitated and easily frightened. Such states often are responsive to antidepressant treatment. Patients who can speak may report delusions; they may believe, for example, that the nursing-home staff is trying to poison them, thus leading the patients to refuse medications. Derogatory auditory hallucinations also can occur.

THE PHENOMENOLOGY OF BIPOLAR DISORDER IN HUNTINGTON DISEASE

In the 10% of patients with HD who also have bipolar disorder, the pattern of the bipolar disorder can vary. In some, episodes of depression alternate with euthymia and with episodes of full-fledged mania. Another common pattern is brief episodes of hypomania alternating with episodes of major depression. We also have observed several patients with mixed affective states; in some cases, elements of major depression occur simultaneously with elements of mania, and in others, elevated mood states alternate with severe depression in the course of a day or even several hours. When patients with HD are manic, they become unrealistically cheerful and confident, tend to exaggerate their self-importance, and can be very irritable. They also sleep and eat less and have high energy and activity levels compared with their normal state.

DIAGNOSIS

The greatest difficulty in diagnosing major depression among patients with HD lies in the readiness with which meaningful explanations can be put forward for depressed mood in those afflicted with this illness. During the course of HD, patients often suffer a long series of losses, ranging from the loss of motor control and cognitive ability to the loss of independence, or even divorce and job termination. When standard criteria are used for diagnosing a depressive syndrome, however, clear-cut major depression will be recognized in patients with HD.

During the early and middle stages of HD, it is appropriate to evaluate patients for major depression using a standard clinical interview and standard diagnostic criteria; the DSM-III-R criteria generally are quite adequate. However, according to the classification schema in the DSM-III-R, major depression should not be diagnosed in a patient with an underlying organic disorder (such as HD) that could initiate or maintain this syndrome; instead, one is supposed to diagnose "organic mood syndrome" in such cases. This diagnosis has far less rigorously defined criteria, and for this reason, and because we disagree on theoretic grounds with the arbitrary division in the DSM-III-R of "organic" and "nonorganic" mood disorders, we advocate the use of the standard DSM-III-R criteria of major depression in HD. The only modification we suggest is that if this syndrome occurs only in the context of a parent's death, the diagnosis of HD, or divorce, the diagnosis should not be made for research purposes. For clinical purposes, the diagnosis of major depression definitely should be considered in these settings. If the patient is not helped by counselling or psychotherapy, and if the full depressive syndrome persists, then treatment with pharmacologic therapy should be undertaken.

To characterize the severity of major depression (and its response to pharmacologic intervention), standard rating scales for major depression that have been well validated in idiopathic affective disorder can be used in the context of a semistructured psychiatric interview. For example, the Hamilton Depression Scale (Hamilton 1960) or the Montgomery Asberg Scale can be employed. Some items on these scales are seen in many patients with HD, regardless of whether they are depressed. These features can become more marked with depression in HD, but they are nonspecific. Nevertheless, a phenomenologic approach can be taken, simply rating what is seen. For example, the Hamilton Scale includes a rating for "fidgetiness;" patients with chorea often look very "fidgety" and can be rated as such. Patients with depression will score higher on these scales, and scores change with the patient's mood. Such rating scales are useful for following and characterizing patients with depression, but they cannot substitute for an experienced clinician who must determine whether the elements of major depression are present.

The differential diagnosis of major depression in HD, as in idiopathic affective disorder, includes adjustment disorders with depressed mood. Demoralization and discouragement can certainly be seen in HD, but as with patients having other serious illnesses, demoralized patients with HD ordinarily do not meet DSM-III-R criteria for major depression. If an adjustment disorder with depressed mood is diagnosed, then the patient deserves careful follow-up, so that if the dysphoric mood does not resolve despite time and appropriate interventions, the possibility of affective disorder can be reconsidered. In some cases, profound apathy also can be difficult to distinguish from depression. Family members sometimes will state that a patient is "depressed" but only describe an apathetic state when questioned, and the patient will report a euthymic mood. Pronounced apathy and irritability can be seen in patients with HD in the absence of depression (Peyser et al. 1990), and such patients do not exhibit low mood or self-attitude. They may have little energy but generally do not have a sleep disturbance. However, when a patient with profound apathy also has several features of depression (such as a sleep disturbance), the diagnosis of affective disorder should be considered, and the clinician may elect to conduct an empiric treatment trial. While irritability is common in patients with HD and affective syndromes, many patients are irritable or even aggressive in the absence of a depressive or manic state. Again, it is necessary to consider the presence or absence of mood change and other features of affective disorder to clarify the psychiatric diagnosis.

The phenomenology of major depression later in HD already has been discussed and thus clearly poses more diagnostic problems than depression early in HD. Careful interviews of the patient, observations of behavior, and questioning of family members and nursing-home staff about the patient's behavior will help the clinician to determine whether a major depressive syndrome is present.

We have covered some of the subtleties and difficulties of diagnosing major depression in HD. What is most striking, however, is how similar the phenomenology of major depression in HD is to the phenomenology of major depression in idiopathic affective disorder.

ASSOCIATED PHENOMENA

As described previously, those patients with HD and affective disorder tend to have a later age at the onset of illness. In one sample (Folstein et al. 1987), their average age at the onset of motor symptoms was 43 years, compared with 39 years for those without affective disorder. This observation appears to conflict with those of Bolt (1970) and Mattson (1974), who reported that patients with HD who presented with psychiatric disorder had a relatively earlier onset. These patients, however, included cases that began with "personality changes" such as apathy or irritability without affective disorder; therefore, the subgroup of HD cases specified is not the same.

The higher prevalence of affective disorder in white patients with HD in contrast to black patients already has been described (Folstein et al. 1987). Analyzing data from the Maryland survey, we have been unable to identify other disease features that characterize the subset of HD cases with affective disorder from those without mood disorder. For example, some patients with HD have more prominent rigidity and others more prominent chorea. Others have more severe dementia earlier in the course of HD, but we have been unable to demonstrate a difference in this pattern in those with mood disorders.

SUICIDE

Huntington (1872) pointed out in his original description of this disease that patients often suffer from "that form of insanity which leads to suicide." In general, empiric studies of suicide in HD have supported Huntington's observation that suicide is more common in those afflicted with HD than in the general population. Morris (1991) provided an excellent review of the literature on suicide in HD, and Farrer (1986) used data from the National Huntington Disease Roster in the United States to study causes of death in a large series of patients with HD. Information on the cause of death was available for 440 of 452 deceased patients; 25 (5.7%) died by suicide. In 1984, the rate of suicide in the United States was estimated at 11.8 per 100,000, or approximately 0.1% (CDC 1985), based on coroners' statistics. The United States suicide rate in general is certainly underestimated from these figures (Dublin 1963), so it cannot be compared directly to the figures given for the apparent suicide rate in HD. However, even using an estimate that approximately 1% of all deaths are because of suicide (not a conservative estimate), the rate of suicide in HD can be seen to be elevated.

Several different issues must be considered when thinking about these findings. It has been documented extensively that affective disorder is a major risk factor for suicide in general (Barraclough et al. 1974, Robins 1981), and suicide attempts in HD often are made in the context of an affective disorder. For example, in a series of 8201 deaths of patients with HD in South Wales (Morris 1991), four were suicides. Three of these four clearly were depressed as well. Minski and Guttman (1938) reported a familial clustering of suicide and attempted suicide, and in some of these families with HD, depression was common. Dimaio (1991) found that 50% of suicides in families with HD occurred in only 28% of the families studied; it would be interesting to investigate whether affective disorder was present in these families. Because depression in HD usually can be treated successfully, one would hope this would decrease the suicide rate, but this has not yet been documented.

A second issue is the impact of chronic disease on suicide rates. In a study that traced cancer patients through the Finnish Cancer Registry, the suicide rate for patients with cancer was 1.3 times higher for men and 1.9 times higher for women than in the general population (Louhivouri and Hakama 1979).

There have been six suicides among patients known to the Baltimore HD Project, and at least three of these had affective disorder. One man was not depressed but shot himself in fulfillment of an earlier vow to do so when he could no longer walk. The other two patients were not under our care, so we have no information about their mental state.

MECHANISM

In our opinion, overwhelming evidence exists that affective disorder in HD cannot be explained as an understandable psychologic reaction to the ravages of this disease but that it rather is related to some aspect of its neurobiology. The question then becomes: what about this neurologic disease produces affective disorder, and why is this seen only in a subset of families with HD?

These questions can be approached in at least two broad ways. First, one may consider what about the characteristic pathophysiology of HD might produce affective disorder. It could be that those cases who do not develop mood disorders have some protective factor, or perhaps something about the timing of the injury produced by HD is different in depressed compared with nondepressed individuals. This line of reasoning focuses on what is characteristic of HD in general and what HD shares with other diseases (such as Parkinson disease) in which major depression is common. Second, one may attempt to find differences in brain structure, biochemistry, or function between depressed and nondepressed cases; if such differences can be found, they might provide clues not only to the mechanism of the mood disorder of HD but also the mechanism of mood disorders in some other neurologic diseases and possibly idiopathic affective disorder as well.

THE CHARACTERISTIC PATHOPHYSIOLOGY OF HUNTINGTON DISEASE AS A CLUE TO MOOD DISORDER

The most evident and consistent neuropathologic change in HD is atrophy and neuronal loss in the neostriatum (Bruyn 1968). The most profound cell losses usually are noted in the caudate, then the putamen, with the ventral striatum affected in a much more subtle fashion. Macroscopic pathologic changes also are present outside the basal ganglia. There can be marked atrophy of the cerebral cortex, particularly in frontal, occipital, and sometimes temporal regions

(Bruyn 1968, Lange 1981, De La Monte et al. 1988), and neuronal loss has been documented in the prefrontal cortex (Sotrel et al. 1991) and in the dorsal prefrontal cortex in HD (Hedreen et al. 1991). Both McHugh (1990) and Folstein (1990) drew attention to the common occurrence of affective disorder in diseases and conditions affecting the caudate, and the basal ganglia more generally, and to the "subcortical triad" of depression, movement disorder, and dementia (Folstein et al. 1991) that so often emerges when a variety of insults damage this critical region of the brain. Evidence from all the literature on depression in Parkinson disease in cerebrovascular accident also supports the notion that the basal ganglia are involved in mood regulation.

Trying to explain findings from studies of depression following cerebrovascular accident, Starkstein and Robinson (1989) suggested that mood disturbances following both cortical and subcortical strokes may be caused by the lesions having interrupted the ascending biogenic amine pathways. However, this is an unlikely explanation for the affective disorder associated with HD, where fibers passing near the striatum are not known to be affected.

Because of the early occurrence of affective disorder in HD, Peyser and Folstein (1990) hypothesized that it might relate to the area of the striatum that is first affected in HD. Vonsattel et al. (1985) provided substantial evidence that the earliest neuronal loss in HD is to be found in the dorsal medial caudate; this portion of the caudate is the target for rich innervation from the frontal cortex and is a major target for fibers originating in the limbic cortex. Thus, damage to caudate disrupts a number of circuits that may be critical for the normal regulation of mood. Well before any neuronal cell loss can be appreciated in this region, neurochemical changes occur. In a striking case report, Albin et al. (1990) studied the brain of a woman who was proven to carry the *HD* gene but who did not yet have a clear movement disorder; she did, however, have a well-documented affective disorder that led to her death through suicide. No macroscopic or microscopic pathologic change could be documented in the brain of this woman, but neurochemical studies showed a marked depletion of one class of glutamate receptor, the *N*-methyl-D-aspartate receptor in putamen (caudate was not assayed). In addition, Albin et al. documented a marked reduction in enkephalinergic projections to the globus pallidus. The caudate is rich in GABAergic, enkephalin-containing neurons, and it is quite reasonable, based on Albin et al's work, to posit that such neurons might be biochemically abnormal even in "presymptomatic" HD. Several of the documented biochemical abnormalities in HD (for instance, in either the glutamatergic, GABAergic, or enkephalinergic neurons) could play a role in the mood disorder of HD (Peyser and Folstein 1990), and given that a variety of insults to caudate can produce mood disorder, perhaps what is critical is not the exact neurochemical disruption but rather a subtle deficit in caudate cellular function, thus disrupting both limbic-caudate and frontal-caudate circuits. We do not propose that caudate dysfunction necessarily underlies mood disorders in all instances (idiopathic, in Parkinson disease, all post-stroke depressants, and so on). Rather, we propose that when caudate is damaged or caudate function disrupted by insults occurring elsewhere (such as in the substantia nigra in Parkinson disease), depression very often will be produced.

BRAIN DIFFERENCES BETWEEN HUNTINGTON DISEASE CASES WITH AND WITHOUT DEPRESSION

It is possible that in this disease, with its marked but variable neuropathology, it might be feasible to identify significant differences in brain pathology or at least brain function between cases with and without a history of affective disorder. We have been able to demonstrate differences in regional cerebral glucose metabolism in between patients with HD who were depressed and those who had never been depressed (Mayberg et al. 1992). We measured regional cerebral glucose metabolism using 2-(18F)-fluoro-2-deoxy-D-glucose and positron emission tomography in nine patients with early HD; four had major depression and five were not depressed. Patient groups were matched for years of duration of motor disorder as well as age and were comparable for severity of dementia and the overall functional disability. Caudate, putamen, and cingulate metabolism were significantly lower in the patients compared with control subjects independent of mood state. Orbital frontal and inferior prefrontal cortex hypometablism differentiated patients with depression from both patients without depression and normal controls. These findings implicate selective dysfunction of the paralimbic regions of the frontal lobes in the mood disorder of HD. The regional localization is similar to that seen in patients with depression and Parkinson disease and is consistent with the pattern of hypometabolism described in primary affective disorders; it could be what the mood disorder of HD shares with the mood disorders seen in several other conditions.

There are a number of possible explanations for the pathogenesis of the cortical hypometabolism in patients with HD and depression; here, we focus on some of the explanations that might separate depressed from never-depressed HD cases. First, depression may be related to the extent of cortical involvement. Frontal cortical atrophy can be seen in HD, although the extent can be quite variable. Neuronal loss in frontal cortex also has been documented (Sotrel et al.

1991, Hedreen et al. 1991), but neuronal counts have not yet been done in the inferior orbital area that was metabolically abnormal in scans. It is possible that the hypometabolism reflects abnormal function of the orbitofrontal neurons, which are injured by the pathologic process of HD; another possibility is that anterograde dysfunction of multisynaptic pathways linking the dorsomedial caudate to the dorsomedial thalamus and orbital-inferior prefrontal cortex that results in remote hypometabolism in the thalamus and this specific region of cortex. If so, there may be a disproportionate dysfunction in the dorsomedial caudate (relative to other affected brain regions) early during the course of HD in patients with affective disorder. There also could be subtle differences in the pattern of medial caudate involvement between cases with and without affective disorder, such as differences in the relative degeneration of patch and matrix compartments (Graybiel and Ragsdale 1978).

There have been a few neuropathologic studies comparing the pathologic findings in the brains of patients with HD who did and did not exhibit affective disorder during the course of their illness. In a morphometric study on the brains of 30 patients with HD (six of whom had clinical histories of depression), De La Monte et al. (1988) showed that depression correlated with more severe global atrophy of the cerebral cortex and white matter. Brains of patients with a history of depression also had more striking atrophy of the basal ganglia at the level of the caudate-putamen-accumbens. This aspect of the De La Monte study is preliminary, however, because the presence of depression was assessed by chart review and no diagnostic criteria for depression reported.

Recent studies of Alzheimer disease have demonstrated a relationship between a history of depression and the severity of neuronal loss within the locus coeruleus and possibly the dorsal raphe nucleus as well (Zweig et al. 1988, Iverson et al. 1983). When these biogenic amine–producing nuclei were studied in HD, cell loss in the locus coeruleus was found in advanced illness (Zweig et al. 1992); however, Zweig et al. found no differences in cell counts at three levels of the locus coeruleus between the 13 patients with a clearly documented history of major depression and the 14 cases who clearly never had affective disorder. In addition, cell counts were done at three levels of the dorsal raphe, a key nucleus in the serotonergic system, and again, no differences were found between depressed and non-depressed HD cases. Figure 8.1 shows these data.

Despite extensive work on the biochemistry of HD, almost no attention has been paid to the psychiatric correlates of biochemical findings. One exception is the study by Kurlan et al. (1988). Prompted by reports of elevated corticotropin-releasing factor and

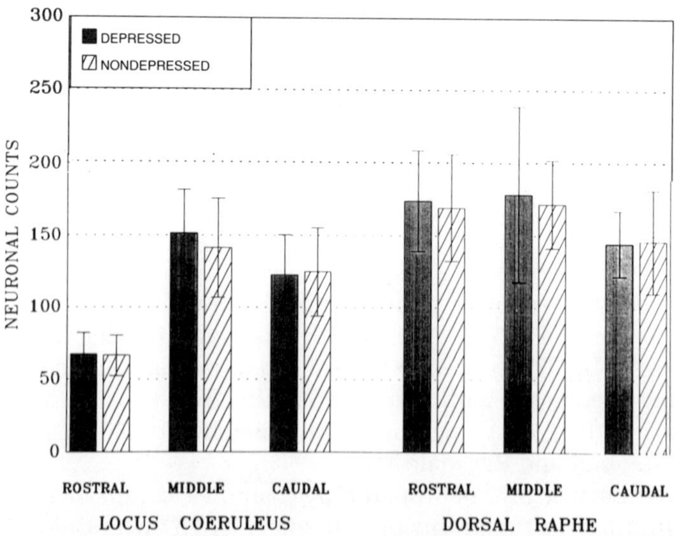

Figure 8.1. Mean numbers of neuronal profiles at three levels of the locus coeruleus and dorsal raphe nucleus in 13 HD cases with clear history of major depression (*dark bars*) and 14 cases with no history of depression (*striped bars*). Error bars indicate standard deviation.

reduced 5-hydroxyindoleacetic acid concentrations in the lumbar CSF of patients with idiopathic major depression, they examined these CSF constituents in 56 unmedicated patients during early stages of HD. Patients with depressive disorders (major depression or dysthymia) did not differ from those without depression in respect to CSF 5-hydroxyindoleacetic or corticotropin-releasing factor concentrations; within the depressed group, however, a positive correlation existed between the severity of major depression and CSF corticotropin-releasing factor concentrations.

In summary, the pathophysiologic basis of depression in HD remains to be elucidated, but good clues are emerging. Pursuing these might lead to a better understanding not just of the depression of HD but of depression in a number of neurologic disorders and in idiopathic affective disorder as well. It is clear that further studies of the neuroanatomic, neuropathologic, and neurochemical correlates of affective disorder in HD are needed. Positron-emission tomography scanning also provides an important tool for the further study of this issue, and it is crucial for studying the early phases of the illness. Evaluating the MRI scans of psychiatrically characterized patients with HD could be used to characterize anatomic differences, and it will be possible to perform more definitive neurochemical studies in patients with HD who are examined regularly for psychiatric illness during life and eventually come to autopsy.

TREATMENT

In the vast majority of cases, major depression in HD can be treated successfully. There are no treatment studies, however, and our conclusions are based on our own clinical experience and discussions of treatment strategies with other clinicians who are expert in the management of HD.

The fundamental principle of treating patients with HD and mood disorder is to approach treatment in the same fashion as a psychiatrist would approach the treatment of idiopathic mood disorder. It is curious that in this genetic disorder, where the mutation appears to involve one locus on chromosome 4, not all patients with depression are responsive to the same antidepressant medication. This is clearly the case, however, and the clinician must take an empiric approach. Tricyclic antidepressants often are effective treatments in the depression of HD, and we use nortriptyline as our first line of treatment. Nortriptyline has fewer anticholinergic side effects than many of the other tricyclics (except desipramine), and it is well documented that there is a "window" of serum levels that tend to be effective in idiopathic affective disorder. Patients with HD often respond to "subtherapeutic" serum levels of nortriptyline and other tricyclics as well, but when they fail to respond, the dosage should be increased until therapeutic serum levels are obtained unless the patient cannot tolerate the side effects. For patients with severe anxiety or agitation in the context of major depression, a more sedating antidepressant (such as amitriptyline or imipramine) can be considered. If low dosages of these antidepressants can be used (e.g., the patient responds at low serum levels, which often is the case), then patients with HD generally can tolerate the side effects of these agents; however, when higher dosages are needed for a response, fatigue, sedation and increased cognitive impairment from the anticholinergic side effects can be troublesome. For this reason, we use nortriptyline or desipramine whenever possible. Tricyclics are particularly useful for patients with HD and depression who have a sleep disturbance; indeed, in a cases of HD where sleep disturbance has been profound in the absence of affective disorder, we also have found tricyclics to be a useful treatment.

During the last few years, we have treated many patients with HD and depression by using the serotonin reuptake blocker fluoxetine (Prozac, Dista Products Company, Indianapolis, Indiana, USA) and achieved very good results. Generally, we have used fluoxetine either after a tricyclic trial has failed or in patients with prominent obsessions and/or compulsions. A very low dose of fluoxetine needs to be used at times because of prominent sedation in patients with HD, and if the insomnia often associated with fluoxetine treatment is problematic, a small dose of trazodone can be added to the regimen.

When treatment with these agents has failed, we have used numerous other antidepressants, including monoamine oxidase inhibitors. Also, we successfully treated several patients with HD and depression using carbamazepine (which we use routinely as a treatment for severe irritability in HD); however, we would not recommend this as a first-line treatment of depression in HD.

In the treatment of refractory depression in HD, and especially for severe agitation or near catatonia, we have employed successfully a course of electroconvulsive therapy. HD poses no contraindication to electroconvulsive therapy, but, as in other patients with dementia, those with HD need to be monitored carefully for delirium during their course of electroconvulsive therapy. Occasionally, the treatment schedule will need to be modified accordingly.

When major depression in HD is accompanied by psychotic features (delusions or hallucinations), treatment with an antidepressant alone generally is insufficient just as in idiopathic affective disorder. We recommend adding either a neuroleptic to the antidepressant regimen or else electroconvulsive therapy.

The main difference in the pharmacologic strategy of treating affectively ill patients with HD compared with patients having idiopathic affective disorder lies in the treatment of bipolar disorder. In our experience, lithium carbonate rarely works for bipolar disorder in HD, but carbamazepine treatment often is very successful. Carbamazepine may be combined with neuroleptics when needed in mania. (In patients with HD and depression not responding to a tricyclic, we have tried a "lithium booster" of the tricyclic on many occasions, but without a single success; we have therefore abandoned this practice.) In patients with bipolar HD who do not tolerate carbamazepine, lithium can be used with caution. Lithium toxicity may occur more commonly as patients with HD can become dehydrated easily.

The effective treatment of affective disorder in HD is of tremendous importance to both patients and their families, and it is extremely gratifying to the clinician who, unfortunately, cannot yet offer any treatment to stop the progression of this fatal disease. In talking about depression in HD, we often are asked, "Aren't *all* patients depressed?" Indeed, they are not; many still are able to get much pleasure from their lives and their families. When you ask such patients if they feel that life is not worth living, they look at you in disbelief, as if to say, "Why would I feel like that?" Effective treatment of affective disorder in HD often makes it possible for patients to enjoy several years when they are not yet terribly disabled, and it makes it possible for their families to continue to care for the patients at home.

CONCLUSIONS

There is a strikingly high rate of affective disorders, including bipolar disorders, in patients with HD. Most evidence suggests it is not plausible to explain the mood disorder in HD as an understandable reaction to adversity; instead, it is likely that biologic factors are involved in the genesis of the mood disorder in HD. We have touched on the evidence that mood disorders are a characteristic feature of diseases of the basal ganglia and have examined in this light the characteristic neuropathology of HD with damage to the caudate and frontal cortex. Our recent glucose positron-emission tomography scan study demonstrated clear differences in glucose metabolism between well-matched depressed and never-depressed patients with HD (Mayberg et al. 1992). The pathophysiologic basis for depression in HD remains unclear, but clues are emerging.

Two differing approaches may be useful in generating hypotheses that can be tested experimentally. The first is to consider both neuropathologic and neurochemical features common to the basal ganglia diseases that produce depression; such an approach may suggest hypotheses that can be applied to studies of the brains of patients who had idiopathic affective disorder (Peyser and Folstein 1990). Second, given the variable pathology of HD, pathologic differences between the brains of patients who had and who never had depression, choosing for examination those structures with some plausible relationship to the brain systems involved in the regulation of emotion.

No evidence exists for damage or interruption of the ascending biogenic amine pathways, either serotonergic or noradrenergic, in HD. This contrasts with some other biologic models for depression, such as some of the stroke literature and some evidence from studies on depression in Alzheimer disease. Given differences in the family-association pattern of depression in HD and Alzheimer disease as well as differences in phenomenology (with bipolar disorder far more prevalent in HD), such differences in neural correlates are not surprising. Each disease may provide different clues worth pursuing in studies of idiopathic affective disorder.

Clinically, once one resists the tendency to use meaningful explanations to "explain away" the phenomena of depression in HD and instead relies on standard diagnostic criteria, diagnosing major depression in HD generally is not difficult. The phenomenology of depression in HD usually is striking, and it is remarkably similar to the phenomenology of idiopathic affective disorder. The mood disorder of HD is treatable often with gratifying results.

REFERENCES

Albin RL, Young AB, Penney JB, et al. 1990. Abnormalities of striatal projection neurons and N-methyl-D-aspartate receptors in presymptomatic Huntington's disease. *N Engl J Med* 322:1293–1298.

American Psychiatric Association. 1980. *Diagnostic and Statistical Manual of Mental Disorders, Third Edition.* Washington, D.C.: American Psychiatric Association.

Barraclough B, Bunch J, Nelson B, et al. 1974. A hundred cases of suicide: clinical aspects. *Br J Psychiatry* 125:355–373.

Bolt JMW. 1970. Huntington's chorea in the west of Scotland. *Br J Psychiatry* 116:259–270.

Bruyn GW. 1968. Huntington's chorea. Historical, clinical and laboratory synopsis. In: *Handbook of Clinical Neurology.* Vinken PJ, Bruyn GW, eds. Amsterdam: Elsevier, pp. 298–378.

Caine ED, Shoulson I. 1983. Psychiatric syndromes in Huntington's disease. *Am J Psychiatry* 140:728–733.

Centers for Disease Control. 1985. *Suicide Surveillance, 1970–1980. Atlanta: United States Department of Health and Human Services, Public Health Service.*

Davenport CB, Muncey EB. 1916. Huntington's chorea in relation to heredity and eugenics. *Am J Insanity* 73:195–222.

De La Monte SM, Vonsattel JP, Richardson EP. 1988. Morphometric demonstration of atrophic changes in the cerebral cortex, white matter and neostriatum in Huntington's disease. *J Neuropathol Exp Neurol* 47:516–525.

Dewhurst K, Oliver JE, McKnight AL. 1970. Socio-psychiatric consequences of Huntington's disease. *Br J Psychiatry* 116:255–258.

Dimaio L, Squittieri F, Napolitano G, et al. 1991. Suicide risk in Huntington's disease. Proceedings of the World Federation of Neurology Research Group on Huntington's Chorea, Abstract #8.

Dublin L. 1963. *Suicide: a Sociological and Statistical Study.* New York: Raven Press.

Dunner DL, Fleiss JL, Addonizio G, et al. 1976. Assortative mating in primary affective disorder. *Biol Psychiatry* 11:43–51.

Farrer LA. 1986. Suicide and attempted suicide in Huntington's disease: implications for preclinical testing of persons at risk. *Am J Med Genet* 24:305–311.

Folstein SE, Folstein MF, Starkstein SE. 1990. Diseases of the caudate as a model for a manic depressive disorder. In: *Function and Dysfunction in the Basal Ganglia.* Franks AJ, et al., eds. Manchester: Manchester University Press, pp. 239–246.

Folstein SE, Abbott MH, Chase GA, et al. 1983. The association of affective disorder with Huntington's disease in a case series and in families. *Psychol Med* 13:537–542.

Folstein SE, Chase GA, Wahl WE, et al. 1987. Huntington's disease: clinical aspects of racial variation. *Am J Hum Genet* 41:168–179.

Folstein SE, Folstein MF. 1983. Psychiatric features of Huntington's disease: recent approaches and findings. *Psychiatr Dev* 2:193–206.

Folstein SE, Peyser CE, Starkstein SE, et al. 1991. The subcortical triad of Huntington's disease: a model for a neuropathology of depression, dementia and dyskinesia. In: Carroll BJ, Barrett JE, eds. *Psychopathology and the Brain*. New York: Raven Press, pp. 65–75.

Graybiel AM, Ragsdale CW. 1978. Histochemically distinct compartments in the striatum of human, monkey and cat demonstrated by acetylocholiesterase staining. *Proc Nat Acad Sci USA* 75:5723–5726.

Hamilton M. 1960. A rating scale for depression. *J Neurol Neurosurg Psychiatry* 23:56–61.

Heathfield KWG. 1967. Huntington's chorea. Investigation into the prevalence of this disease in the area covered by the North East Metropolitan Regional Hospital Board. *Brain* 90:203–232.

Hedreen JC, Peyser CE, Folstein SE, et al. 1991. Neuronal loss in lamina VI of cerebral cortex in Huntington's disease. *Neurosci Let* 133:257–261.

Huntington G. 1872. On chorea. *Adv Neurol* 1:33–35.

Iversen LL, Rosser MN, Reynolds GP. 1983. Loss of pigmented dopamine-B-hydroxylase positive cells from locus coeruleus in senile dementia of Alzheimer's type. *Neurosci Lett* 39:95–100.

Kraepelin E. 1915. Organic dementias. In: Deifendorf AR, ed. *Clinical Psychiatry: A Textbook for Students and Physicians*. New York: MacMillan.

Kurlan R, Caine E, Rubin A, et al. 1988. Cerebrospinal fluid correlates of depression in Huntington's disease. *Arch Neurol* 45:881–883.

Lange HW. 1981. Quantitative changes of telencephalon, diencephalon, and mesencephalon in Huntington's chorea, post-encephalitic and idiopathic Parkinsonism. *Verhandlungen Anatomische Gesellschaft* 75:923–925.

Louhivouri KA, Hakama M. 1979. Risk of suicide among cancer patients. *Am J Epidemiology* 109:59–65.

Mattson B. 1974. Huntington's chorea in Sweden. II. Social and clinical data. *Acta Psychiatr Scand Suppl* 255:221–235.

Mayberg HS, Starkstein SE, Peyser CE, et al. 1992. Paralimbic frontal lobe hypometabolism in depression associated with Huntington's disease. *Neurology* 42:1791–1797.

McHugh PR. 1990. The basal ganglia: the region, the integration of its systems and implications for psychiatry and neurology. In: Franks AJ, ed. *Function and Dysfunction in the Basal Ganglia*. Manchester: Manchester University Press, pp. 259–269.

McHugh PR, Folstein MF. 1975. Psychiatric syndromes of Huntington's chorea: a clinical and phenomenologic study. In: Benson DF, Blumer D, eds. *Psychiatric Aspects of Neurologic Disease*. New York: Grune and Stratton, pp. 267–286.

Merikangas KR, Spiker DG. 1982. Assortative mating among in-patients with primary affective disorder. *Psycholog Med* 12:753–764.

Mindham RHS, Steele C, Folstein MF, et al. 1985. A comparison of the frequency of major affective disorder in Huntington's disease and Alzheimer's disease. *J Neurol Neurosurg Psychiatry* 48:1172–1174.

Minski L, Guttmann E. 1938. Huntington's chorea: a study of 34 families. *J Mental Sci* 84:21–96.

Morris M. 1991. Psychiatric aspects of Huntington's disease. In: Harper P, ed. *Huntington's Disease*. London: W.B. Saunders Company Ltd.

Oliver JE. 1970. Huntington's chorea in Northamptonshire. *Br J Psychiatry* 116:241–253.

Pearlson GD, Ross CA, Lohr WD, et al. 1990. Family history of affective disorder is associated with the depressive syndrome of Alzheimer's disease. *Am J Psychiatry* 147:452–456.

Peyser CE, Folstein SE. 1990. Huntington's disease as a model for mood disorders: clues from neuropathology and neurochemistry. *Mol Chem Neuropathol* 12:99–119.

Peyser CE, Starkstein SE, Folstein SE, et al. 1990. Apathy and irritability in Huntington's disease. American Psychiatric Association 43rd Annual Meeting Proceedings, Symposium 87B:250.

Pflanz S, Besson JA, Ebmeier KP, et al. 1991. The clinical manifestation of mental disorder in Huntington's disease: a retrospective case record study of disease progression. *Acta Psychiatr Scand* 83:53–60.

Robins E. 1981. *The Final Months.* New York: Oxford University Press.

Robins LN, Helzer JE, Croughan J, et al. 1981. The NIMH diagnostic interview schedule, version III. Public Health Service, publication ADM-T-42-3(5-81, 8-81).

Robins LN, Helzer JE, Weissman MM, et al. 1984. Lifetime prevalence of specific psychiatric disorders in three sites. *Arch Gen Psychiatry* 41:949–958.

Rosenbaum D. 1941. Psychosis with Huntington's chorea. *Psychiatr Q* 15: 93–96.

Sotrel A, Paskevich PA, Kiely DK, et al. 1991. Morphometric analysis of the prefrontal cortex in Huntington's disease. *Neurology* 41:1117–1123.

Starkstein SE, Robinson RG. 1989. Affective disorders in cerebral vascular disease. *Br J Psychiatry* 41:949–958.

Thompson WD, Orvaschel H, Prusoff BA, et al. 1982. An evaluation of the family history method for ascertaining psychiatric disorders. *Arch Gen Psychiatry* 39:53–60.

Vonsattel JP, Meyers RH, Stevens TJ, et al. 1985. Neuropathological classification of Huntington's disease. *J Neuropathol Exp Neurol* 44:559–577.

Weissman MW, Merikangas KR, Boyd JH. 1989. Epidemiology of affective disorder. In: Michels R, ed. *Psychiatry.* Philadelphia: J.B. Lippincott.

Zweig RM, Ross CA, Hedreen JC, et al. 1988. The neuropathology of aminergic nuclei in Alzheimer's disease. *Ann Neurol* 24:233–242.

Zweig RM, Ross CA, Hedreen JC, et al. 1992. Locus coeruleus involvement in Huntington's disease. *Arch Neurol* 49:152–156.

9

DEPRESSION IN TRAUMATIC BRAIN INJURY

J. Paul Fedoroff, M.D.
Ricardo E. Jorge, M.D.
Robert G. Robinson, M.D.

Many neurologists and psychiatrists have described an association between brain injury and depression (Meyer 1904, Babinski 1914, Kraepelin 1921, Denny-Brown et al. 1952, Gainotti 1972), but despite these clinical associations, literature regarding the frequency and nature of depression following brain injury has been inconsistent. The reasons for these inconsistent findings are numerous; perhaps the most important is the inconsistencies between the populations studied; some studies have included soldiers injured during World War I (Goldstein 1948) or World War II (Lishman 1968), and others have included children (Brown et al. 1981); patients with mild (Rutherford et al. 1979), moderate (Rimel et al. 1982), or severe head injury (Tate et al. 1989); or open (Tellier et al. 1989) or closed (Denny-Brown 1945) head injuries. Studies also have differed in terms of the time of evaluation, ranging from inhospital (Fedoroff et al. 1992) to many years following the injury (Thompsen 1984). Finally, there have been differing methods to assess the clinical state, with some studies using depression rating scales and others diagnostic criteria. (Prigatano [1987] reviewed methodologic issues regarding research into the psychiatric aspects of head trauma.)

Several facts underline the clinical importance of depression following head trauma. First, the number of people surviving head trauma has increased dramatically in the last two decades, and these survivors are now living longer. Therefore, an increased likelihood exists that any predisposition of patients with head trauma toward depression will be expressed. As a result, clinicians can expect to see more patients with head trauma and serious depression. Second, of all the changes that occur in the lives of individuals with head trauma, those affecting psychologic functioning and social behavior are rated by family members as the most consistently distressing and are predictive of whether individuals may live independently (Livingston et al. 1985, Wedell 1980, Thompsen 1984).

Individuals and their relatives frequently complain that symptoms of apathy, poor concentration, irritability, social withdrawal, and hopelessness about the future are particularly distressing. These are all symptoms that occur frequently in populations having major depression without head injury, and they are responsive to treatment. Systematic efficacy studies regarding the treatment of depressive disorders in patients with head trauma are needed.

Finally, information that is now available from neuroradiologic techniques makes possible the investigation of the relationship between depressive disorders and both structural and functional brain abnormalities. These techniques include single photon emission CT, MRI, and positron-emission tomography scan methodologies.

PREVALENCE

In a review of epidemiologic studies concerning depression among patients with head trauma, Gualtieri (1991) estimated that major depression occurred in 25% to 50% of patients with traumatic brain injury, and another 15% to 30% showed symptoms compatible with the diagnosis of dysthymia. Kinsella et al. (1988) reported a series of 39 patients within 2 years of severe head injury; 33% were classified as depressed and 26% as suffering from anxiety. Rutherford et al. (1977) found that 6% of 145 patients with minor head injury had a significant number of depressive symptoms within 6 weeks after injury. In addition, the rate of suicide in soldiers with head injury has been reported to be increased compared with uninjured soldiers (Vauhkonen 1959), and these rates increased with time from injury (Achte and Anttinen 1963). We found that 17 of 66 patients (26%) admitted to a trauma unit with a closed head injury had a diagnosis of major depression, while another 11 patients (16%) developed a major depression at some time during a 1-year follow-up period (Fedoroff et al. 1992, Jorge et al. 1992a).

DIAGNOSIS

Individuals with traumatic brain injury who develop a persistent mood change that is unattributable to delirium satisfy the DSM-III-R criteria for the diagnosis of organic mood syndrome (American Psychiatric Association 1987). These diagnostic criteria have the advantage of simplifying the diagnosis of mood disorders in this population; organic mood syndrome diagnostic criteria, however, have the disadvantage of a considerable loss of consistency in clinical presentation. For example, in patients with stroke, we have found significant differences between those satisfying diagnostic symptom criteria for major depression and those satisfying symptom criteria for dysthymic disorder in terms of the duration of depression or the frequency of a positive DST (Lipsey et al. 1985).

In addition to the issue of whether different types of depression should be recognized, a more fundamental question is whether the symptoms used for diagnosing depression in populations without brain injury are applicable to depression in patients with traumatic brain injury. For example, many symptoms of major depression and dysthymia, such as decreased interest and changes in weight, sleep, appetite, energy, or ability to concentrate, are symptoms that might be attributable to causes other than depression. It is reasonable to be concerned that depressive disorders easily could be overdiagnosed in populations with head injuries because of both these and other nonspecific symptoms. However, patients might deny the presence of a depressed mood as part of a general unawareness deficit or denial syndrome; this would result in the underdiagnosis of depression.

We longitudinally examined the specificity of depressive symptoms used in the diagnosis of depression following traumatic brain injury (Jorge et al. 1992c). We found that the mean frequency of both autonomic and psychologic symptoms was more than three times higher in patients who reported a depressed mood ($n = 19$) compared with those without a depressed mood ($n = 47$). Both autonomic and psychologic symptoms distinguish patients with from patients without depression following traumatic brain injury, but the number and type of symptoms associated with depression change over time. The psychologic symptoms that consistently discriminated patients with traumatic brain injury who were and were not depressed at both the initial evaluations and at 1-year follow-up were those related to changes in self-attitude (feelings of hopelessness, suicidal ideation, loss of interest, self-deprecation, lack of self-confidence). The only autonomic symptom that was significantly related to depression during the entire 1-year period was lack of energy (i.e., subjective anergia). Anxiety symptoms were significantly associated with depression only during the first 6 months following closed head trauma; at the 1-year follow-up, their frequency was not significantly different in patients with or without depressed mood. Autonomic symptoms such as decreased appetite, weight loss, difficulty falling asleep, and diurnal mood variation (with morning depression) appeared to be significantly associated with depression only during the initial and 3-month evaluations and not at the 1-year follow-up. However, early morning awakening, loss of libido, difficulty concentrating, and inefficient thinking distinguished patients with depression from those without only after 6 months or 1 year elapsed; increased appetite, weight gain, and hypersomnia did not differentiate depressed from nondepressed groups at any time.

We then examined whether diagnostic criteria for major depression should be altered to include only those symptoms that were significantly associated with depression. If we required that three of the symptoms significantly associated with depression (including depressed mood) be present as criteria for diagnosing major depression, then standard DSM-III-R criteria had a 100% sensitivity and 94% specificity at the initial evaluation, 88% sensitivity and 94% specificity at 3 months, 91% sensitivity and 96% specificity at 6 months, and 80% sensitivity and 100% specificity at the 1-year follow-up. Thus, the standard diagnostic criteria (DSM-III-R) for major depression have a high sensitivity and specificity compared with alternative diagnostic criteria that use only those symptoms specific to depression. Standard diagnostic criteria may be used for the diagnosis of depression in this population.

Finally, the frequency of "masked" depressions (i.e., patients who presented with at least three specific symptoms of depression but denied a depressive mood) was impressively low. At the 1-year follow-up, "masked" depressions occurred in only two patients.

ASSOCIATED VARIABLES

One problem facing most studies of head trauma is that trauma, by its nature, generally is unexpected, and it often is difficult to ascertain what individuals were like before their injury. In a follow-up study comparing twins in which one had sustained a head injury, Denker (1960) concluded that the symptoms of headache, vertigo, dizziness, and photophobia were more closely related to constitutional factors than to the nature of the injury. In addition, head-injured, dizygotic twins were more likely to be accident-prone and antisocial, and to have had a lower social position than the uninjured co-twin. Other researchers have reported that patients with head trauma may be "maladjusted" (Fahy et al. 1967), have a higher incidence of previous trauma (Jamieson 1971), and have poorer premorbid academic performance (Haas et al. 1987). These premorbid constitutional factors may play an important role in symptomatic outcome following head injury, and they may influence the development of depressive disorders.

We examined 66 consecutive admissions to a head trauma unit of patients with acute closed head injury approximately 1 month after injury (Fedoroff et al. 1992). Patients were entered in the study only if their primary injury was traumatic brain injury and they did not have significant injury to another body system, such as multiple fractures, ruptured spleen, lung collapse, and so on; in addition, only patients who were able to comprehend and answer questions during a verbal interview were included. Patients were divided into those who met DSM-III criteria for major depression ($n = 17$) and those with no mood disorder ($n = 47$). Two additional patients meeting symptom criteria for dysthymic (minor) depression were excluded from further analysis because of their small number.

There were no significant differences between the major-depression and the nondepressed groups in terms of age, gender, race, education, marital status, socioeconomic class, neurologic findings, type of brain injury, or acute Glasgow Coma scores; on psychiatric examination, patients with depression had significantly higher PSE and Hamilton Depression Scale scores. There were no significant between-group differences in cognitive impairment as measured by the Mini-Mental State Examination (Folstein et al. 1975), in ADLs as measured by the Johns Hopkins Functional Inventory (Robinson and Szetela 1981), or in degree of premorbid social support as measured by the Social Ties Checklist (Starr et al. 1983). The acute major-depression group, however, had a significantly greater frequency of previous personal history of psychiatric disorders (including alcohol or other substance abuse). In addition, the acute major-depression group showed significantly increased (i.e., more impaired) Social Functioning Examination scores. The social function exam during the initial evaluation measured satisfaction with social functioning during the period before brain injury; this suggests that patients with poor social adjustment and social dissatisfaction before injury are more prone to develop depression following traumatic brain injury.

Descriptions regarding the course of recovery from traumatic brain injury consistently note that mood disorders may occur at any time, often years after the injury, and that the course of recovery does not appear to be related directly to the seriousness of the injury (Levin et al. 1979). In fact, emotional problems appear to increase during the first year after injury while neurologic symptoms resolve (McKinlay et al. 1981, Fordyce et al. 1983, Dunlop et al. 1991).

Bond (1984) proposed a useful categorization, consisting of three stages, of the recovery from severe head injury. Stage 1 generally is several days in duration and characterized by unconsciousness and maximum severity of neurologic deficits. Stage 2 usually occurs over the next 3 to 6 months; it is characterized by a return to full consciousness and the gradual recovery of both physical function and memory. Stage 3 occurs over the following 3 to 6 months and is characterized by a stabilization of physical recovery and mental ability. Depressive disorders have been reported during time periods corresponding to all three stages (McKinlay et al. 1981); however, because the first is characterized by an altered level of consciousness, delirium is a more common diagnosis during stage 1. Diagnosis of depressive disorders becomes more frequent as consciousness returns (Bond 1984).

We also cross-sectionally analyzed our data at 3, 6, and 12 months of follow-up (Jorge et al. 1992a). Of the original 66 patients, 54 were evaluated at 3 months; major depression was diagnosed in 12 (22.2%), and four (7.7%) had minor depression. Among the patients who were not depressed during the inhospital period (i.e., at the initial evaluation), major depression had occurred in 17% by 3-months follow-up. At 6-months posttrauma, 43 patients were reevaluated, and 11 met DSM-III diagnostic criteria for either major or minor depression. Of these, 10 patients (23.2%) were diagnosed as having major and one (2.3%) as having minor depression. Among patients who were not depressed either initially or at the 3-month follow-up, the incidence of major depression was 15%. Finally, of the original 66 patients, 43 were interviewed at the 1-year follow-up, and 11 of these patients (25.6%) met DSM-III-R criteria for either major or minor depression (eight with major and three with minor depression). Among the patients who had not developed depressive disorders at the time of the preceding evaluations, the incidence of major depression was 12%. Thus, 15 patients developed delayed-onset major or minor depressions during the follow-up period. Of the 41 patients initially without depression who were seen at follow-up, 11 (26.8%) were later diagnosed with major depressive disorder (four patients at the 3-month follow-up evaluation, four at the 6-month evaluation, and three at the 1-year follow-up evaluation); the four remaining patients of those 15 with delayed-onset depression received a diagnosis of minor (dysthymic) depression. In summary, even though some patients were getting better and others developing new depressions, the overall frequency of major depression remained relatively stable at approximately 25% throughout the first year following traumatic brain injury.

Merskey and Woodforde (1972) followed patients with head injury and compared the outcome of patients who both had and had not sought financial compensation. They found no differences between the two groups in terms of symptoms profiles; however, patients with poor outcome also appeared to have symptoms of "endogenous depression." Merskey and Woodforde concluded that the symptoms frequently attributed to neuroticism or malingering (such as headache, dizziness, depressed mood, and anxiety) were not always psychogenic in origin. The possibility that depression affected outcome was raised as well, and Bornstein et al. (1989) found a positive relationship between the degree of neuropsychologic impairment and the level of emotional disturbance in a group of 124 patients who suffered work-related closed head injuries.

In our studies, depression was unrelated to the degree of cognitive or physical impairment, but we found a consistent relationship between depression and impaired social functioning. We have noted that patients already having poor social adjustment are more prone to develop depression following traumatic brain injury; in addition, however, social functioning and depression appear to interact in such a way that, after the brain injury, patients with previous social functioning impairment remained depressed and, perhaps, the social functioning of the patients with depression deteriorated. One might infer from these findings, therefore, that social intervention as well as the treatment of depression may be necessary to alleviate these severe and long-lasting mood disorders.

PATHOGENESIS

In his review of traumatic brain injury, Lishman (1987) identified 10 factors that may contribute to the development of psychiatric disturbances following brain injury. These factors were mental constitution and premorbid personality, emotional impact of the injury, environmental factors, compensation and litigation, response to intellectual impairments, development of epilepsy, and the amount and location of brain injury.

The most important physical factors determining extent of brain damage in traumatic head injuries are the force and site of impact, brain exposure, and the degree of head motion before and after impact. After impact, brain lesions are most marked at the impact site and the opposite pole ("contre coup" injury); the brain areas most frequently affected are the ventral aspects of the frontal and temporal lobes. Unconsciousness most commonly is associated with closed head injury that results in trauma or shearing of the subcortical and brainstem areas. Secondary sequelae of traumatic brain injury include vascular lesions, changes in blood perfusion, and cerebral edema which in turn may lead to varying degrees of anoxia.

Head injury also has been associated with neurotransmitter and neurohormonal changes. Van Woerkom et al. (1977) found that patients with traumatic brain injury and frontal-temporal contusions had decreased levels of 5-hydroxyindoleacetic acid in their CSF compared with patients having diffuse traumatic injuries and evidence of brainstem dysfunction. Hamill et al. (1987) serially measured plasma levels of epinephrine, norepinephrine, and dopamine in 33 patients with traumatic brain injury and proposed that highly elevated circulating catecholamines may be excellent endogenous markers of the amount of brain damage as well as predictors of long-term outcome. In addition, Prigatano (1987) hypothesized that the important changes in adrenocorticotropic hormone and cortisol levels that occur in patients with traumatic brain injury may mediate changes in mood as well.

In a study comparing stroke and trauma in a population with chronic brain injury (Robinson and Szetela 1981), we found that patients with stroke were more severely depressed than patients with traumatic injury. Differences in the anterioposterior location of CT-visualized lesions in the left hemisphere, however, explained this difference in the severity of depressive symptoms. When the two groups were matched for lesion location, there was no difference in the severity of depression. In addition, there was a significant correlation for both groups between the proximity of the largest left hemisphere lesion to the frontal pole and the severity of depression, thus suggesting that depression in both groups (at least among those with left anterior lesions) may have similar pathogenesis.

In our previously described study of traumatic brain injury (Fedoroff et al. 1992) 56 (85%) of the original 66 patients had brain abnormalities on CT scan. Twenty-two patients had single focal lesions, and 23 had multiple or bilateral lesions. The remaining 11 patients had either extraparenchymal hemorrhages (epidural, subdural, or subarachnoid) or neuroradiologic evidence of brain edema, brain atrophy, or hydrocephalus. Most patients in both the depressed and nondepressed groups had CT-scan evidence of brain contusions (i.e., 71% with and 62% without depression). There were no significant differences in the frequency of the various types of injury between the depressed and nondepressed groups, and to analyze the relationship between lesion location and the presence of major depression, a logistic regression procedure was used. The model included the following location variables: left, right, cortical, subcortical, single, multiple, frontal, orbitofrontal, temporal, temporobasal, left anterior (i.e., left dorsolateral frontal cortex and/or left basal ganglia lesions), and parietal-occipital. We found an overall significant association between lesion location and the development of major depression ($\chi^2 = 33.64$, df $= 12$, $P = 0.0008$). A backward selection procedure was performed to remove the nonsignificant variables ($P < 0.05$), and after their removal the reduced model included the following: left (i.e., left hemisphere lesions only), right (i.e., right hemisphere lesions only), cortical, frontal (i.e., right, left, or bilateral frontal lesions excluding orbitofrontal involvement), left anterior, and parietal-occipital lesions ($\chi^2 = 31.394$, df $= 6$, $P = 0.0001$).

The presence of a left anterior lesion was by far the strongest correlate of major depression (Wald $\chi^2 = 12.97$, $P = 0.0003$). To a lesser degree, parietal-occipital (Wald $\chi^2 = 6.91$, $O = 0.008$) and right hemisphere (Wald $\chi^2 = 4.75$, $P = 0.03$) lesions increased the probability of developing major depression; however, the presence of left (Wald $\chi^2 = 4.08$, $P = 0.04$), cortical (Wald $\chi^2 = 6.28$, $P = 0.01$) and frontal (Wald $\chi^2 = 6.56$, $P = 0.01$) lesions decreased the probability of developing brain depression. Comparing the predicted and observed events, this model (based on lesion location) showed a 70% sensitivity and 83% specificity for major depression. This finding is consistent with that of Lipsey et al. (1983) that patients with left anterior strokes had a higher frequency of depression regardless of whether they had lesions in other locations as well.

The association between major depression and lesion location appears to be restricted to the initial stage of traumatic brain injury, however. At the 3-month evaluation, this association was no longer significant (Jorge et al. 1992a), and this finding contrasts with the evidence gathered among patients with stroke. The association between major depression and location of brain damage, however, was significant up to 1 year of follow-up.

We also have found that although both acute- and delayed-onset depressions share the same factors of previous personal psychiatric history as well as social vulnerability in the development of depression (Jorge et al. 1992b), there are important differences between these disorders. Some acute-onset depressions are related to lesion characteristics; delayed-onset depressions appear to be related to social factors or previous history of psychiatric disorder. We hypothesize that acute-onset depressions may have their etiology in the biologic responses of the injured brain and that delayed-onset depressions may be mediated by psychosocial factors with psychologic reaction as a possible mechanism.

TREATMENT

Using a retrospective research design, O'Shanick et al. (1984) compared the treatment received by patients with head trauma and left or right cerebral injuries. They found that patients with left cerebral injuries were five times more likely to have received antidepressant medications than those patients with right cerebral lesions. Unfortunately, there have been no double-blind controlled studies comparing the efficacy of various pharmacologic treatments of depression in patients with closed head injury; successful treatment of depression in such patients has been reported with psychostimulants (primarily methylphenidate) (Gualtieri 1988), trazodone (Gualtieri 1991), fluoxetine (Cassidy 1989), and buspirone (Gualtieri 1991). Tricyclic antidepressants, however, remain the mainstay of pharmacologic treatment in patients with head injuries (Fedoroff and Robinson 1989), and because no one antidepressant has been shown to be superior to others in relieving depression, medication choices tend to be made based on side effect profiles. In patients with head injury, low sedation, minimal effect on seizure threshold, and low anticholinergic activity are important.

Electroconvulsant therapy is not contraindicated in patients with traumatic brain injury. This method of treatment should be considered if others have not been successful.

Whether or not pharmacologic treatment is undertaken, psychotherapy and social support for the patient and the patient's relatives and caregivers is crucial (O'Shanick 1986). For example, at 1 year of follow-up, Rosenbaum and Najenson (1976) found a high incidence of depressive disorders in the wives of soldiers with head injuries. Thus, the current empiric evidence regarding the clinical importance of depressive disorders that follow traumatic brain injury emphasizes the need of assuring that not only the patient but the patient's family and caregivers receive both evaluation and treatment not only for the head injury but for possible depression as well.

CONCLUSIONS

Depression is only one of many psychiatric disorders that may occur following traumatic brain injury. It may, however, be one of the most easily overlooked and misunderstood conditions, because its symptoms are easily confused with the expected physical symptoms or psychologic reactions to the injury. Our studies of patients with traumatic brain injury found that major depression occurred in 42% at some point during a 1-year follow-up period; these depressions were associated with social functioning, previous psychiatric history, and location of brain injury. Other investigators also have identified clinical correlates, including previous personality, epilepsy, and severity of impairment. How these factors interact or may lead independently to depression is unknown. Preliminary evidence suggests that failure to recognize and treat depression may interfere with the rate and degree of recovery as well as decrease the chance of returning to independent living in the community. Further studies of the phenomenology, course, pathogenesis, and efficacy of the treatment of depression following traumatic brain injury are needed to improve our understanding and care of these patients.

REFERENCES

Achte KA, Anttinen EE. 1963. Suizide bei hirngeschadigten des krieges in Finland. *Fortshr Neurologie Psychiatrie* 31:645–667.
American Psychiatric Association. 1987. *Diagnostic and Statistical Manual*

of Mental Disorders, Third Edition (Revised). Washington, D.C.: American Psychiatric Association.

Babinski J. 1914. Contributions a l'etude des troubles mentaux dans l'hemiplegie organique cerebral (anosognosie). *Rev Neurol (Paris)* 27:845–848.

Bond MR. 1984. The psychiatry of closed head injury. In: Brooks N, ed. *Close Head Injury: Psychological, Social, and Family Consequences*. Oxford: Oxford University Press, pp. 148–178.

Bornstein RA, Miller HB, Van Schoor JT. 1989. Neuropsychological deficit and emotional disturbance in head injured patients. *J Neurosurg* 7:509–513.

Brown G, Chadwick O, Schaffer D, et al. 1981. A prospective study of children with head injuries: 111 psychiatric sequelae. *Psychol Med* 11:63–78.

Cassidy JW. 1989. Fluoxetine: a new serotonergically active antidepressant. *J Head Trauma Rehabil* 4:67–69.

Denny-Brown DE. 1945. Disability arising from closed head injury. *JAMA* 127:429.

Denny-Brown DE, Meyer JS, Horenstein S. 1952. The significance of perceptual rivalry resulting from parietal lesions. *Brain* 75:434–471.

Denker SJ. 1960. Closed head injury in twins. *Arch Gen Psychiatry* 2:569–575.

Dunlop TW, Udvarhely GB, Steden AFA, et al. 1991. Comparison of patients with and without emotional behavioral deterioration during the first year after traumatic brain injury. *J Neuropsychiat Clin Neurosci* 3: 150–156.

Fahy TJ, Irving MH, Millac P. 1967. Severe head injuries. *Lancet* ii:475–479.

Fedoroff JP, Robinson RG. 1989. Tricyclic antidepressants in the treatment of post-stroke depression. *J Clin Psychiatry* 50(suppl):1823.

Fedoroff JP, Starkstein SE, Forrester AW, et al. 1992. Depression in patients with acute traumatic brain injury. *Am J Psychiatry*, 149:918–923.

Folstein MF, Folstein SE, McHugh PR. 1975. Mini-Mental State: a practical method for grading the cognitive state of patients for the clinician. *J Psychiatr Res* 12:189–198.

Fordyce DJ, Roueche JR, Prigatano GP. 1983. Enhanced emotional reactions in chronic head trauma patients. *J Neurol Neurosurg Psychiatry* 46:620–624.

Gainotti G. 1972. Emotional behavior and hemispheric side of lesion. *Cortex* 8:4155.

Goldstein K. 1948. *After-Effects of Brain Injuries in War*. New York: Grune and Stratton.

Gualtieri CT. 1988. Pharmacotherapy and the neurobehavioral sequelae of traumatic brain injury. *Brain Inj* 2:101–129.

Gualtieri CT. 1991. *Neuropsychiatry and Behavioral Pharmacology*. New York: Springer-Verlag.

Haas JF, Cope DN, Hall K. 1987. Premorbid prevalence of poor academic performance in severe head injury. *J Neurol Neurosurg Psychiatry* 50:52–56.

Hamill RW, Woolf PD, McDonald JV, et al. 1987. Catecholamines predict outcome in traumatic brain injury. *Ann Neurol* 21:438–443.

Jamieson KG. 1971. Prevention of head injury. In: Caveness W, Walker E, eds. *Head Injuries*. Edinburgh: Churchill Livingstone.

Jorge RE, Robinson RG, Arndt SV, et al. 1992a. Depression and traumatic brain injury: a longitudinal study. *J Nerv Ment Dis* (in press).

Jorge RE, Robinson RG, Arndt SV, et al. 1992b. Comparison between acute and delayed onset depression following traumatic brain injury. *J Neuropsychiat Clin Neurosci* (in press).

Jorge RE, Robinson RG, Arndt SV. 1992c. Are there symptoms which are specific for a depressed mood in patients with traumatic brain injury? *J Nerv Ment Dis* (in press).

Kinsella G, Moran C, Ford B, et al. 1988. Emotional disorder and its assessment with the severe head injured population. *Psychol Med* 18:57–63.

Kraepelin E. 1921. *Manic Depressive Insanity and Paranoia*. Edinburgh: E and S Livingstone.

Levin HS, Grossman RG, Rose JE, et al. 1979. Long-term neuropsychologic outcome of closed head injury. *J Neurosurg* 50:412–422.

Lipsey JR, Robinson RG, Pearlson GD. 1985. Dexamethasone suppression test and mood following stroke. *Am J Psychiatry* 142:318–323.

Lipsey JR, Robinson RG, Pearlson GD, et al. 1983. Mood change following bilateral hemisphere brain injury. *Br J Psychiatry* 143:366–373.

Lishman WA. 1968. Brain damage in relation to psychiatric disability after head injury. *Br J Psychiatry* 114:373–410.

Lishman WA. 1987. *Organic Psychiatry: the Psychological Consequences of Cerebral Disorder*. Oxford: Blackwell.

Livingston M, Brooks N, Bond M. 1985. Patient outcome in the year following severe head injury and relative's psychiatric and social functioning. *J Neurol Neurosurg Psychiatry* 48:876–881.

McKinlay WW, Brooks DN, Bond MR, et al. 1981. The short-term outcome of severe blunt head injury as reported by relatives of the injured person. *J Neurol Neurosurg Psychiatry* 44:527–533.

Merskey H, Woodforde JM. 1972. Psychiatric sequelae of minor head injury. *Brain* 95:521–528.

Meyer A. 1904. The anatomical facts and clinical varieties of traumatic insanity. *Am J Insanity* 60:373.

O'Shanik G, Scott R, Peterson LG. 1984. Psychiatric referral after head trauma. *Psychiatr Med* 2:131–137.

O'Shanick GJ. 1986. Neuropsychiatric complications in head injury. *Adv Psychosom Med* 16:173–193.

Prigatano GP. 1987. Psychiatric aspects of head injury: problem areas and suggested guidelines for research. In: Levin HS, Grafman J, Eisenberg HM, eds. *Neurobehavioral Recovery from Head Injury*. New York: Oxford University Press.

Rimel EW, Giordani B, Barth JT, et al. 1982. Moderate head injury: completing the clinical spectrum of brain trauma. *Neurosurgery* 11:344–351.

Robinson RG, Szetela B. 1981. Mood change following left hemisphere brain injury. *Ann Neurol* 9:447–453.

Rosenbaum M, Najenson J. 1976. Changes in life pattern and symptoms of low mood as reported by wives of severely brain injured soldiers. *J Consult Clin Psychol* 44:881–888.

Rutherford WH, Merrett JD, McDonald JR. 1977. Sequelae of concussion caused by minor head injury. *Lancet* ii:1–4.

Rutherford WH, Merrett JD, McDonald JR. 1979. Symptoms at one year following concussion from minor injuries. *Injury* 10:225–230.

Starr LB, Robinson RG, Price TR. 1983. Reliability, validity, and clinical utility of the social functioning exam in the assessment of stroke patients. *Exp Aging Res* 9:101.

Tate RL, Lulham JM, Broe GA, et al. 1989. Psychosocial outcome for the survivors of severe blunt head injury: the results from a consecutive series of 100 patients. *J Neurol Neurosurg Psychiatry* 52:1128–1134.

Tellier A, Adonis KM, Walker AE, et al. 1990. Long-term effects of severe penetrating head injury on psychosocial adjustment. *J Consult Clin Psychol* 58:531–537.

Thompsen IV. 1984. Late outcome of very severe blunt head trauma: a 10–15 year second follow-up. *J Neurol Neurosurg Psychiatry* 47:260–268.

Van Woerkom TC, Teelken AW, Minderhoud JM. 1977. Difference in neurotransmitter metabolism in frontotemporal lobe contusion and diffuse cerebral contusion. *Lancet* i:812–813.

Vauhkonen K. 1959. Suicide among the male disabled with war injuries to the brain. *Acta Psychiatr Neurolog Scand Suppl* 137:90–91.

Wedell R, Oddy M, Jenkins D. 1980. Social adjustment after rehabilitation: a two year follow-up of patients with severe head injury. *Psychol Med* 10:257–263.

10

DEPRESSION IN APHASIA

D. Frank Benson, M.D.
Alfredo Ardila, Ph.D.

Aphasia ranks among the most psychologically devastating neurologic conditions, with serious psychiatric implications that are significant not only for the patient but also for relatives and caregivers. Aphasia has been recognized for over a century and has undergone a broad range of psychologic studies, including a treatment procedure based primarily on psychologic support. Despite this background, however, relatively little attention has been given to the psychiatric complications that often prove crucial to the evolution and ultimate outcome of the aphasic condition.

By definition, *aphasia* is an impairment in verbal communication (specifically, the loss or impairment of language) resulting from brain damage (Benson 1979, Hécaen 1972). Aphasia is common, and approximately 100,000 Americans become aphasic each year (Albert et al. 1981) as a result of cerebrovascular accidents, traumatic brain injury, or intracranial neoplasms. Many additional cases also result from degenerative brain diseases, infections to the central nervous system, and other destructive brain processes.

The term *depression* indicates a far more common disorder, with estimates that up to 25% of the general population suffer psychiatrically significant depression at some period of their life (Siever et al. 1991). An overlap of these two disorders would appear reasonable, but depression is considerably more common in patients with aphasia. Depression also appears to be related to the etiology and/or the site of the lesion. Few studies have been devoted to the analysis of depression in aphasia, at least in part because of the obvious difficulty of performing in-depth psychiatric interviews with patients suffering a partial or total loss of language function.

Depression is also frequent in speech disorders (as distinguished from language disorders). Stuttering has been associated with depression and social withdrawal (Perello 1970, Rosenfield 1982), and depression is a common complicating factor in various types of dysarthria (Tanner and Gerstenberger 1988). In fact, depression is a frequent behavioral complication of several primary neurologic disorders that produce speech problems, including Huntington disease, multiple sclerosis, and Parkinson disease (McHugh and Folstein 1975, Whitlock and Siskind 1980).

A direct correlation between the severity of aphasia (as represented by the size of brain lesion) and depression has not been possible. Some concurrence between lesion size and the degree of depression can be seen in global aphasia, but a direct association is not present in other aphasic syndromes. For instance, in cases of Broca aphasia, the location of the lesion as well as the direction of the lesion extension represent critical factors; in Wernicke aphasia, an inverse correlation between lesion size and depression exists: the smaller the lesion, the more evident the depression (Robinson and Benson 1981).

TYPES OF DEPRESSIVE REACTIONS

Depression is a complex, heterogenous phenomenon, and differences in the type of depression seen in patients with aphasia could be anticipated. Unfortunately, investigation into the characterization of depression in aphasia is sparse, but several studies reporting the overall occurrence of depression following cerebrovascular accident are available (Benson 1973; Charatan and Fisk 1978; Folstein et al. 1977; Gainotti 1969, 1972, 1983; Robinson and Benson 1981; Robinson and Chait 1985; Robinson and Price 1982; Robinson and Szetela 1981; Robinson et al. 1984a, 1984b; Ruckdeschel-Hibbard et al. 1986; Starkstein et al. 1987; Starkstein and Robinson 1988). Data from these studies as well as personal observations (Benson 1973, 1992) suggest that at least three distinct types of depressive reaction can occur in aphasic subjects. Table 10.1 presents these and a fourth significant complication of depression in aphasia.

Table 10.1. Affective Problems of Aphasia

Grief, psychosocial loss
Organic affective syndrome
Frustration, depression, catastrophic reaction syndrome
Suicide

GRIEF

The obvious psychosocial factor that affects most patients with aphasia stems from the sudden, unexpected onset of a calamitous alteration in lifestyle. Language is so basic to human existence that its loss ranks with acute blindness or quadriplegia in the degree of psychic shock. The magnitude of the problem appears almost overwhelming; anyone who has lived in an alien linguistic environment recognizes the solitude and helpless feeling produced by the inability to understand or communicate everyday events with others. An intense frustration can develop in the patient with aphasia (Herrmann and Wallesch 1989), and in addition, destabilizing changes occur in the patient's employment status, social and family position, recreational opportunities, and so on. The onset of aphasia produces severe psychosocial problems.

Among these important psychosocial problems, the alteration in economic status ranks as a major concern. Aphasia usually occurs at a stage when the individual has become comparatively independent and self-sufficient. This pleasant status suddenly disappears, and those with aphasia may realize that their economic independence is permanently lost, which is a matter of deep and realistic concern for both the patient and family. To complicate the situation, paranoid concerns about money may arise. Some with aphasia express fear that their relatives are trying to take their money (which is sometimes realistically based), and many fear a state of fiscal dependency. Loss of the ability to generate income can lead to a feeling of uselessness.

A similar alteration occurs in the patient's social position. Most with aphasia have developed fixed patterns in both their employment and social affairs by the time the disorder strikes. They have firm relationships with relatives, co-workers, employees, neighbors, social and recreational associates and others; that status is abruptly changed. Neither the actual change nor the realization of the degree of change is recognized immediately, but it eventually becomes an important psychosocial consideration. Many patients, not by plan or choice, are forced to retire and must face all the problems of retired individuals.

The patient with aphasia often experiences an altered family status as well. The patient's role in the family, either as leader or significant contributor, is jeopardized. If the disability is comparatively mild, the patient's previous status may be regained, but when the language disturbance and associated motor impairments are severe, the spouse or some other family member must assume the leadership role. Needing help in everyday activities and finding that most decisions are made by the spouse or children, the patient may be forced into a passive, child-like position within the family. Reaction to the downgrading of family position may be violent, with negative, hostile, paranoid, and even cruel behavior directed toward close family members. Realization of the altered position often is delayed following the onset of symptoms, and aphasia may be perceived initially as a transient problem. Relatives frequently overestimate anticipated improvement and misinterpret the patient's potential for psychosocial adjustment (Herrmann and Wallesch 1989, Müller et al. 1983). Only with time does the family accept the permanent alteration in lifestyle. Many families are not capable of gracefully effecting this alteration, and if the patient is isolated from family activities or the family members express anger or hostility based on decreased income, altered social position, and many new responsibilities, then an additional psychologic burden is created.

Many patients also suffer alterations in their physical capability. A previously active, self-caring individual may be hemiparetic, must learn to stand and walk, and can never again participate in vigorous activities. Physical impairment represents yet another demoralizing loss for those with aphasia.

Additionally, real or imagined loss of sexual capability can produce considerable anguish. Aphasia-producing pathology does not affect sexual competency in most individuals, but paralysis and the inability to communicate create obvious hindrances to normal sexual relationships. Even in elderly individuals, jealousy (either real or imagined) often is an additional complication to the patient's relationship with the spouse.

Physical incompetence, economic dependence, altered social and employment status, and impaired family relationships represent significant losses, and it would be natural for the patient to undergo a mourning reaction or period of bereavement. The combination of losses produces a disturbance of self-image, often with self-deprecation, including a hopeless and worthless feeling in the patient that may lead to psychologically significant depression.

The psychosocial losses are real, and while a period of grief would appear inevitable, it is not seen consistently. Most patients with aphasia do not show the anticipated grief reaction, at least not during the early postonset stages of their disorder. Rather, grief may appear suddenly many weeks or even months after the onset of aphasia and be characterized by a general anhedonia and a tendency to complain of personal losses; to discuss worries concerning family, business, finances, and so on; to withdraw from full participation in physical and language therapies; and to avoid nursing and rehabilitation staff and family members. The onset of this reactive depression is a matter of concern and demands intelligent, coordinated efforts. While transient and usually nonthreatening, the grief reaction may be intense and produce considerable discomfort for the patient, family, and rehabilitation staff. It is a very real form of depression.

ORGANIC AFFECTIVE SYNDROME

In addition to the obvious, socially produced psychologic difficulties, some patients with aphasia appear to suffer emotional responses that vary with the location of pathology. Two behavioral reactions to the aphasic condition correlate with the anatomic locus: one accompanies nonfluent (anterior) aphasia, and a second appears in fluent (posterior) aphasia (Alxander and Benson 1991; Benson 1973, 1979; Robinson and Benson 1981).

Depression is the emotional disturbance most often observed during nonfluent aphasia, with severe aphasic depression most often reported in global aphasia, Broca aphasia (Robinson and Benson 1981), or subcortical aphasia with anterior extension (Alexander and LoVerme 1980, Starkstein et al. 1987). Robinson and Szetela (1981) conjecture that at least part of this depression is a result of left hemisphere damage, not simply a reaction to psychosocial loss. Severe depression after left hemisphere damage appears to correlate most strongly with involvement of the deep frontal regions, particularly the junction of the anterior limb of the internal capsule and the frontal isthmus (Robinson et al. 1984a, Starkstein et al. 1987). In fact, depression following a left hemisphere lesion is not necessarily associated with aphasia; among patients with left hemisphere damage tested during an initial post-stroke period, no significant difference in depression scores was noted between those with and those without aphasia (Robinson and Szetela 1981). Instead, it appears that during the early stages, the closer to the left frontal pole the damage was located, the more severe the depression regardless of the presence or severity of aphasia. After the first few months, however, a steadily increasing correlation was demonstrated between depression scores and the severity of both physical and language impairment. By the sixth month, the correlation between impaired activities of daily living and depression was as strong as the relationship between the lesion location and the depression severity during the first 2 months (Robinson et al. 1984a, 1984b). These results suggest that while the presence of depression during the initial months reflects lesion location, as the status stabilizes, a stronger correlation develops between the level of impairment and the depression scores; post-stroke depression has been found to have a duration of approximately 12 months (Starkstein and Robinson 1988).

The psychologic features of this acquired depression are somewhat difficult to characterize; the aphasia obscures clear presentation by the patient. Psychomotor retardation, apathy, and decreased motivation are obvious, and hypophonia further obscures verbal interchange. Feelings of hopelessness, worthlessness, and concern about being a burden to the family may be presented, negativity is common, and suicidal ideation also may be expressed.

Multiple studies demonstrate that depression is far more common following left than right frontal stroke (Gainotti 1972, 1983; Robinson and Cahit 1985). It has been conjectured that interruption or damage to the frontal catecholamine pathways may explain the depression that occurs after left frontal damage (Morrison et al. 1979, Robinson et al. 1975, Welch et al. 1977, Zervas 1974), but this theory depends on an asymmetry of catecholamine activity between the two hemispheres (the left greater than the right). Evidence to support an asymmetric catecholamine distribution, however, is not robust, but the clinical observations are strong. Therefore, the existence of an organically based affective disorder complicating aphasia based on left hemisphere damage appears real.

Patients with a fluent (posterior) aphasia suffer a dramatically different psychiatric problem. Some (but not all) have difficulty comprehending spoken language, may be unaware of the deficit, and fail to realize that their own verbal output is incomprehensible (jargon). Some patients with posterior aphasia are fully anosognosic, actively denying their defect in comprehension and verbalization (Benson 1979, 1992). When unaware of their own disturbances, such patients tend to blame communication difficulties on others, suggesting the other individual is not speaking clearly enough to be understood or is not paying sufficient attention to what the patient is saying; patients with posterior aphasia may even believe that individuals whom they see talking together (but whom they cannot understand) are using a special code to discuss them. This tendency to misinterpret and to blame others produces a paranoia that may become serious. The paranoia of posterior aphasia is similar, if not identical, to the long-recognized paranoia of acquired deafness, and it is particularly evident in patients with word-deaf aphasia (Benson 1973, 1979).

The two serious psychiatric complications of aphasia described here (apathy/depression and anosognosia/paranoia) occur in different types of aphasia (nonfluent and fluent) based on different neuroanatomic sites of damage (anterior and posterior). Thus, separate from psychosocial bereavement, a significant depression that occurs in some patients with aphasia appears to be related to the location of the aphasia-causing lesion, and deserves classification as an organic affective disorder.

FRUSTRATION/DEPRESSION/CATASTROPHIC REACTION SYNDROME

During their course of recovery, many patients with aphasia (particularly those with anterior lesions) demonstrate frustration and depression, problems that may advance to a catastrophic level. The frustration/depression syndrome is more longlasting than the transient reactive depression, but it may be related at least in part to the organic affective syndrome described earlier.

Patients with the frustration/depression syndrome recognize their problems and are irritated by their inability to handle what previously were easily performed tasks. Their sense of failure is augmented by a feeling of helplessness and social isolation; the resulting dysphoria may become pervasive, with withdrawal or a listless and half-hearted participation in rehabilitation activities, decreased communication with family and ward personnel, poor appetite, little interest in activities, and carelessness about personal appearance. Patients may ruminate on their feelings of uselessness, appear to lack motivation, are unable to fight the disappointments of therapy failure, and may question the advisability of continued effort. They also may mention suicide. Frustration/depression syndrome should be recognized as a serious problem deserving remedial management (Benson 1979, Gainotti 1972, Robinson and Benson 1981, Starkstein and Robinson 1988).

Some individuals suffering frustration/depression syndrome if improperly managed, can develop a powerful emotional breakdown, a psychotic reaction in aphasia termed *catastrophic reaction* by Goldstein (1948). When fully developed, this catastrophic reaction is characterized by an aggressive refusal to cooperate (negativity), incessant crying, and total withdrawal. Gainotti (1969, 1972) demonstrated a frequent association between negative utterances, outbursts of tears, anxiety, refusal to cooperate, and aphasia; he found that the highest frequency of catastrophic reaction was in patients with Broca aphasia and lowest in those with Wernicke aphasia. Gainotti suggested that the catastrophic reaction resulted from the frustration associated with defects in verbal communication as well as impaired ability to use the preferred right hand. Patients with a fully developed catastrophic reaction stop eating, no longer care for themselves, and refuse all attempts to socialize. Sleep patterns, diet, and personal hygiene deteriorate, and the patient must be considered dangerously ill. Most catastrophic reactions are short lived, however, sometimes lasting only a few hours, but they may continue for a number of days.

Rigid administration of psychologic- and language-assessment batteries, producing repeated failure on material the patient previously easily mastered, is particularly dangerous. Careful monitoring of the patient's mood with alterations in formal therapy and general management to emphasize success is a significant ploy to avoid catastrophic reaction. Modern, well-monitored rehabilitation units rarely allow a catastrophic reaction to develop, and the full clinical picture is rare.

Frustration and depression are common, however, even almost ubiquitous in patients with anterior aphasia, and they appear to represent an independent disturbance only partially related to the psychosocial grief reaction and to the organic affective problem. Frustration, depression, and catastrophic reaction can be considered a spectrum of affective disorder in aphasia. Proper attention to the frustrations of the patient decreases the severity of this spectrum and avoids the catastrophic reaction.

SUICIDE

The incidence of suicide is relatively small in aphasia, but the possibility must be considered seriously. It would be natural to anticipate that the depression/frustration/catastrophic spectrum of anterior aphasia would provide a strong potential for suicide, and some patients with anterior aphasia do discuss or even threaten suicide. Suicide itself, however, rarely is reported in this group. It is more common in patients with posterior, fluent aphasia, particularly when both paranoia and impulsive behavior are present. Suicide is sufficiently infrequent that statistics concerning its overall frequency and division into anterior/posterior or other aphasia classifications are not meaningful.

In the authors' experience, two suicides occurred in approximately 4500 aphasics that were under management; in each instance, the suicide occurred in individuals with Wernicke-type aphasia. Both were in stable status months following an initial stroke and were in active language therapy. Both were known to be depressed, had major concern about their altered psychosocial status, and were under active psychiatric management. In both instances, the suicide attempt was carefully planned and executed. During a period when these patients gained increasing awareness of their disability, its probable permanence, and the profound alterations demanded for their lifestyles, premeditated self-destruction occurred.

Treatment of potential suicide is difficult in patients with posterior aphasia. The aphasia (particularly the comprehension difficulties) makes free communication difficult, and it precludes most traditional person-to-person psychotherapeutic measures. In all instances where the possibility exists, however, standard suicide precautions should be put into effect. Potential self-destructive devices should be removed and the activities of the patient carefully monitored, and if the threat is considered significant, the patient should be transferred to a secure situation (e.g., locked ward or seclusion room). Considerable effort should be made to establish and maintain close interpersonal relationships and to minimize frustration. Antidepressant pharmaceuticals should be instituted (if they are not already in use), but too great a reliance on their efficacy may be dangerous. Even when the potential for suicide is recognized and appropriate measures taken, a well-planned, life-ending act may still occur. Management of a potentially suicidal patient with aphasia is a considerable burden, but the possibility must be recognized. Nursing staff, rehabilitation team, physicians, and family members all should actively participate in preventive measures.

MANAGEMENT AND TREATMENT

During the past few decades, neurologic rehabilitation has become a strong discipline. Both physical and language rehabilitation are now available for most individuals with brain damage. While demanding, tiring, time-consuming, and expensive, rehabilitation produces positive responses, and such measures probably represent the single most effective therapeutic modality for the patient with aphasia and depression (Benson, 1992). Whenever possible, management of the depression should be coordinated with rehabilitation efforts.

Two approaches can be suggested for the treatment of affective disorder in aphasia: pharmacologic management, and traditional psychotherapy. To a certain extent, both have proved successful.

PHARMACOLOGIC MANAGEMENT

Antidepressant medications, usually administered in low doses, may be advisable for patients with aphasia and depression. Patients with stroke treated with tricyclic antidepressants show a significant improvement in depression scores (Reding et al. 1986), but the potential side effects of most antidepressant medications (particularly the anticholinergic effects of the tricyclic antidepressants) must be recognized and their use carefully monitored in elderly or atherosclerotic patients. One antidepressant, fluoxetine (Prozac, Dista Products Company, Indianapolis, Indiana, USA), is said to alter serotonin metabolism and through this action, combines both antidepressant and stimulating properties; its use in the elderly, however, demands caution as it can produce anxiety, insomnia, and gastrointestinal upset. Stimulants are infrequently prescribed in aphasia, but in well-selected cases, methylphenidate (Ritalin, CIBA Pharmaceutical Company, Summit, New Jersey, USA) or amphetamine may be appropriate. When brain damage is sufficient to cause lethargy and decreased drive (psychomotor retardation), judicious use of a stimulant may be helpful (Benson 1992).

Crucial to the pharmacologic treatment of aphasic depression is the possibility of adverse reactions or cross-reactions. Most patients, particularly those of older age, will take one or more medications (polypharmacy is almost universal in elderly patients), many of which have powerful effects. The treating physician must be aware of all medications currently taken by the patient as well as the possibility of cross-complications with drugs added to ameliorate depression. In general, drugs should be recognized as adjuncts and not primary treatment modalities (Benson 1992), but they may be of tremendous, even life-saving value in selected cases.

PSYCHOTHERAPY

The most powerful psychotherapy used for patients with aphasia and depression is the emotional support provided by family members, nursing staff, therapists, physicians, and others in contact with the patient. Although they rarely express appreciation for such encouragement, most patients depend on these interpersonal considerations.

Powerful antidepressant measures can be obtained from formal rehabilitation efforts, and active physical and occupational training, eventually producing noticeable gains, provides both a meaningful purpose and sense of accomplishment for the patient. Encouragement by the therapist along with demonstrations of accomplishment can alleviate feelings of hopelessness, and the language therapist offers an even more significant antidepressant effect through a direct, goal-oriented treatment of the aphasia. The presence of an expert dedicated to the treatment of aphasia, the accomplishment of goals in language therapy, and the encouragement that others with aphasia have improved with this therapy provide considerable solace for the patient. The language therapist can be a major provider of supportive psychotherapy.

The wide variations in the language deficits makes group psychotherapy difficult. In large rehabilitation centers, aphasic groups can be developed and, if properly managed, provide both language and psychiatric therapy. The individual bereft of language often considers the disturbance unique; most patients and their families have never heard of aphasia before its onset. Association with others having aphasia can be helpful as it tends to decrease the feeling of isolation. In addition, the patient sees the improving status of other group members and, finally, sees their own status improve in comparison with others. In a properly managed aphasic group, these factors can be manipulated and used as positive measures for the management of depression.

The use of family members to provide psychotherapy also deserves attention. Family members should be taught to communicate with the patient; to avoid crossed communications, to diminish background noises and voices (television, radio, and so on); to speak clearly and simply; to present information in a redundant way; and to avoid repeatedly asking the patient to repeat himself. An intelligent, well-motivated spouse or child can provide support and encouragement, but unfortunately, a disturbed family member is a far-too-frequent problem. Family members are often upset by the altered circumstances caused by the patient's aphasia, and they may provide a serious negative influence. Family counselling, distancing of certain family members from the patient, and/or suggestions for their own psychiatric counseling may be needed. Management of the family, while difficult, may be crucial to the successful management of aphasia. Isolation of the patient from family support is disturbing, but integration into the family's decisions, plans, and activities helps to overcome emotional difficulties.

The role of psychiatrists in the management of aphasic depression is uncertain. Their expertise in pharmacologic management may be invaluable, but the communication disorder effectively impedes in-depth interpersonal psychotherapy. It is preferable in many instances for the psychiatrist to act as a consultant and not the active therapist. As already noted, patients with aphasia frequently derive considerable support from the language therapist; a strong positive transference, a valuable psychotherapeutic phenomenon, almost always occurs. Most language therapists, however, are not trained in psychiatric management, may feel intimidated by the psychiatric problems, and often request referral of the patient away from language therapy. This represents a negative backslide for an already depressed individual. Language therapists need coaching and encouragement to continue treatment of a psychiatrically disturbed patient, but whenever possible, the bulk of psychotherapy provided to those with aphasia should be performed by the language therapist.

MANAGEMENT OF CATASTROPHIC REACTION

The preferred treatment for the catastrophic reaction is prophylactic (Benson 1979). The patient with frustration, depression, and anterior aphasia should not be pushed too hard in either language testing or therapy. Continual failure is unpleasant for anyone, and even worse for someone with nonfluent aphasia who knows the correct response but cannot express it. It is obviously desirable to avoid humiliating the patient, something easily achieved by attending to the individual's feelings and not merely recording their responses. Catastrophic reactions should never occur, but if one does take place, the prime treatment modality is sympathy and concern. This, along with the healing course of time, will eventually prove successful.

REFERENCES

Albert ML, Goodglass H, Helm NA, et al. 1981. *Clinical Aspects of Dysphasia*. New York: Springer-Verlag.

Alexander MP, Benson DF. 1991. Aphasia and related disturbances. In: Joynt RJ, ed. *Clinical Neurology*. Philadelphia: J.B. Lippincott, in press.

Alexander MP, LoVerme SP. 1980. Aphasia after left hemispheric intracerebral hemorrhage. *Neurology* 30:1193–1202.

Benson DF. 1973. Psychiatric aspects of aphasia. *Br J Psychiatry* 123:555–566.

Benson DF. 1979. *Aphasia, Alexia, and Agraphia*. Boston: Churchill Livingstone.

Benson DF. 1992. Neuropsychiatric aspects of aphasia and related language impairments. In: Yudofsky SC, Hales RE, eds. *Textbook of Neuropsychiatry, 2nd Ed*. Washington, D.C.: American Psychiatric Press, pp. 311–322.

Charatan FB, Fisk A. 1978. The mental and emotional results of strokes. *NY State J Med* 78:1403–1405.

Folstein MF, Maiberger R, McHugh PR. 1977. Mood disorder as a specific complication of stroke. *J Neurol Neurosurg Psychiatry* 41:470–473.

Gainotti G. 1969. Réactions "catastrophiques" et manifestations d'indifference au cours des arteintes cérébrales. *Neuropsychologia* 7:195–204.

Gainotti G. 1972. Emotional behavior and hemisphere side of the lesion. *Cortex* 8:41–55.

Gainotti G. 1983. Laterality of affect. The emotional behavior of right and left brain damaged patients. In: Mislobodski M, ed. *Hemisyndromes: Psychobiology, Neurology and Psychiatry*. New York: Academic Press, pp. 175–192.

Goldstein K. 1948. *Language and Language Disturbances*. New York: Grune & Stratton.

Hécaen H. 1972. *Introduction à la neuropsychologie*. Paris: Larousse-Université.

Herrmann M, Wallesch CW. 1989. Psychosocial changes and psychosocial adjustment with chronic and severe nonfluent aphasia. *Aphasiology* 6:513–526.

McHugh PR, Folstein MF. 1975. Psychiatric syndromes of Huntington's chorea: a clinical and phenomenologic study. In: Benson DF, Blumer D, eds. *Psychiatric Aspects of Neurologic Disease*. New York: Grune & Stratton, pp. 267–286.

Morrison JH, Molliver ME, Grzanna R. 1979. Noradrenergic innervation of cerebral cortex: widespread effects of focal cortical lesions. *Science* 205:313–316.

Müller DJ, Code C, Mugdorf J. 1983. Predicting psychosocial adjustment to aphasia. *Br J Commun Disord* 18:23–29.

Perello J. 1970. *Transtornos del habla [Speech impairments]*. Barcelona: Editorial Cientifico-Médica.

Reding MJ, Orto LA, Winter SW, et al. 1986. Antidepressant therapy after stroke: a double-blind trial. *Arch Neurol* 43:763–765.

Robinson RG, Benson DF. 1981. Depression in aphasic patients: frequency, severity, and clinical-pathological correlations. *Brain and Language* 14:282–291.

Robinson RG, Chait RM. 1985. Emotional correlates of structural brain injury with particular emphasis on post-stroke mood disorders. *CRC Crit Rev Clin Neurobiol* 4:285–318.

Robinson RG, Kubos KL, Starr LB, et al. 1984a. Mood disorders in stroke patients: importance of location of lesion. *Brain* 107:81–93.

Robinson RG, Price TR. 1982. Post-stroke depressive patients: a follow-up study of 103 patients. *Stroke* 13:635–641.

Robinson RG, Shoemaker WJ, Schlumpf M, et al. 1975. Effects of experimental cerebral infarction in rat brain catecholamines and behaviour. *Nature* 255:332–334.

Robinson RG, Starr LB, Lipsey JR, et al. 1984b. A two-year longitudinal study of post-stroke mood disorders: dynamic changes and associated variables over the first six months of follow-up. *Stroke* 15:510–517.

Robinson RG, Szetela B. 1981. Mood change following left hemisphere brain injury. *Ann Neurol* 9:447–453.

Rosenfield DB. 1982. Neuropsychiatric aspects of stuttering. In: Benson DF, Blumer D, eds. *Psychiatric Aspects of Neurologic Disease, Volume 2.* New York: Grune & Stratton, pp. 301–314.

Ruckdeschel-Hibbard M, Gordon WA, Diller L. 1986. Affective disturbances associated with brain damage. In: Filskov S, Boll T, eds. *Handbook of Clinical Neuropsychology, Volume 2.* New York: John Wiley, pp. 305–337.

Siever LJ, Davis KL, Gorman LK. 1991. Pathogenesis of mood disorders. In: Davis KL, Klar H, Coyle JT, eds. *Foundations of Psychiatry.* Philadelphia: W.B. Saunders, pp. 254–262.

Starkstein SE, Robinson RG, Berthier ML, et al. 1987. Comparison of cortical and subcortical lesions in the production of post-stroke mood disorders. *Brain* 110:1045–1059.

Starkstein SE, Robinson RG. 1988. Aphasia and depression. *Aphasiology* 2:1–20.

Tanner C, Gerstenberger DL. 1988. The grief response in neuropathologies of speech and language. *Aphasiology* 2:79–84.

Welch KMA, Chabi E, Buckingham J, et al. Cathecholamine and 5-hydroxytryptamine levels in ischemic brain, influence of *p*-chlorophenylalanine. *Stroke* 8:341–346.

Whitlock FA, Siskind MM. 1980. Depression as a major symptom of multiple sclerosis. *J Neurol Neurosurg Psychiatry* 43:861–865.

Zervas NT, Hori H, Negora M, et al. 1974. Reduction of brain dopamine following experimental cerebral ischemia. *Nature* 247:283–284.

11

DEPRESSION IN MULTI-INFARCT DEMENTIA

Jeffrey L. Cummings, M.D.
David L. Sultzer, M.D.

After Alzheimer disease, ischemic brain injury with subsequent cognitive impairment (multi-infarct dementia [MID]) is the second most common cause of intellectual decline in elderly people. MID accounts for between 10% and 25% of dementia cases in elderly persons (Cummings and Benson 1992), and in addition to cognitive impairment and motor dysfunction, MID produces considerable neuropsychiatric morbidity. Delusions, personality alterations, and mood disorders are all common concomitants of MID as well (Cummings et al. 1987, Dian et al. 1990, Ishii et al. 1986). This chapter presents the relationship of depression to MID, discusses the definitions and classifications of MID and depression, summarizes the prevalence of MID and of mood alterations in MID, and reviews the literature describing the frequency of depression in MID. Factors that potentially contribute to the occurrence of mood changes in MID are considered, and the treatment of depression in MID also is summarized. New data regarding depressive symptoms in MID, as revealed by the Hamilton Depression Rating Scale (Hamilton 1960) and the Neurobehavior Rating Scale (Levin et al. 1987), are reported as well.

PREVALENCE

Multi-infarct dementia results from cerebrovascular disease, and the prevalence of MID closely follows the prevalence of stroke. MID increases in frequency with age, and it afflicts approximately 2.5% of individuals after the age of 65 years (Table 11.1). The reported frequency varies with the study methodology, sensitivity of the screening instruments, and the specificity of diagnostic criteria. The average prevalence rate for depression in MID is approximately 25%, but the rate differs in the various subsyndromes of MID.

Table 11.1. Epidemiologic Studies of the Prevalence of Multi-Infarct Dementia

Study	Patients, *n*	Patient Age, *years*	Prevalence of MID, %	Study Methodology/Location
Kay et al. (1964)	309	>65	3.9	Community dwelling; England; random sample
Kay et al. (1964)	154	>65	12.9	Complete sample of institutionalized elderly in designated electoral wards; England
Akesson (1969)	4198	>70	0.21 (severe)	Rural Sweden; all elderly patients with suspected dementia
Broe et al. (1976)	808	>65	1.9	Random sample; urban Scotland
Sulkava et al. (1985)	8000	>65	2.7	Stratified cluster sample; Finland
Shibayama et al. (1986)	3106	>65	2.8	Stratified random sample; Japan
Brayne and Calloway (1989)	270	70 to 74	2.2	Women; stratified random sample; England
	207	75 to 79	2.8	
Rocca et al. (1990)	778	>59	2.2	Door-to-door survey; Italy

DIAGNOSIS: DEFINITIONS AND CLASSIFICATIONS

MULTI-INFARCT DEMENTIA

The most widely used criteria for the diagnosis of MID are presented in the DSM-III-R (American Psychiatric Association 1987). In summary, these criteria include:

Memory disturbance;
At least one of the following: impaired abstract thinking, abnormal judgment, aphasia, apraxia, agnosia, constructional disturbances, or personality change;
Intellectual changes severe enough to interfere with work, social activities, or interpersonal relationships;
Absence of delirium;
Stepwise deterioration;
"Patchy" distribution of intellectual deficits early in the clinical course;
Focal neurologic signs and symptoms; and
Evidence from history, physical examination, or laboratory tests of cerebrovascular disease that is judged to be related etiologically to the disturbance.

These criteria are applicable to the majority of patients with MID, but clinical experience suggests that further revisions are necessary to ensure their sensitivity and specificity. For example, memory impairments are required for a diagnosis of MID, but multifocal lesions could produce a dementia syndrome with relatively preserved memory; to include such syndromes, memory loss should be included among the list of possible cognitive deficits but not specifically required for the diagnosis. In other cases, MID could result from several strokes occurring more or less simultaneously and no stepwise deterioration would be observed. Stepwise progression would best be regarded as supportive of but not critical to the diagnosis of MID. Another difficulty is these criteria do not include some of the most common behavioral manifestations of MID. Most vascular lesions involve subcortical structures and the resulting disorder has features of subcortical dementia (Wallin et al. 1991), but these features are not included in the definition. The diagnostic approach to MID could be more sensitive by adding characteristics of subcortical dementia, such as psychomotor retardation and executive function deficits, to the list of possible intellectual manifestations (Cummings and Benson 1992). Neuroimaging also plays an increasingly important role in supporting the diagnosis of MID, and findings on CT or MRI that are required for the diagnosis should be specified. In addition, the clinical criteria are not operationalized to indicate the requisite extent of memory, language, judgement, or social disability, and development of such operationalized criteria would increase the reliability of the definition. These observations indicate that current diagnostic approaches to MID are relatively insensitive and that MID is probably underrecognized.

Multi-infarct dementia is not a homogenous entity. The profile of cognitive impairment and both the motor- and sensory-system changes reflect the distribution of ischemic lesions, and it is recognized increasingly that the neuropsychiatric manifestations of cerebrovascular disease also have regional relationships (Beckson and Cummings 1991). Table 11.2 summarizes the principal types of currently recognized MID syndromes, the distribution of the ischemic lesions, the arteries that irrigate the injured structures, and the commonly associated neurologic and neuropsychiatric manifestations. Lacunar state and Binswanger disease typically co-occur, producing injury to the deep gray and white matter structures of the cerebral hemispheres (Roman 1987); the patients may manifest subcortical dementia, pyramidal and extrapyramidal motor dysfunction, gait abnormalities, pseudobulbar palsy, and mood alterations (Celesia and Wanamaker 1972, Ishii et al. 1986). Patients with bilateral thalamic infarction evidence subcortical dementia, apathy, and marked amnesia. However, they are rarely depressed (Katz et al. 1987, Stuss et al. 1988). Occlusion of the major intracranial vessels (anterior, middle, posterior cerebral) produces hemiparesis, hemisensory loss, hemianopsia, and cortical dementia with aphasia, amnesia, agnosia, apraxia, and constructional disturbances. Mood changes vary with the location of the lesions, and they are particularly common with strokes involving anterior hemispheric structures (Robinson and Starkstein 1990). Extracranial occlusion of the carotid arteries results in ischemic injury to the borderzone regions between the principal intracranial arteries, in turn resulting in proximal arm and leg weakness, transcortical aphasia, and constructional impairment. Mood changes have not been studied in this syndrome, but most anatomic or radiologic investigations have found deep hemispheric lacunar or Binswanger-type lesions in most patients with MID and a variable number who exhibit co-occurring cortical infarctions (Erkinjuntti 1987, Meyer et al. 1988, Parnetti et al. 1990). Thus, there is considerable clinical variability among patients with vascular syndromes, although a few major syndromes are evident within the MID complex. The vessels involved and the structures injured determine the clinical manifestations of the syndrome, and depression is most frequent in patients with basal ganglia lesions, white matter damage, and specific cortical infarctions.

Table 11.2. Multi-Infarct Dementia Syndromes

Syndrome	Distribution of Ischemic Lesions (Vessels Occluded)	Depression	Common Neurologic and Neuropsychiatric Features
Lacunar state*	Basal ganglia, thalamus, internal capsule, deep white matter (lateral lenticulostriate arteries)	Common	Gait disturbance, pyramidal and extrapyramidal motor dysfunction, pseudobulbar palsy, subcortical dementia, apathy, irritability, delusions
Binswanger disease*	Hemispheric white matter, periventricular and corona radiata (medullary arteries penetrating from cortical surface toward the corner of the lateral ventricle)	Common	Indistinguishable from lacunar state
Thalamic dementia	Medial dorsal nuclei of thalamus bilaterally and adjacent structures (thalamoperforant branches of posterior cerebral or posterior communicating arteries)	Rare	Subcortical dementia, apathy, severe amnesia
Multiple large strokes	Infarctions in bed territories of anterior, middle, or posterior cerebral arteries (major intracranial arteries)	Variable	Hemiparesis, hemisensory loss, hemianopsia, cortical dementia (aphasia, amnesia, agnosia, apraxia constructional disturbances), delusions
Borderzone ischemia	Infarction in the regions between the major cortical arterial distributions (carotid arteries)	Unknown	Proximal arm and leg weakness, transcortical aphasia, constructional disturbances

*Lacunar state and Binswanger disease usually co-exist.

DEPRESSION

Depressed mood occurring in conjunction with MID would necessarily be diagnosed as an organic mood disorder of the depressed type according to DSM-III-R criteria (American Psychiatric Association 1987). The criteria for this syndrome, however, are relatively unrestrictive, requiring only that the patient exhibit prominent and persistent depressed mood, have no evidence of delirium, and have an identifiable etiologic disorder. To provide additional clinical substance to a diagnosis of depression, many investigators studying the neuropsychiatric manifestations of neurologic illness have used the DSM-III-R criteria for major depressive episode, excluding the stipulation that the disorder not have an organic factor that initiated or maintained the mood disturbance. These criteria require that the patient have a syndrome that persists for at least 2 weeks, represents a change from previous functioning, and includes depressed mood or loss of interest or pleasure as well as four of the following: significant weight change, sleep disturbance, psychomotor retardation or agitation, fatigue or loss of energy, feelings of worthlessness or inappropriate guilt, indecisiveness or inability to think or concentrate, and recurrent thoughts of death or suicide. In addition, the criteria require that the disturbance is not a normal reaction to the death of a loved one, there have been no prolonged periods of hallucinations or delusions in the absence of mood disorder, and that the mood symptoms are not superimposed on another major psychiatric illness such as schizophrenia, schizophreniform disorder, delusional disorder, or other psychotic disorder. When the mood changes in MID are less severe, the criteria for dysthymia may be utilized, excluding the requirements for a duration of 2 years and the absence of an etiologic factor to allow the occurrence of a recent stroke. These modified criteria require that patients have depressed mood and exhibit at least two of the following: appetite change, sleep disturbance, low energy or fatigue, low self-esteem, poor concentration or difficulty making decisions, and feelings of hopelessness. In addition, patients with dysthymia do not meet criteria for a major depressive episode, have no evidence of a past manic episode, and have no chronic psychotic disorder such as schizophrenia or delusional disorder.

Application of these criteria to patients with MID involve several difficulties. First, the criteria were developed explicitly for patients without neurologic disease, and their validity, sensitivity, and specificity in patients with MID or other neurologic disorders have not been assessed thoroughly. Second, many of the identification criteria for a depressive disorder (weight change, sleep disturbance, low energy, poor concentration, agitation, or retardation) are common in patients with MID without associated mood changes. These overlapping symptoms may lead to either underdiagnosis of depression, by ascribing mood-related symptoms to dementia, or overdiagnosis by ascribing dementia-related symptoms to a mood disorder. This difficulty also accompanies the use of rating scales, such as the Hamilton Depression Rating Scale (Hamilton 1960), that assess symptoms common to both dementia and depression. Most important, however, is that a majority of studies fail to specify the criteria used in the diagnosis of depression in MID, and they have not distinguished between syndromes of different severity such as major depressive episodes and dysthymia. Taken together, these shortcomings indicate that verifying the occurrence of mood changes in MID and characterizing the mood and affect of patients with MID constitute an important research agenda.

REVIEW OF THE LITERATURE

Table 11.3 presents a summary of 19 studies reporting on the frequency of depression in patients with MID. The reported prevalence of depression among these patients ranged from 0% to 71% (mean, 29%). The mean frequency among the four largest studies (each having over 50 patients) was 24%, but the range remained large even among these studies (5.8% to 45%). The study with the lowest frequency reported only the presenting characteristics and may have found a higher rate if the patients had been followed or a history of depression (after the onset of MID but not evident at the time of presentation) had been investigated. Few studies defined their criteria for the diagnosis of MID, and even fewer had specific criteria for the diagnosis of depression. Most were based on populations referred to dementia clinics for the evaluation of intellectual decline: none used an epidemiologic design. All are subject to referral biases, and most were cross-sectional in design, thus providing little insight into the course of depression in MID. With few exceptions, however, the studies are consistent in suggesting that depression is common among patients with MID.

Four studies have reported depression rating scale scores of patients with MID. Cummings et al. (1987) used the Hamilton Depression Rating Scale (Hamilton 1960) and found the mean score among 15 patients with MID was 12.7 (range, 3 to 32). Greenwald et al. (1989) also used the Hamilton Depression Rating Scale as well as a comprehensive inventory of depressive symptoms derived from other scales; 20% of the patients with MID were considered to be depressed. (Their rating scale scores, however, are not reported.) Fisher et al. (1990) applied the same instrument and found a mean score of 10.3 (range, 3 to 19) among 37 patients with MID, and Bucht

Table 11.3. Studies Reporting the Frequency of Depression in Multi-Infarct Dementia

Study	Frequency of Depression, %	Comments
Clow (1940)	24.0	100 institutionalized patients with cerebral arteriosclerosis; no specific diagnostic criteria
Rothschild (1941)	14.0	Autopsy-based study of 29 patients with "arteriosclerotic psychoses;" 14% exhibited depression with "pronounced suicidal tendencies;" no specific criteria
Celesia and Wanamaker (1972)	50.0	6 patients with arteriosclerotic parkinsonism; depression graded as mild, moderate, or severe
Bernheimer et al. (1973)	17.0	6 patients with arteriosclerotic parkinsonism and dementia; autopsy confirmation; no specific clinical criteria
Loizou et al. (1981)	27.0	15 patients with Binswanger disease; diagnosis based on clinical and CT features
Bucht and Adolfsson (1983)	0.0	20 patients; DSM-III criteria for MID; rating scale assessment of depression
Reding et al. (1985)	6.0	At study onset, 1 of 16 patients with MID were depressed; clinical criteria for dementia and depression
	25.0	After 3 years of follow-up; 5 of 20 patients with MID were depressed
Barclay et al. (1985)	5.8	69 patients with MID referred to a dementia clinic; criteria for dementia but not depression
Ishii et al. (1986)	67.0	Autopsy study of 30 patients with multiple lacunes; clinical features based on chart review; patients had "mood changes"

Hershey et al. (1986)	71.0	Longitudinal study of 7 patients with vascular dementia diagnosed by clinical and MRI findings; no criteria for depression
Babikian and Ropper (1987)	21.0	Review of 47 cases of pathologically verified cases of Binswanger disease; depression was noted to be "overt" and 3 had attempted suicide
Cummings et al. (1987)	27.0	Major depressive episode based on DSM-III criteria for MID and depression; 15 patients
	13.0	Dysthymia based on DSM-III criteria
Mathers et al. (1987)	4.0	Depression with suicidal gesture presenting feature in 1 of 22 patients with Binswanger disease
Erkinjuntti (1987)	42.9	14 patients with subcortical infarctions; DSM-III criteria
	24.6	65 patients with cortical infarctions, some of whom also had subcortical infarctions
Thal et al. (1988)	22.2	18 patients referred for evaluation of dementia; diagnoses based on clinical information; no specific criteria
Erkinjuntti et al. (1988)	17.4	23 pathologically verified cases; DSM-III criteria for dementia; no specific criteria for depression
Lechner et al. (1988)	45.0	94 patients; diagnosis based on clinical and CT evidence; no specific criteria
Greenwald et al. (1989)	20.0	54 patients; diagnosis based on DSM-III-R criteria; rating scale assessment of mood
del Ser et al. (1990)	61.0	28 pathologically verified cases; retrospective chart review of clinical assessment without specific criteria

Note: CT = computed tomography; DSM-III = *Diagnostic and Statistical Manual of Mental Disorders, Third Edition*; DSM-III-R = *Diagnostic and Statistical Manual of Mental Disorders, Third Edition (Revised)*; MID = multi-infarct dementia; MRI = magnetic resonance imaging.

and Adolfsson (1983) reported that none of their 20 patients with MID had a score over 1 (mild) on the "apparent sadness" item of the Comprehensive Psychopathological Rating Scale. More experience is necessary with these instruments to distinguish the effects of dementia from those of depression, to relate the score to clinical diagnoses of mood disorders, and to establish the most valid means of assessing the characteristics of depression in patients with MID.

Two studies explored the association between depression and dementia severity. Cummings et al. (1987) found no correlation between the Hamilton Depression Rating Scale scores and dementia severity as assessed by the Mini-Mental State Examination (Folstein et al. 1975). Likewise, Fischer et al. (1990) found no significant relationship between Hamilton Scale and Mini-Mental State Examination scores. These preliminary observations suggest that depression is unrelated to the severity of intellectual impairment in MID.

RATING SCALE ASSESSMENT OF MOOD IN MULTI-INFARCT DEMENTIA

We extended our own studies using the Hamilton Depression Rating Scale to evaluate mood changes in patients with MID. Twenty-nine patients met DSM-III-R criteria for MID and had neuroimaging confirmation of at least one lesion on CT or MRI scan. Hachinski Ischemia Scale (Hachinski et al. 1975) scores ranged from 6 to 16, above the range that is consistent with degenerative dementia, and the age of the patients ranged from 60 to 85 years (mean age, 73 years). Severity of dementia was assessed using the Mini-Mental State Examination; the mean score was 20 (range, 8 to 28). Table 11.4 lists the scores of the 17 items of the Hamilton Depression Rating Scale for these patients. Seventeen of the 29 patients had scores of at least 1 on the item regarding depressed mood, nine expressed feelings of guilt, and six "felt that life was not worth living." The eight items most commonly endorsed were depressed mood, middle insomnia, loss of interest in work, retardation, psychic anxiety, general somatic symptoms, genital symptoms, and impaired insight (all items had a mean score over 0.6). Examining the scores of patients with total Hamilton scores of 18 or above (the range consistent with major depressive episodes), the eight items forming the core elements of the dementia–depression syndrome were depressed mood; early, middle, and late insomnia; loss of interest in activities; retardation; psychic anxiety; genital symptoms; hypochondriasis; and impaired insight (all items had a mean score of at least 1). On the basis of this sample, the depression syndrome of MID most commonly appears to be an anxious depression with prominent insomnia, psychomotor retardation, and somatic symptoms.

Table 11.4. Scores on the Hamilton Depression Rating Scale of 29 Patients with Multi-Infarct Dementia

Item	Mean Score	Range
Depressed mood	0.76	0.3
Guilt	0.34	0.2
Suicidal ideation	0.21	0.1
Insomnia, initial	0.48	0.2
Insomnia, middle	0.62	0.2
Insomnia, terminal	0.34	0.2
Loss of interest in work	3.0	0.4
Retardation	0.83	0.4
Agitation	0.31	0.2
Psychic anxiety	1.21	0.4
Somatic anxiety	0.21	0.2
Gastrointestinal symptoms	0.10	0.2
General somatic symptoms	0.62	0.2
Genital symptoms	0.69	0.2
Hypochondriasis	0.34	0.2
Weight loss	0.10	0.2
Loss of insight	1.00	0.2
Total	11.16	

Depression also was assessed in this group of patients by the Neurobehavior Rating Scale (Levin et al. 1987). This measures each of 27 cognitive, psychiatric, and behavioral symptoms on seven-point scales of severity (0 = not present, 6 = extremely severe impairment). Ten of the 29 patients with MID (34%) had at least mild impairment on the depressed-mood item of the Neurobehavior Rating Scale; in addition, 12 patients (41%) had at least mild anxiety, 11 (38%) at least mild somatic concern, eight (28%) at least mild tension, and five (17%) at least mild guilt feelings. Preliminary analysis revealed no correlations between the extent of cognitive impairment and the scores on the depressed-mood item of the Neurobehavior Rating Scale.

Results from both the Hamilton Depression Rating Scale and the Neurobehavior Rating Scale support the validity of a depression syndrome in patients with MID. Prominent features include depressed mood, anxiety, and somatic symptoms. There was a trend for Hamilton scores to be higher in patients with more advanced dementia, but no relationship between depressed mood as measured by the Neurobehavior Rating Scale and severity of dementia was evident. This may reflect the greater weight given to neurovegetative symptoms on the Hamilton Scale as well as the tendency for such symptoms to appear later in the course of MID.

DIFFERENTIAL DIAGNOSIS

Two principal clinical symptoms should be considered in the differential diagnosis of depression in MID. These are pseudobulbar palsy and the dementia syndrome of depression.

Pseudobulbar palsy is a complex behavioral disturbance that includes loss of control over emotional affect, dysarthria, dysphagia, exaggerated gag reflex, and brisk jaw and facial reflexes (Langworthy and Hesser 1940). In elderly individuals, the most common pseudobulbar affect is forced weeping, a disorder that easily can be mistaken for depression. Pseudobulbar affect is distinguished from major depression by the presence of the accompanying neurologic signs (Dysarthria, dysphagia, abnormal reflexes) as well as the absence of significantly depressed mood. Pseudobulbar crying is precipitated when the patient experiences a minor emotional stimulus, and it has an immediate and exaggerated display of weeping and distress out of proportion to the event. In some cases, no precipitant may be identifiable; the sham emotion appears spontaneously. Pseudobulbar palsy most commonly reflects bilateral lesions of the descending corticobulbar tracts.

The dementia syndrome of depression is a disorder of acquired cognitive impairment that occurs in conjunction with depression, and it resolves with successful treatment of the mood disorder. The disorder affects primarily older individuals and produces psychomotor retardation and memory dysfunction. The depression syndrome usually includes anxiety and mood-congruent delusions (La Rue et al. 1986, Rabins et al. 1984); in patients with stroke or vascular risk factors, it might be misidentified as MID with depression. Several features help distinguish the two syndromes, however (Table 11.5). The dementia syndrome of depression may occur in the absence of stroke or after a single cerebrovascular event, whereas multiple strokes are more characteristic of MID. The dementia of this syndrome also follows the onset of depression, whereas the depression accompanying MID typically follows the onset of dementia. The depression of this syndrome frequently includes mood-congruent delusions, but these psychotic manifestations have been rare in the depression accompanying MID. A family history of psychiatric illness or a past personal history of depression would support a diagnosis of dementia syndrome of depression. Its dementia improves with successful treatment of the depression. The depression occurring with MID improves with antidepressant treatment, but cognitive impairment is unaffected or, at best, is only partially ameliorated. These guidelines usually can differentiate the two syndromes.

Table 11.5. Distinguishing Features of Multi-Infarct Dementia with Depression and the Dementia Syndrome of Depression

Feature	Multi-Infarct Dementia with Depression	Dementia Syndrome of Depression
Course	Dementia before depression	Depression before dementia
History of stroke	Multiple	Absent or single
Family history of depression	Variable	Yes
Past history of depression	Variable	Yes
Mood-congruent delusions	No	Yes
Neurologic examination	Multiple pyramidal or extrapyramidal signs	Normal or few focal signs
Dementia responds to antidepressant therapy	No	Yes

FACTORS POSSIBLY CONTRIBUTING TO DEPRESSION IN MULTI-INFARCT DEMENTIA

The pathogenesis of depression in MID is unknown. The lack of correlation between depression severity and the degree of cognitive impairment suggests that mood changes are not simply a reaction to declining intellect (Cummings et al. 1987, Fischer et al. 1990). Table 11.6 lists a number of factors that may play a role in determining which patients with MID exhibit mood changes and which are spared this complication. Robinson and Starkstein (1990) emphasized the importance of lesion location in determining post-stroke depression, and their investigations suggest that lesions involving the left frontal lobe (either cortical or subcortical structures) are particularly likely to be associated with depressive mood changes. The high frequency of depression in patients with lacunar state and Binswanger disease may reflect the tendency of these disorders to affect the frontal lobe and frontal-subcortical structures (Ishii et al. 1986) as well.

In addition to local effects, ischemic injuries also may have distant effects that could influence mood. For example, deep white matter lesions may reduce cortical activity through the interruption of fiber tracts and the disconnection of remote structures (Fig. 11.1) (Metter et al. 1985). Lesion size also may contribute to the occurrence of mood changes; Schwartz et al. (1990) found a significant correlation between depression severity and the volume of dysfunctional brain tissue as revealed by single photon-emission CT. In ad-

Table 11.6. Factors Potentially Contributing to Depression in Multi-Infarct Dementia

- Vascular and lesion effects
  - Local effects of infarction
  - Remote effects of infarction
  - Volume of infarction
  - Global cerebral hypoperfusion
  - Serum protein deposits and compromise of the blood–brain barrier
- Biochemical alterations
  - Decreased dopamine
  - Decreased serotonin
- Person-specific effects
  - Age effects
  - Gender effects
  - Hereditary vulnerability
  - Premorbid personality
- Toxic-metabolic effects
  - Systemic vascular disease effects
  - Drug treatment of vascular disease and depression
- Psychosocial contributions

dition to the local perfusion defects associated with stroke, global cerebral perfusion has been shown to be reduced in patients with MID, and this reduction occurs before the emergence of cognitive impairment (Rogers et al. 1986). This global hypoperfusion may limit reparative activities following stroke and increase vulnerability to post-stroke mood changes. Finally, immunocytochemical studies have revealed deposits of plasma proteins around numerous capillaries in layers I through IV of the frontal cortex in patients with MID (Alafuzoff et al. 1985), and these deposits impugn the integrity of the blood–brain barrier of the cortical capillaries. This deposition of material associated with blood–brain barrier dysfunction could play a role in mood changes during MID.

Neurochemical alterations may contribute to the occurrence of depression in MID as well. Wallin et al. (1989) found that serotonin was reduced in the hippocampus and parahippocampal gyrus in patients with MID, and 5-hydroxyindoleacetic acid (the principal metabolite of serotonin) was reduced in the caudate nucleus, putamen, mesencephalon, hippocampus, and parahippocampal gyrus. Dopamine and its metabolite homovanillic acid have been found to be reduced in the caudate nucleus and putamen of patients with MID (Bernheimer et al. 1973, Wallin et al. 1989), but the only study that assessed levels of noradrenalin and its metabolite 3-methoxy-4-hydroxyphenylglycol found no alterations in transmitter levels in the tissues assessed (caudate, putamen, mesencephalon, hippocampus, parahippocampal gyrus, temporal gyrus) (Wallin et al. 1989). Also, information regarding cholinergic function in patients with

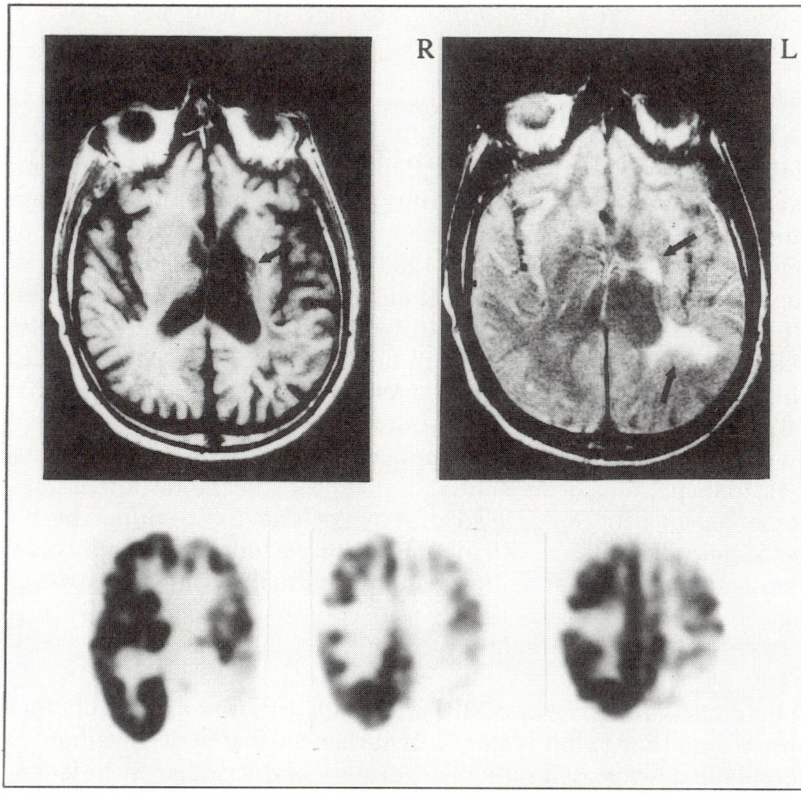

Figure 11.1. Brain T_1-weighted MRI scan (*top left*), T_2-weighted MRI scan (*top right*), and fluorodeoxyglucose positron-emission tomogram (*bottom*) of a patient with subcortical infarctions and dementia. The MRI scans reveal infarction of the left thalamus and left posterior periventricular white matter, the frontal and superior parietal cortex appear unaffected. The positron-emission tomogram demonstrates marked hypometabolism of the left thalamus and caudate nuclei as well as widespread patchy hypometabolism in the cortex of the left hemisphere. A focal hypometabolic region also is evident in the right superior postcentral gyrus.

MID is conflicting. Wallin et al. (1989) found significant reductions of choline acetyltransferase in the hippocampus, parahippocampus, and temporal gyrus; Rinne et al. (1988) found no changes in choline acetyltransferase levels in the frontal, temporal, and hippocampal cortex of patients with MID compared to control subjects. The variability in findings may reflect the variability in lesion location, with some strokes interrupting the ascending transmitter transport systems while others spare these connections. Sufficient information is available, however, to document that neurotransmitter changes are common during MID. Mood disorders are associated with abnormalities of neurochemical systems, including disturbances of norepinephrine, serotonin, and dopamine, and the neurochemical abnormalities of MID may contribute to the mood symptoms of this disorder.

Individual factors also may contribute to vulnerability to depression in conjunction with MID. Age-related changes in cerebral perfusion, neurotransmitter availability, neuronal numbers, and neuronal function may determine a margin of safety, symptom threshold, or physiologic resiliency that increase the likelihood of depression (Katzman and Terry 1983). Gender may affect the rate of depression as well; Cummings et al. (1987) noted that women with MID were more likely than men to exhibit depressive symptoms. Hereditary factors may have a role in determining which patients with MID develop depression, and Starkstein et al. (1989) reported that patients with depression following right hemisphere strokes were significantly more likely to have a family history of psychiatric illness than patients with similar lesions and no mood alterations. Some personality styles also may make one more vulnerable to depression than others. MID represents a personal loss of physical, intellectual, and social abilities, and individuals with narcissistic or borderline character structure as well as those with chronically fragile self-esteem are susceptible to depression in response to such losses.

Patients with stroke and MID often have vascular disease of other organs, and they suffer systemic disturbances that may contribute to depression. Arteriosclerotic heart disease and vascular disorders of the kidney lead to cardiac or renal failure; both disorders are associated with increased rates of depression (Cohen-Cole 1989, Robin and Craven 1989). In addition, drugs commonly are used to treat the associated conditions, and these pharmacologic agents may increase the risk of depression. Hypertension is the most common cause of MID, and several antihypertensive agents are known to induce or precipitate depression, including α-methyldopa, propranolol, reserpine, and clonidine. Digitalis and thiazide diuretics, two other agents commonly used in patients with vascular disease, have been implicated in the production of depression as well (Pascualy and Veith 1989). Thus, when assessing mood changes in patients with MID, both the physical status and treatment regimen must be considered as potential contributing factors.

Psychosocial factors should not be ignored in the patient with MID and depression. Occupational disability, physical illness, interpersonal isolation, dramatic changes in social and family role and status, loss of income, relocation to a convalescent facility, and impaired sexual functioning are among the events that affect patients with dementia, and these contribute to lowered self-esteem and a sense of personal helplessness and worthlessness. These experiences may facilitate the occurrence or magnify the effects of depression.

TREATMENT OF DEPRESSION IN MULTI-INFARCT DEMENTIA

Little systematic research has been devoted to the treatment of depression in MID, and only a limited number of anecdotal observations have been recorded. No double-blind, controlled trials of antidepressant treatment of depression in MID have been conducted. Venna et al. (1988) reported three patients with Binswanger disease that improved following treatment with phenelzine and maprotiline (case 1, one agent used in each of two depressive episodes), imipramine (case 2), and imipramine and desipramine (case 4, one agent used in each of two depressive episodes). Joyce and Levy (1989) also reported the successful treatment of depression in a patient with Binswanger disease using a combination of lithium (800 mg/day) and mianserin (120 mg/day). When this regimen was discontinued, depression recurred and responded to lithium (800 mg/day) and amitriptyline (150 mg/day); no improvement in cognition accompanied the mood changes. These preliminary observations must be interpreted with caution, but they suggest that tricyclic and tetracyclic antidepressant medications, monoamine oxidase inhibitors, and lithium may be efficacious in the treatment of depression accompanying MID.

Depression following stroke in patients without major cognitive compromise has been reported to respond to nortriptyline (Lipsey et al. 1984), trazodone hydrochloride (Reding et al. 1986), methylphenidate (Lingam et al. 1988), and dextroamphetamine (Masand et al. 1991). These observations indicate that depression in patients with cerebrovascular disease responds to treatment with pharmacologic agents, and a therapeutic trial of antidepressant treatment is warranted in patients with MID and depression.

CONCLUSIONS

Multi-infarct dementia is a syndrome of intellectual impairment that results from multifocal ischemic brain injury. There are several clinical types of MID, including lacunar state, Binswanger disease, and multiple large infarctions associated with intracranial and extracranial vascular occlusion. Depression is common in lacunar state and Binswanger disease and variable in other MID syndromes. The prevalence of major depression in MID has been noted to be in the range of from 20% to 30% by most investigators, and preliminary studies suggest that the depressive syndrome of MID is characterized by sadness, anxiety, insomnia, psychomotor retardation, and somatic symptoms. MID with depression must be distinguished from pseudobulbar palsy and the dementia syndrome of depression. There are many factors that may contribute to the occurrence of depression in MID, including both the site and size of lesion, biochemical alterations, individual characteristics (age, gender, personality style, family history of psychiatric illness), associated physical illness and medication effects, and the social and interpersonal circumstances of the patient. Treatment of the depression with conventional antidepressant medications usually has been successful, and a therapeutic trial is warranted in depressed patients with MID.

ACKNOWLEDGMENT

This project was supported in part by the Department of Veterans Affairs and by the National Institute of Mental Health (K07MH00910), and by a National Institute on aging Alzheimer's Disease Care Center grant.

REFERENCES

Akesson HO. 1969. A population study of senile and arteriosclerotic psychoses. *Hum Heredity* 19:546–566.

Alafuzoff I, Adolfsson R, Grundke-Jqbal I, et al. 1985. Perivascular deposits of serum proteins in cerebral cortex in vascular dementia. *Acta Pathol* 66:292–298.

American Psychiatric Association. *Diagnostic and Statistical Manual of Mental Disorders, Third Edition (Revised).* Washington, D.C.: American Psychiatric Press.

Babikian V, Ropper AH. 1987. Binswanger's disease: a review. *Stroke* 18:2–12.

Barclay LL, Zemcov A, Blass JP, et al. 1985. Survival in Alzheimer's disease and vascular dementias. *Neurology* 35:834–840.

Beckson M, Cummings JL. 1991. Neuropsychiatric aspects of stroke. *Intl J Psychiatry Med* 21:1–15.

Bernheimer H, Birkmayer W, Hornykiewicz O, et al. 1973. Brain dopamine and the syndromes of Parkinson and Huntington. Clinical, morphological and neurochemical correlations. *J Neurol Sci* 20:415–455.

Brayne C, Calloway P. 1989. An epidemiological study of dementia in a rural population of elderly women. *Br J Psychiatry* 155:214–219.

Broe GA, Akhtar AJ, Andrews GR, et al. 1976. Neurological disorders in the elderly at home. *J Neurol Neurosurg Psychiatry* 39:362–366.

Bucht G, Adolfsson P. 1983. The Comprehensive Psychopathological Rating Scale in patients with dementia of Alzheimer type and multiinfarct dementia. *Acta Psychiatr Scand* 68:263–270.

Celesia GG, Wanamaker WM. 1972. Psychiatric disturbances in Parkinson's disease. *Dis Nerv Syst* 33:577–583.

Clow HE. 1940. A study of one hundred patients suffering from psychosis with cerebral arteriosclerosis. *Am J Psychiatry* 97:16–26.

Cohen-Cole SA. 1989. Depression and heart disease. In: Robinson RG, Rabins PV, eds. *Aging and Clinical Practice: Depression and Coexisting Disease*. New York: Igaku-Shoin, pp. 27–39.

Cummings JL, Benson DF. 1992. *Dementia: a Clinical Approach, 2nd Ed.* Boston: Butterworths.

Cummings JL, Miller B, Hill MA, et al. 1987. Neuropsychiatric aspects of multi-infarct dementia and dementia of the Alzheimer type. *Arch Neurol* 44:389–393.

del Ser T, Bermejo F, Portera A, et al. 1990. Vascular dementia. A clinicopathological study. *J Neurol Sci* 96:1–17.

Dian L, Cummings JL, Petry S, et al. 1990. Personality alterations in multi-infarct dementia. *Psychosomatics* 31:415–419.

Erkinjuntti T, Haltia M, Palo J, et al. 1988. Accuracy of the clinical diagnosis of vascular dementia: a prospective clinical and post-mortem neuropathological study. *J Neurol Neurosurg Psychiatry* 51:1037–1044.

Erkinjuntti T. 1987. Types of multi-infarct dementia. *Acta Neurol Scand* 75:391–399.

Fischer P, Simanyi M, Danielczyk W. 1990. Depression in dementia of the Alzheimer type and in multi-infarct dementia. *Am J Psychiatry* 147:1484–1487.

Folstein MF, Folstein SE, McHugh PR. 1975. "Mini-Mental State." A practical method for grading the cognitive state of patients for the clinician. *J Psychiatr Res* 12:189–198.

Greenwald BS, Kramer-Ginsberg E, Marin DB, et al. 1989. Dementia with coexistent major depression. *Am J Psychiatry* 146:1472–1478.

Hachinski VC, Iliff LD, Zilhka E, et al. 1975. Cerebral blood flow in dementia. *Arch Neurol* 32:632–637.

Hamilton M. 1960. A rating scale for depression. *J Neurol Neurosurg Psychiatry* 23:56–61.

Hershey LA, Modic MT, Jaffe DF, et al. 1986. Natural history of the vascular dementias: a prospective study of seven cases. *Can J Neurol Sci* 13:559–565.

Ishii N, Nishara Y, Imamura T. 1986. Why do frontal lobe symptoms predominate in vascular dementia with lacunes? *Neurology* 36:340–345.

Joyce EM, Levy R. 1989. Treatment of mood disorder associated with Binswanger disease. *Br J Psychiatry* 154:259–261.

Katz DI, Alexander MP, Mandell AM. 1987. Dementia following strokes in the mesencephalon and diencephalon. *Arch Neurol* 44:1127–1133.

Katzman R, Terry R. 1983. Normal aging of the nervous system. In: Katzman R, Terry R, eds. *The Neurology of Aging*. Philadelphia: F.A. Davis, pp. 15–50.

Kay DWK, Beamish P, Roth M. 1964. Old age mental disorders in Newcastle upon Tyne. Part I: a study of prevalence. *Br J Psychiatry* 110:146–158.

La Rue A, Spar J, Hill CD. 1986. Cognitive impairment in late-life depression: clinical correlates and treatment implications. *J Affect Dis* 11:179–184.

Langworthy OR, Hesser FH. 1940. Syndrome of pseudobulbar palsy an anatomic and physiologic analysis. *Arch Intern Med* 65:106–121.

Lechner H, Bertha G, Ott E. 1988. Results of a five-year prospective study of 94 patients with vascular and multi-infarct dementia. In: Meyer JS, Marshall J, Lechner H, et al., eds. *Vascular and Multi-infarct Dementia*. New York: Futura Publishing Co., pp. 101–111.

Levin H, High WM, Goethe KE, et al. 1987. The neurobehaviour rating scale: assessment of the behavioural sequelae of head injury by the clinician. *J Neurol Neurosurg Psychiatry* 50:183–193.
Lingam VR, Lazarus LW, Groves L, et al. 1988. Methylphenidate in treating poststroke depression. *J Clin Psychiatry* 49:151–153.
Lipsey JR, Robinson RG, Pearlson GD, et al. 1984. Nortriptyline treatment of post-stroke depression: a double-blind study. *Lancet* i:297–300.
Loizou LA, Kendall BE, Marshall J. 1981. Subcortical arteriosclerotic encephalopathy: a clinical and radiological investigation. *J Neurol Neurosurg Psychiatry* 44:294–304.
Masand P, Murray GB, Pickett P. 1991. Psychostimulants in post-stroke depression. *J Neuropsychiatry Clin Neurosci* 3:23–27.
Mathers SE, Chambers BR, Merory JR, et al. 1987. Subcortical arteriosclerotic encephalopathy: Binswanger disease. *Clin Exp Neurol* 23:67–70.
Metter EJ, Mazziotta JC, Itabashi HH, et al. 1985. Comparison of glucose metabolism, x-ray CT, and postmortem data in a patient with multiple cerebral infarct. *Neurology* 35:1695–1701.
Meyer JS, McClintic KL, Rogers RL, et al. 1988. Aetiological considerations and risk factors for multi-infarct dementia. *J Neurol Neurosurg Psychiatry* 51:1489–1497.
Parnetti L, Mecocci P, Santucci C, et al. 1990. Is multi-infarct dementia representative of vascular dementia? A retrospective study. *Acta Neurol Scand* 81:484–487.
Pascualy M, Veith RC. 1989. Depression as an adverse drug reaction. In: Robinson RG, Rabins PV, eds. *Aging and Clinical Practice: Depression and Coexisting Disease*. New York: Igaku-Shoin, pp. 132–151.
Rabins PV, Merchant A, Nestadt G. 1984. Criteria for diagnosing reversible dementia caused by depression: validation by 3-year follow-up. *Br J Psychiatry* 144:488–492.
Reding M, Haycox J, Blass J. 1985. Depression in patients referred to a dementia clinic. A three-year prospective study. *Arch Neurol* 42:894–896.
Reding MJ, Orto LA, Winter SW, et al. 1986. Antidepressant therapy after stroke. A double-blind trial. *Arch Neurol* 43:763–765.
Rinne JO, Sako E, Paljarvi L, et al. 1988. A comparison of brain choline acetyltransferase activity in Alzheimer's disease, multi-infarct dementia, and combined dementia. *J Neurol Transmission* 73:121–128.
Robin G, Craven J. 1989. Depression and endstage renal disease. In: Robinson RG, Rabins PV, eds. *Aging and Clinical Practice: Depression and coexisting disease*. New York: Igaku-Shoin, pp. 61–72.
Robinson RG, Starkstein SE. 1990. Current research in affective disorders following stroke. *J Neuropsychiatry Clin Neurosci* 2:1–14.
Rocca WA, Bonaiuto S, Lippi A, et al. 1990. Prevalence of clinically diagnosed Alzheimer's disease and other dementing disorders: a door-to-door survey in Appignano, Macerata Province, Italy. *Neurology* 40:626–631.
Rogers RL, Meyer JS, Mortel KF, et al. 1986. Decreased cerebral blood flow precedes multi-infarct dementia, but follows senile dementia of Alzheimer type. *Neurology* 36:1–6.
Roman GC. 1987. Senile dementia of the Binswanger type. *JAMA* 258:1782–1788.
Rothschild D. 1941. The clinical differentiation of senile and arteriosclerotic psychoses. *Am J Psychiatry* 98:324–333.
Schwartz JA, Speed NM, Mountz JM, et al. 1990. ^{99m}Tc-Hexamethylpropyleneamine oxime single photon emission CT in poststroke depression. *Am J Psychiatry* 147:242–244.

Shibayama H, Kasahara Y, Kobayashi H. 1986. Prevalence of dementia in a Japanese elderly population. *Acta Psychiatr Scand* 74:144–151.
Starkstein SE, Robinson RG, Honig MA, et al. 1989. Mood changes after right-hemisphere lesions. *Br J Psychiatry* 155:79–85.
Stuss DT, Guberman A, Nelson R, et al. 1988. The neuropsychology of paramedian thalamic infarction. *Brain Cognition* 8:348–378.
Sulkava R, Wikstrom J, Aromaa A, et al. 1985. Prevalence of severe dementia in Finland. *Neurology* 35:1025–1029.
Thal LJ, Grundman M, Klauber MR. 1988. Dementia: characteristics of a referral population and factors associated with progression. *Neurology* 38:1083–1090.
Venna N, Mogocsi S, Jay M, et al. 1988. Reversible depression in Binswanger's disease. *J Clin Psychiatry* 49:23–26.
Wallin A, Alafuzoff I, Carlsson A, et al. 1989. Neurotransmitter deficits in a non-multi-infarct category of vascular dementia. *Acta Neurol Scand* 79:397–406.
Wallin A, Blennow K, Gottfries C-G. 1991. Subcortical symptoms predominate in vascular dementia. *Intl J Geriatr Psychiatry* 6:137–145.

12

NEUROIMAGING STUDIES OF DEPRESSION IN NEUROLOGIC DISEASE

Helen S. Mayberg, M.D.

Depression is a common feature of many neurologic conditions. Despite the etiologic diversity of these disorders, mood symptoms in such patients are clinically indistinguishable from those seen during primary affective illness, and these clinical similarities suggest that neurologic depressions may be appropriate and useful models to study the pathophysiology of mood disorders in general. A number of hypotheses have, in fact, been proposed and supported by both descriptive and experimental studies, suggesting the involvement of specific neural pathways and a variety of neurotransmitters in depression associated with particular neurologic syndromes (Bear 1983; Cantello et al. 1989; Fibiger 1984; Holcomb 1985; Mayberg et al. 1988, 1990a; Mayeux et al. 1988; McHugh 1990; Mesulam 1985; Zubenko et al., 1990a). A single unifying mechanism for these depressions has not yet been established, but the strong association of depression with specific neurologic diseases continues to provide a framework for examining the neuroanatomic and neurochemical systems that regulate mood and emotions.

CLINICAL STUDIES

Clinical observations of patients with neurodegenerative diseases (Caine and Shoulson 1983, Cummings and Victoroff 1990, Folstein and Folstein 1983, Gotham et al. 1986, Jagust et al. 1989, Knesevich et al. 1983, Lazarus et al. 1987, Mayeux et al. 1981, Mayeux 1983, Shoulson 1990, Starkstein et al. 1990b, Zubenko and Moossy 1988), immunologic disorders (Goodstein and Ferrell 1977, Mathews 1979), and systemic illnesses involving the central nervous system (Hietaharju et al. 1990, Nemeroff 1989, Omdal et al. 1988) have noted mood symptoms in subsets of patients. Classical lesion-deficit correlations in patients with depression and Alzheimer disease (Zubenko et al. 1990b), multiple sclerosis (Honer et al. 1987), and in the depressed elderly (Coffey et al. 1990, Rabins et al. 1991) however, are often difficult to interpret in part because of the generalized or random distribution of pathologic abnormalities. These limitations have led to studies of depression in diseases where the neurochemical or neurodegenerative changes are better defined, such as Parkinson disease (Cantello et al. 1989, Mayeux et al. 1988, Rogers et al. 1987, Starkstein et al. 1990b, Taylor et al. 1986), Huntington disease (Folstein et al. 1983b, Peyser and Folstein 1990), progressive supranuclear palsy (Albert et al. 1974), Fahr-Volhard disease (Seidler 1985), Wilson disease (Dening and Berrios 1989), and carbon monoxide poisoning (Laplane et al. 1989), or in patients with discrete brain lesions as occur with trauma (Damasio and Van Hoesen 1983, Grafman et al. 1986, Lishman 1966, Stuss and Benson 1986), ablative surgery (Eslinger and Damasio 1985), stroke (Gainotti 1972; Mendez et al. 1989; Robinson et al. 1984; Robinson 1988; Ross and Rush 1981; Starkstein et al. 1987, 1988a), and tumors or focal epilepsy (Altshuler et al. 1990, Bear and Fedio 1977, Flor-Henry 1969, Mendez et al. 1986, Perini and Mendius 1984, Robertson et al. 1987).

A prominent role for both the frontal and temporal lobes in the expression and modulation of mood and emotions has emerged from these studies (Bear 1983, Blumer and Benson 1975, Damasio and Van Hoesen 1983, Mesulam 1985); there is less agreement, however, on whether the left or right hemisphere is dominant in these behaviors. Observations of patients with traumatic brain injury report a high correlation between affective disturbances and nondominant hemisphere pathology, especially in those with frontal lobe lesions (Grafman et al. 1986). Studies concerning stroke, however, suggest that left-sided lesions are more likely to result in depressive symptoms than right lesions, where displays of euphoria or indifference are more characteristic (Gainotti 1972, Robinson et al. 1984, Starkstein et al. 1987). Still, not all authors agree (Ross and Rush 1981, Sinyor et al. 1986), but lateralization of emotional behaviors is supported further by studies of pathologic crying and laughing. Crying is more common with left hemisphere lesions, while laughter is seen in patients with right lesions (Sackheim et al. 1982). Analogous studies of depression in patients with temporal lobe epilepsy have been conducted and are also somewhat contradictory; affective disorders have been described with left (Altschuler et al. 1990, Mendez et al. 1986, Perini and Mendius 1984), right (Flor-Henry 1969) and nonlateralized temporal lobe foci (Robertson et al. 1987).

ANATOMIC STUDIES

Quantitative studies of lesion size and location using anatomic imaging methods such as x-ray CT or MRI complement and expand on many of the previously reported behavioral, electrical, surgical, and postmortem observations. Lesion-deficit studies in stroke patients both with and without mood disorders demonstrated a high association of mood changes with infarction of the frontal lobe and basal ganglia (Mendez et al. 1989, Robinson 1988, Starkstein et al. 1988). Similarly, depression observed in patients with complex partial seizures occurs with lateralized temporal lobe foci (Altshuler et al. 1990), but there have been no supplementary anatomic studies that define the critical sites within the temporal lobe associated with these mood changes. Studies of plaque loci in multiple sclerosis also have suggested an association of depression with lesions in the temporal lobe (Honer et al. 1987); however, these studies have not shown lateralized effects.

Despite the many similarities among different neurologic conditions, considerable variability in the localization of lesions associated with depression exists. In part, this variability arises from the methodologic and theoretic limitations of anatomic imaging techniques, which restrict lesion identification to those brain areas that are structurally damaged. Functional imaging can complement structural imaging in that the consequences of anatomic or chemical lesions on both global and regional brain function can be directly assessed. These methods provide an alternative strategy to test how similar mood symptoms occur with anatomically or neurochemically distinct disease states or, conversely, why comparable lesions do not always result in comparable behavioral phenomena.

FUNCTIONAL IMAGING STUDIES

METHODS

Positron emission tomography involves the measurement of tissue concentrations of physiologically active compounds labeled with positron emitting isotopes (Links 1990, Phelps et al. 1982). This technique can measure a variety of physiologic variables (Phelps et al. 1982, 1983) including regional brain blood flow (Frackowiak et al. 1980, Raichle et al. 1983), oxygen metabolism (Baron et al. 1981, Frackowiak et al. 1980), glucose utilization (Phelps et al. 1979, Reivich et al. 1979, Sokoloff 1981), blood-brain barrier permeability (Yen and Budinger, 1981), tissue pH, and amino acid transport (Comar et al. 1976), as well as quantify receptor density and affinity for a variety of neurotransmitters and neuropeptides (Dannals et al. 1990,

Frost 1986, Gjedde and Wong 1990, Luciagnani et al. 1989, Sedvall et al. 1986).

In brief, this imaging method involves the detection of positrons (positively charged electrons) as they are emitted from the nucleus of a radionuclide. Once emitted, the unstable positron loses kinetic energy and is eventually annihilated by its interaction with a nearby electron. Each positron-electron interaction results in the production of two gamma rays or photons of equal energy (511 keV) that travel in opposite directions. Coincident detection of these photon pairs is accomplished using a series of opposing detectors, arranged in a circular array, around the head or body (Phelps et al. 1975). Electronic sensors ensure that only the simultaneous or near-simultaneous arrival of photons at detector pairs arranged 180° apart will register as a positron-emission event. Using standardized computer back-projection algorithms for image reconstruction, the initial location of the ligand and its attached positron-emitting isotope can be approximated theoretically to within 1 to 3 mm (the distance traveled by the positron before its annihilation). Spatial resolution on the order of 5 mm can be obtained currently using commercially available positron-emission tomography instruments.

Positron-emitting isotopes exist for oxygen (^{15}O; t½ = 2 minutes), nitrogen (^{13}N; t½ = 10 min), carbon (^{11}C; t½ = 20 minutes), and fluorine (^{18}F; t½ = 10 minutes). The availability and short half-lives of these isotopes allow the development of ligands with a wide variety of biologic applications, including ^{15}O-O_2 for measuring oxygen metabolism, ^{15}O-H_2O for cerebral blood flow, ^{18}F-fluoro-2-deoxyglucose for brain glucose utilization, and ^{11}C-carbon for the labelling of many psychoactive pharmaceuticals (Dannals et al. 1990). The sensitivity of the positron-emission tomography instruments allows detection of physiologic (picomolar range) brain concentrations of these compounds. Methods for quantifying regional blood flow, glucose utilization, receptor densities (b_{max}) and affinities (k_d) also have been developed and validated using a variety of analysis strategies (Gjedde and Wong 1990, Huang et al. 1986, Logan et al. 1987, Mintum et al. 1984, Patlak and Blasberg 1985).

STUDIES IN PRIMARY DEPRESSION

Cerebral glucose metabolism and blood flow have been measured in patients with primary affective disorders by several investigators (Baxter et al. 1985, 1989; Buchsbaum et al. 1986; Drevets et al. 1989; Martinot et al. 1990; Post et al. 1987). Caudate and frontal hypometabolism have been identified in patients with depression of varying etiologies, including those with unipolar depression, bipolar depression, and obsessive compulsive disorder with depression (Baxter et al. 1985, 1989; Buchsbaum et al. 1986); similarly, changes in orbital-inferior frontal cortex and caudate blood flow have been described that identify a "state" and "trait" pattern in two groups of patients with unipolar depression (Drevets et al. 1989). Decreased caudate and increased frontal polar cortex flow were present in both the patients with euthymia and those with depression ("trait"). An additional flow abnormality (increased flow in bilateral inferior frontal-pars orbitalis) was found only in the patients with depression ("state"). These studies, however, did not compare the same patients in different behavioral states; increased caudate metabolism following antidepressant therapy in patients with depression also has been reported (Baxter et al. 1989, Martinot et al. 1990), which suggests the existence of state and trait metabolic markers. Temporal cortex hypometabolism has been described (Post et al. 1987) as well, and a more widespread decrease in relative cerebral blood flow (measured with single photon emission computed tomography involving bilateral limbic regions (orbital-inferior frontal, anterior temporal, and cingulate cortex) has been reported in a group of patients with refractory familial unipolar depression (Mayberg et al. 1991a). All of these studies support a role of specific frontal cortical-striatal-thalamic loops (Alexander et al. 1986, 1990) or paralimbic pathways (Mesulam 1985) in the pathophysiology of depression, but no common abnormality has been identified consistently. Prompted by the variability of findings in patients with primary affective disorder, an approach was developed to examine depression in association with specific neurologic diseases.

STUDIES IN DEPRESSION ASSOCIATED WITH NEUROLOGIC DISEASES

Changes in both mood and cognitive performance are common in patients with Parkinson disease, Huntington disease, and following ischemic lesions of the striatum. In particular, the relationship between depression and cognitive impairment has become a topic of increasing interest, as there appears to be clinical heterogeneity in the manifestations of mood and cognitive symptoms in these patient groups (McHugh 1990; Mendez et al. 1989; Starkstein et al. 1989; Taylor et al, 1986, 1988). Bradyphrenia with impaired psychomotor and cognitive performance often is present in patients both with and without depression. In addition, those with depression show deficits in attention and motivation as well as more profound impairment on tasks classically localized to the frontal lobes. Depression in patients without neurologic impairment shares many of the clinical features characteristic of basal ganglia disease, including apathy, bradyphrenia, psychomotor slowing, and disturbed frontal lobe function (Cantello et al. 1989, Rogers et al. 1987); these clinical similarities may indicate the involvement of common neurochemical and neuroanatomic systems in the genesis of both idiopathic depression and depression associated with basal ganglia disease.

Some of these hypotheses can be tested directly using positron-emission tomography. Studies of patients with basal ganglia strokes, Parkinson disease, and Huntington disease illustrate how regional abnormalities measured with positron-emission tomography can provide clues to the neural circuits involved in the mood disorders seen in patients with specific diseases and perhaps to normal emotional processing as well.

STROKE STUDIES

Clinicians have recognized for years that depression is a frequent consequence of stroke, but investigators only recently have examined systematically the relationship between changes in mood, alterations in specific neurotransmitters, and discrete lesion locations. The prevalence of clinically significant depression appears to be dependent on two variables: the location of the brain injury, and the time elapsed since the stroke (Robinson et al. 1984). Patients with any lesion location can have severe depression; however, it has been shown that those with left frontal and left basal ganglia lesions are more likely to develop severe depression that patients with any other lesion location (Robinson 1988, Starkstein et al. 1987).

It has been hypothesized that the mechanisms of biologic depressions following stroke are due to the direct involvement of midbrain catecholamine neurons or disruption of their cortical projections. Experimental stroke lesions in rats, gerbils, and monkeys demonstrated decreased norepinephrine, dopamine, and serotonin concentrations early after brain injury; changes in central monoamines and their metabolites also have been measured in the spinal fluid of patients with stroke (Meyer 1974, Robinson et al. 1988). Decreased 3-methodxy-4-hydroxyphenylglycol levels in patients having left compared with right hemisphere strokes have been demonstrated that correlate to clinical measures of depression severity (Robinson et al. 1988). These neurochemical changes are of great interest, because they support a long-held, unproven theory that mood disorders result from changes in functionally available biogenic amines (Schildkraut 1965).

Alternatively, it has been hypothesized that mood changes result from disconnection of remote brain areas by strategically placed lesions, a phenomenon termed *remote diaschisis* (Baron 1989). This hypothesis might help to explain the high association of both basal ganglia and frontal lesions with depression. Functional imaging methods such as positron-emission tomography and single photon emission computed tomography can test directly this disconnection hypothesis and offer a complementary approach to lesion-mapping studies in the evaluation of brain areas critical for maintaining normal mood after brain injury. With these methods, one can ask what pattern of cortical or subcortical dysfunction is common in patients with similar phenomena and different brain lesions or, alternatively, what is different about patients with seemingly similar lesions but with discordant mood symptoms.

Patterns of Remote Hypometabolism in Patients with Subcortical Strokes. A possible strategy to find such patients is examining the secondary changes that occur in the uninjured areas of cortex in patients with small, discrete subcortical lesions and specific clinical deficits. This approach expands on previous reports of cortical hypometabolism in morphologically intact brain distant from the site of subcortical lesions (Baron 1985, 1989; Pappata et al. 1987); in these previous studies, the pattern of cortical hypometabolism correlated with persistent disturbances of language, memory, and attention (Baron 1989, Metter et al. 1988). This tactic (using subcortical lesions) has definite advantages over studies of patients with cortical infarctions, because there are no confounding effects of direct tissue damage or atrophy in brain areas where metabolism measurements are of the greatest interest, such as the frontal cortex. The high association of behavioral sequelae, including mood disorders, with lesions of the basal ganglia, particularly those involving the head of the caudate, make these patients highly suitable for these types of studies. In addition, the known pathways linking the basal ganglia and specific areas of frontal cortex studied in primates (Alexander et al. 1986, 1990; Goldman-Rakic and Selemon 1984) provide a logical analysis strategy. Whether disruption of specific motor and nonmotor loops linking the basal ganglia, thalamus, and cortex account for specific clinical deficits can be tested by examining the patterns of regional glucose metabolism in relation to specific lesions.

Mayberg et al. (1989) measured regional cerebral glucose metabolism in the resting condition in patients with well-defined subcortical vascular lesions. As in all of the fluorodeoxyglucose studies in patients with neurologic diseases that will be discussed later, an x-ray CT scan was performed in each patient to determine the precise imaging plane, parallel to the anterior commissure–posterior commissure line, to be used for the positron-emission tomography studies (Fox 1985). Patients were studied in the awake, resting condition in a quiet room with their eyes closed and covered. Absolute metabolic rates for glucose were calculated for average whole brain and individual cortical and subcortical regions using standard methods, and all intersubject comparisons were made using regional metabolic rates normalized to the whole brain average. Individual regions of interest were grouped into functional cortical subdivisions derived from human and primate anatomic and physiologic studies (Alexander et al. 1986, 1990; Talairach and Tournoux 1988); these groupings were selected specifically to differentiate primary sensory-motor and premotor areas from the two basic subdivisions of prefrontal cortex: the more rostral heteromodal lateral prefrontal region, and the more caudal orbital-frontal-inferior frontal (paralimbic) cortex (Fig. 12.1). Subcortical regions were placed in the head of the caudate, lenticular nucleus, and thalamus.

Patients with chronic unilateral basal ganglia strokes (more than 30 days after the initial onset of symptoms) with lesions localized by either x-ray CT or MRI were categorized to one of two groups: lesions of motor loop nuclei (putamen alone, putamen and posterior internal capsule), or non-motor loop nuclei (head of the caudate alone, caudate and anterior limb of internal capsule, anterior or dorsal-medial thalamus) (Fig. 12.2).

Patients with putamen lesions had widespread ipsilateral cortical and thalamic hypometabolism, and they were identified clinically

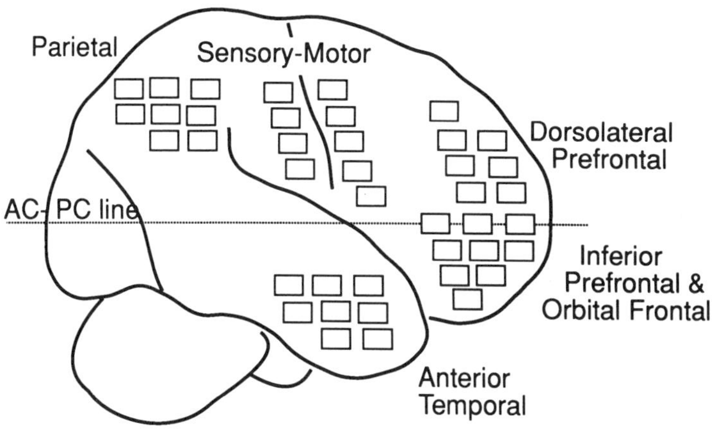

Figure 12.1. Positron-emission tomography region-of-interest template, lateral cortex view. Metabolic rates are measured in various brain regions using each patient's x-ray CT scan as an anatomic template. Regions of interest are placed as shown. Individual cortical regions are combined into functional groups using standardized landmarks and classification schemes. *Note:* AC-PC = anterior-posterior commissure line.

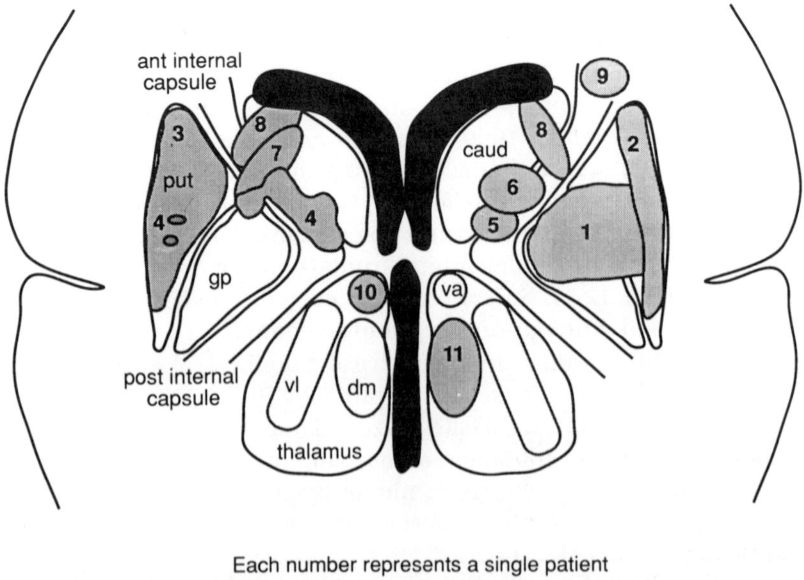

Figure 12.2. Lesion locations of patients with motor and nonmotor subcortical strokes. Motor strokes: lesions of the putamen (*put*) and posterior (*post*) internal capsule (patients 1 through 4). Nonmotor strokes: lesions of the caudate (*caud*), anterior (*ant*) or dorsomedial (*dm*) thalamus, and anterior internal capsule (patients 5 through 11). *Note:* gp = globus pallidus; va = ventral anterior; vl = ventral lateral.

by the presence of motor deficits (Fig. 12.3). In contrast, patients with lesions of the caudate had focal ipsilateral hypometabolism involving very localized regions of frontal, temporal, or cingulate cortex (Fig. 12.3). The pattern of remote cortical hypometabolism was not identical among the individual patients in this group; all, however, had focal rather than hemispheric changes in metabolism ipsilateral to their lesions. As a group, these patients had selective disturbances of cortical function without motor impairment, and the clinical and metabolic phenomenology seen is consistent with segregated motor and nonmotor behavioral circuits described in primates. The data strongly suggest that precise localization of structural lesions using MRI, combined with mapping of remote metabolic phenomena using positron-emission tomography, may be useful in differentiating functionally separate pathways connecting the basal ganglia and cortex, and it may also contribute to understanding the mechanisms underlying lesion-induced disturbances of motor control, mood, and cognition.

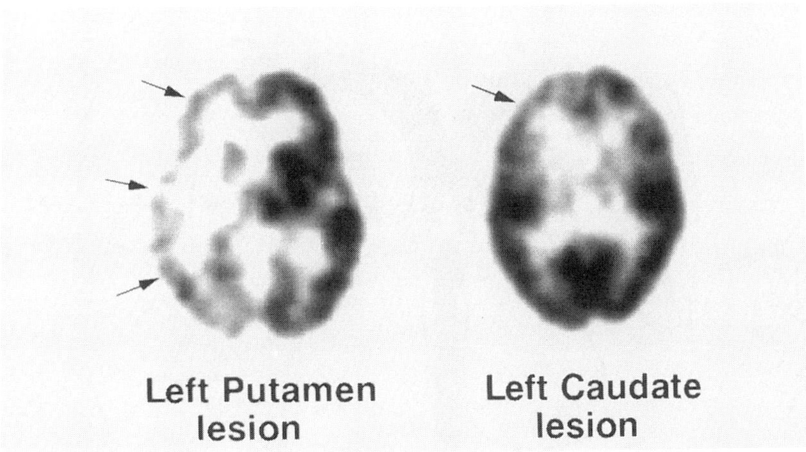

Figure 12.3. Fluorodeoxyglucose PET scans in two patients with motor and nonmotor basal ganglia strokes. The putamen lesion (motor stroke) is associated with diffuse hypometabolism involving the entire ipsilateral hemisphere (*arrows*); note changes in the ipsilateral thalamus as well. The caudate lesion (nonmotor stroke) is associated with a more focal change in cortical metabolism involving prefrontal cortex (*arrow*).

Studies in Patients with Caudate Lesions. A similar strategy can be used to examine patients with comparable basal ganglia lesions but variable mood symptoms. Regional cerebral glucose metabolism was measured using fluorodeoxyglucose and positron-emission tomography in patients without aphasia but with chronic unilateral ischemic lesions both with and without mood changes (Mayberg 1991b, Starkstein 1990a). A group of patients with chronic strokes in whom regional glucose metabolism had been measured previously using fluorodeoxyglucose and positron-emission tomography as part of a clinical study of post-stroke mood disorder were screened by lesion location using CT and MRI scans; patients with single lesions of the basal ganglia (restricted to the head of the caudate, with or without extension into the anterior limb of the internal capsule) were identified. Neurologic and psychiatric exams performed on the day of the positron-emission tomography study were used to subdivide patients by DSM-III mood disorder diagnosis into three groups: those with euthymia, those with depression, and those with mania. Patients in the euthymic and depressed groups all had left-sided lesions, whereas patients with mania all had right-sided lesions (Fig. 12.4).

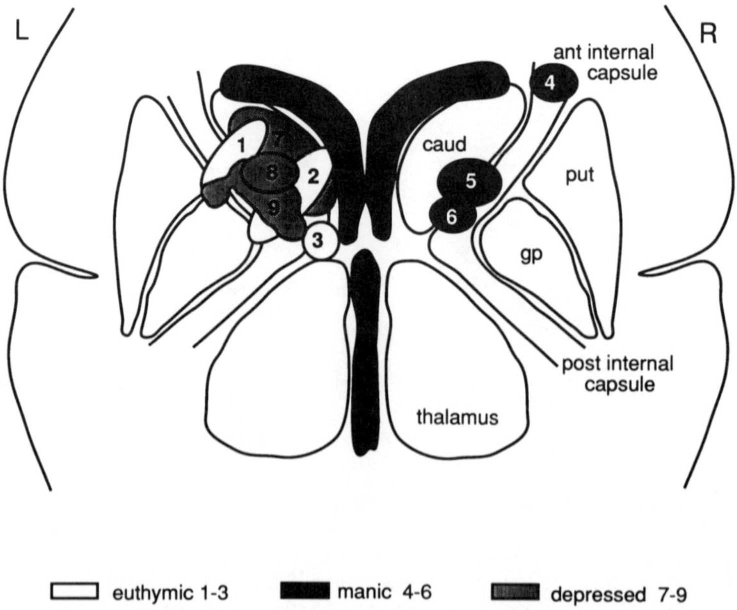

Figure 12.4. Basal ganglia lesion locations in nine patients with and without mood change. *Note:* ant = anterior; caud = caudate; gp = globus pallidus; post = posterior; put = putamen.

All patients had diffuse cortical hypometabolism ipsilateral to the lesion. This is similar to previous findings in patients with a variety of subcortical lesion locations (Baron 1989). When patients with mood change (those with depression and with mania) were compared to patients with euthymia, bilateral hypometabolism was seen in all the limbic regions of interest: orbital-inferior frontal cortex, anterior temporal cortex, and cingulate cortex. The most pronounced changes occurred in the temporal lobes, and metabolism in this region differentiated patients by mood diagnosis (Fig. 12.5). Patients with mania showed temporal hypometabolism ipsilateral to the lesion only, and those with depression had bilateral temporal as well as cingulate hypometabolism. Patients with euthymia had normal temporal and cingulate metabolism. Interestingly, lesion location did not predict mood change, but precision of lesion localization was limited by the structural imaging techniques that were used. Furthermore, the role of lesion side was not fully addressed,

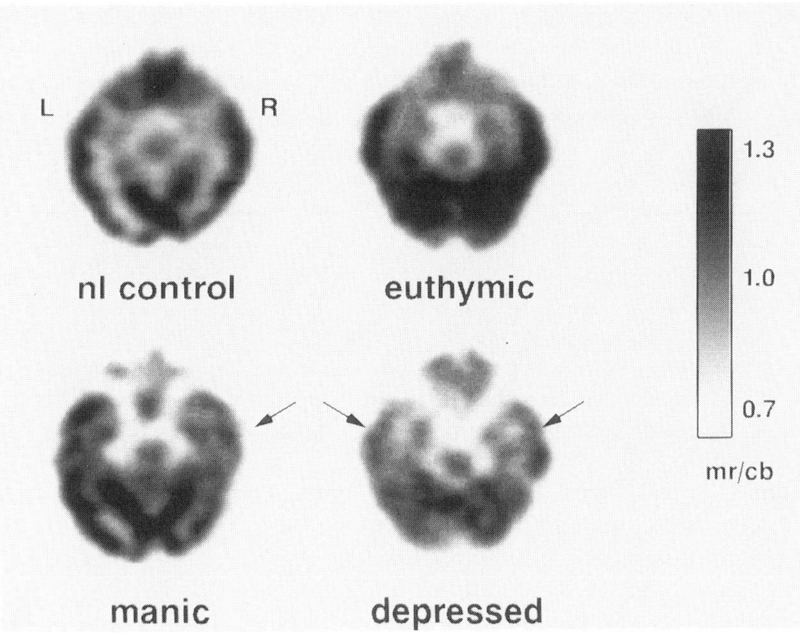

Figure 12.5. Fluorodeoxyglucose PET scans in patients with single caudate lesions and varying mood states. Scans at the level of the temporal lobe are shown in four subjects. Patients with euthymia have normal and symmetric temporal lobe metabolism; in contrast, patients with mania show unilateral (right-sided) temporal hypometabolism and patients with depression show bilateral temporal hypometabolism. *Note:* nl = normal.

because patients with right-sided lesions and depression were unavailable for this study.

The mechanisms underlying these cortical changes still are uncharacterized. It can be postulated, however, that the remote metabolic effects occurring in the orbital-inferior frontal, cingulate, and temporal cortex in patients with isolated basal ganglia lesions may be caused by selective disruption of specific basotemporal limbic pathways or orbital frontal-striatal-thalamic circuits in patients with mood disorders. Undercutting of the medial forebrain bundle as it passes ventral to the caudate, with disruption of selective ascending monaminergic cortical projections, also might result in secondary changes in regional limbic metabolism. Further studies, including selective lesions studies in animals, are necessary to test these hypotheses.

Neurochemical Imaging Studies in Post-Stroke Depression. As region-specific changes are identified using chemically nonspecific mapping methods, such as glucose metabolism, studies may expand to investigate transmitter-specific changes in these same brain regions. Animal models of lateralized post-stroke behavioral changes provide precedent to examine brain catecholamines in human patients with stroke, and findings from these studies were adapted to test similar hypotheses in patients with post-stroke depression using positron-emission tomography measurements of cortical S_2-serotonin receptors.

Animal Stroke Models of Post-Stroke Depression. Using a focal lesion model of stroke in the rat, several groups demonstrated that a small lesion or infarct of the cortex will produce widespread depletions of norepinephrine, serotonin, and dopamine throughout uninjured as well as injured areas of the brain (Brown et al. 1988; Finklestein et al. 1983, 1985; Pearlson et al. 1984; Robinson and Coyle 1980; Starkstein et al. 1988b). In addition, these neurochemical responses appears to be lateralized (Robinson 1979), that is, the degree of catecholamine depletion depends on which hemisphere is injured. This suggests that catecholaminergic depletion may be involved in some of the mood disorders that occur in patients with stroke. It also suggests that the differences between mood disorders associated with left anterior brain lesions (depression) and right anterior lesions (undue cheerfulness and indifference) may be caused by differential neurochemical response to injury depending on which hemisphere is involved.

To assess whether lateralized changes in cortical S_2-serotonin receptors could be demonstrated in response to brain injury in the rat, Mayberg et al. (1990a) performed ^{3}H-spiperone autoradiography 30 days after unilateral cortical suction lesions. Right-side lesions produced bilateral increases in total spiperone binding in frontal cortex (excluding the lesion site), 48% greater than after left-side lesions and 23% greater than shams. Left-side lesions led to bilateral decreases in S_2-receptors in the frontal and perirhinal cortex, and these decreases were asymmetric. The decrease was greater in the hemisphere contralateral to the lesion than in the side with the lesion, and frontal S_2-receptor binding correlated positively with running wheel activity in all animals with lesions regardless of lesion side. These results suggest there is a lateralized receptor and behavioral response to focal injury in rats, perhaps analogous to that observed in humans.

Positron-emission Tomography Measures of S_2-Serotonin Receptors after Stroke. A role for serotonin and other brain monoamines in depression long has been hypothesized (Asberg and Traskman 1981, Van Praag and De Haan 1979). Combined with the findings from lesion studies in animals, this provided the background to examine remote chemical changes in patients with post-stroke depression using positron-emission tomography. Cortical S_2-serotonin receptors were imaged in 17 patients with unilateral strokes (eight left, nine right) using positron-emission tomography and ^{11}C-*N*-methyl-spiperone (Mayberg et al. 1988). Patients with left and right hemisphere strokes were not significantly different in background demographic characteristics, medications taken at the time of positron-emission tomography scanning, or in time since stroke. In addition, the two groups were comparable in motor, sensory, and visual symptoms as well as anterior-posterior lesion location and volume. Four patients met diagnostic criteria for major depressive disorder, but the frequency of major or minor depression and mean depression scores did not differ significantly between groups. *N*-Methyl-spiperone binding was measured in symmetrical frontal, temporal, and parietal regions in both hemispheres, excluding the lesion site.

Patients with right hemisphere strokes had significantly greater ipsilateral to contralateral S_2-serotonin receptor binding than did normal patients or those with either left hemisphere strokes or normal controls (Fig. 12.6). This increased binding ratio in the patients with right-sided stroke arose from increased binding in the right hemisphere as opposed to decreased binding in the left hemisphere (Fig. 12.7). In addition, the ipsilateral-to-contralateral-binding ratio in the temporal cortex correlated negatively with depression severity in patients having left-sided lesions (Fig. 12.8). These data demonstrate that the biochemical response of the brain is different depending on which hemisphere is injured, and based on previous studies, patients with left frontal brain injury are significantly more likely to develop depression than patients with any other lesion location. The positron-emission tomography results further suggest that depression is most severe in the patients with left hemisphere lesions with the lowest spiperone-binding ratios; failure of the left hemisphere to upregulate S_2-serotonin receptors after stroke may play a role in the development of depression in these patients.

This study left several questions unanswered. Two of the most critical concerned the time course of S_2-serotonin receptor changes postinjury and whether receptor binding changes normalized as mood symptoms resolved. These issues were addressed preliminarily by the examination of a patient with post-stroke depression following infarction of the left basal ganglia (Mayberg et al. 1991c). This patient's depression remitted during a 6-week, double-blind treatment trial while receiving placebo medication. Cortical S_2-serotonin receptor binding in the left temporal cortex increased by 25%, par-

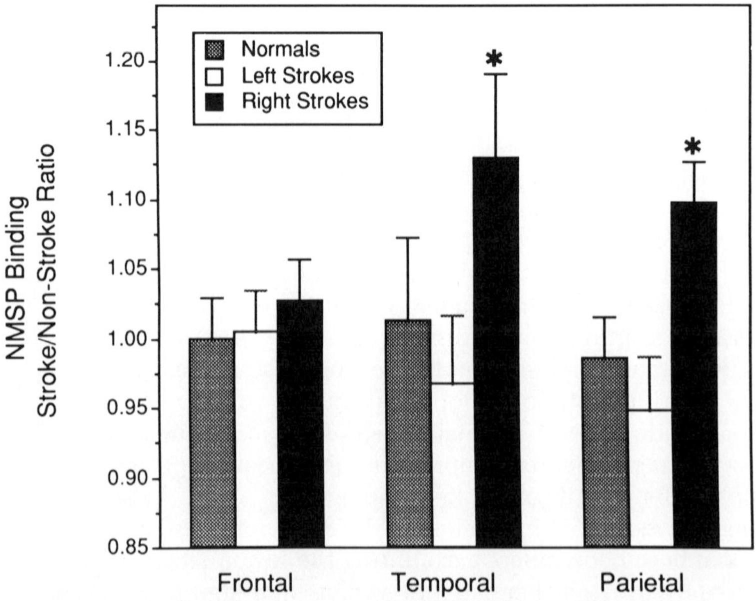

Figure 12.6. Positron-emission tomography measurements of S_2-serotonin receptors in stroke. ^{11}C-*N*-methyl-spiperone binding to cortical S_2-serotonin receptors in patients with right- and left-sided strokes were compared to an age-matched group of normal control subjects. The side of the stroke lesion significantly affected the stroke-to-nonstroke binding ratio. Temporal and parietal S_2-serotonin receptor binding was significantly higher (stroke:nonstroke ratio $>$ 1) in patients with right-sided strokes than those with left-sided strokes or control subjects.

alleling the improvement in mood (Fig. 12.8). This increase contrasted with cortical binding changes of less than 5% in two patients studied twice in the euthymic state, 1 year apart, although any conclusions obviously are limited by lack of a large patient sample. Therefore, the utility of cortical S_2-serotonin receptor binding to predict the onset of depression in a given patient with stroke has yet to be determined, these findings do however, suggest that regional receptor binding may be a useful complement to measures of regional glucose metabolism in elucidating the mechanisms responsible for depression following focal brain injury.

BASAL GANGLIA DISORDERS

Parkinson Disease. Depression is the most common behavioral disturbance seen in patients with Parkinson disease (Gotham et al. 1986). The mean prevalence of depression (both major and minor) is

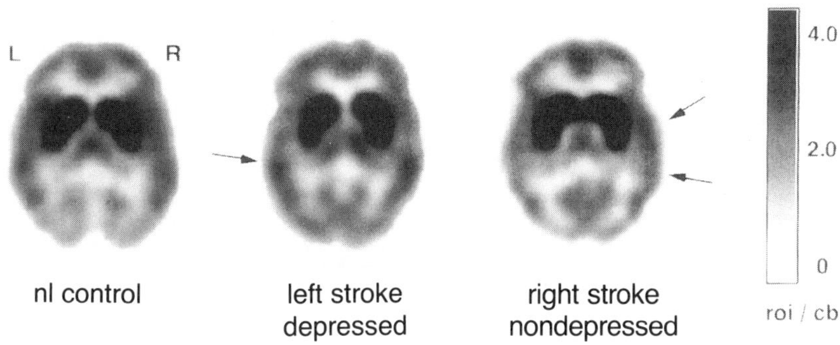

Figure 12.7. *N*-methyl-spiperone PET scans of patients with left- and right-sided strokes. There is symmetric cortical *N*-methyl-spiperone binding in the control subject (*left*) and asymmetric binding (12% lower on the left than on the right) in the patient with depression and a left-sided stroke (*center*). Binding asymmetry is greater in the patient with a right-sided lesion (25% higher on the right than left), illustrating the group findings (*right*). The scale represents the total-to-nonspecific-binding ratio (region:cerebellum) and has been lowered to optimize visualization of changes in the cortex, which accounts for the exaggerated appearance of *N*-methyl-spiperone binding to D_2 receptors in the striatum.

estimated to be approximately 50%, with a range of 20% to 90% among the various clinical series reported.

The cause of depression in Parkinson disease is unknown. Hypotheses implicating the degeneration of mesocortical and mesolimbic dopamine connections to frontal lobe and disruption of monoaminergic afferents from the mesencephalon have been proposed, and these are supported by reduced brain serotonin, nigral and ventral tegmental area dopamine, and locus ceruleus norepinephrine in patients who die from this disease. Degeneration of brainstem monoaminergic neurons with known projections to specific sites in both the striatum and frontal cortex suggests a possible causal role for these specific pathways in the clinical manifestations of depression in Parkinson disease (Mayeux et al. 1988, Sano et al. 1989, Rogers et al. 1987, Taylor et al. 1986, Torrack and Morris 1988, Holcomb 1985).

No anatomic differences between patients with Parkinson disease either with or without depression have been identified using structural imaging methods. However, a large literature exists concerning positron-emission tomography in these patients (Kuhl et al. 1984, Martin et al. 1984, Metter et al. 1984, Perlmutter and Raichle 1985, Wolfson et al. 1985). Increases in cerebral blood flow and glucose

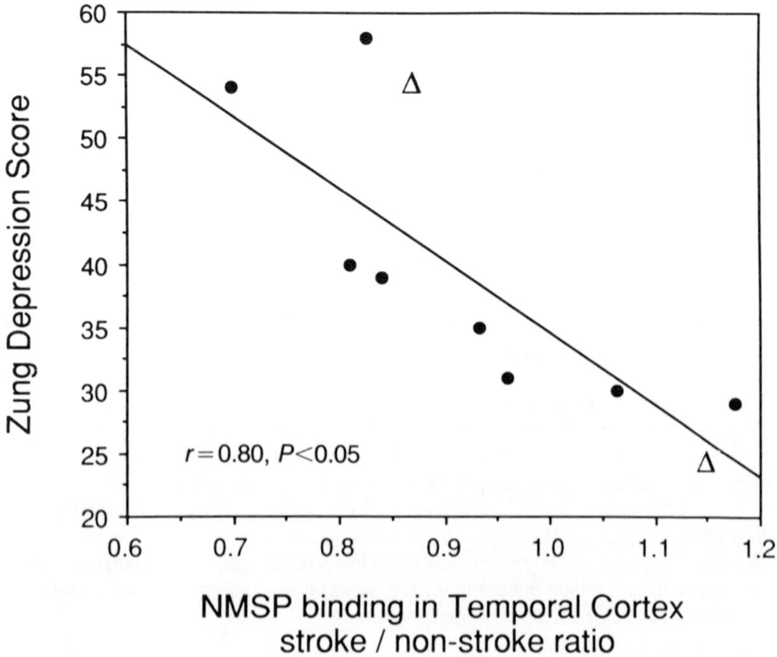

Figure 12.8. Correlation between depression severity and S_2-serotonin receptors in temporal cortex. There is a significant negative correlation between binding asymmetry and depression severity in patients with left-sided lesions. Patients with the lowest ratios (low binding in the left temporal lobe) were the most depressed. One patient with spontaneous remission of depression had a change in *N*-methylspiperone binding between two PET studies performed 6 weeks apart (Δ).

metabolism have been demonstrated in the posterolateral basal ganglia, and these changes, proportional to the severity of motor symptoms, are thought to reflect disinhibition of striatal neurons associated with loss of dopamine cell bodies in the substantia nigra. Cortical changes also have been observed, including global decreases in metabolism and more selective blood flow decreases in dopamine-innervated regions of frontal cortex. Hypometabolism involving temporal-parietal cortex (a pattern similar to that seen in Alzheimer disease) also has been identified in patients with Parkinson disease and dementia (Kuhl et al. 1985). None of these early studies, however, correlate cortical metabolic changes with specific cognitive or emotional deficits.

The relationship between mood, frontal lobe deficits, and patterns of regional glucose metabolism was examined recently in patients with Parkinson disease. Regional cerebral glucose metabolism was measured in two carefully matched groups of such patients without dementia but with or without major depression using FDG and positron-emission tomography (Mayberg et al. 1990b). These studies were performed to determine if an abnormal pattern of regional glucose metabolism could be identified in Parkinson disease that would discriminate patients with depression from both those without depression and age-matched normal volunteers. Using the methods described in the post-stroke section, bilateral caudate, orbital-inferior frontal hypometabolism was found in the patients who were depressed compared to those without depression and control subjects (Fig. 12.9). In addition, the magnitude of the metabolic change in the inferior-orbital frontal lobe region correlated inversely with depression severity as rated by the Hamilton Depression Scale but not with any measures of cognitive performance.

The metabolic changes present in the patients with depression suggested a focal abnormality of orbital frontal-basal ganglia connections, one of the five so-called "complex basal ganglia loops" (Alexander et al. 1986, 1990). This regional localization was consistent, but not identical, with patterns of hypometabolism described in pri-

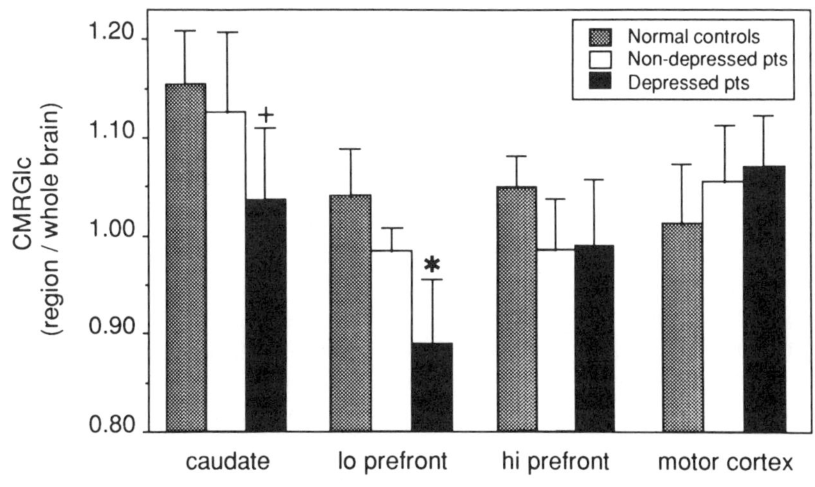

Figure 12.9. Regional glucose metabolism in Parkinson disease both with and without depression. Orbital frontal-inferior prefrontal (*lo prefront*) and caudate hypometabolism differentiated patients with PD and depression from those patients without and from control subjects. $^*P<0.01$: depressed<nondepressed, $p<0.001$: depressed<controls; $^+P<0.02$: depressed<nondepressed and controls. *Note:* nCMRGlc = normalized cerebral metabolic rate for glucose.

mary affective disorders (Baxter et al. 1989) and with lesion location in patients having post-stroke depressions (Robinson et al. 1984, Starkstein et al. 1987), and it implicated a frontostriate defect in Parkinson disease that differentiates patients with from those without depression.

Huntington Disease. George Huntington, in his 1872 description of hereditary chorea, observed that "the tendency to insanity and sometimes to that form of insanity which leads to suicide is marked" (Huntington 1872). Depression occurs in as many as 40% of patients with Huntington disease (Folstein et al. 1983, Shoulson 1990, Caine & Shoulson, 1983) and often precedes the more familiar motor and cognitive symptoms that characterize the illness (Folstein and Folstein 1983, Mayeux et al. 1986). The consistent association of involuntary movements, dementia, and mood change with striatal degeneration has fostered hypotheses that implicate dysfunction of specific motor and nonmotor basal ganglia-thalamic-cortical pathways in the pathogenesis of these symptoms (Albin et al. 1989, McHugh 1990). Motor pathways have been studied in the most detail; studies have focused on selective loss of spiny neurons in the caudate and putamen as well as neurochemical changes in the pallidum and substantia nigra (Albin et al. 1990, Beal and Martin 1986, Young et al. 1988). While the mechanisms underlying both the cognitive and the mood disorders are less well understood, selective involvement of limbic and prefrontal striatal pathways have been proposed.

There have been no systematic anatomic studies of regional atrophy and mood disturbance in Huntington disease, but recent CT studies showed correlations between cognitive performance and subcortical atrophy as measured using the bicaudate ratio (Starkstein et al. 1988c, 1989b). In contrast, a number of published studies have used positron-emission tomography with such patients, and decreases in striatal, cingulate, and frontal cortex glucose metabolism have been described (Berent et al. 1988, Hayden et al. 1986, Kuhl et al. 1982, Kuwert et al. 1989, Leenders et al. 1986, Young et al. 1986). The relationship between the mood disorder and regional metabolic abnormalities only recently has been assessed; using a tactic similar to that reported in the study of patients with Parkinson disease with or without depression, regional cerebral glucose metabolism was measured using fluorodeoxyglucose and positron-emission tomography in patients with early Huntington disease with or without depression (Mayberg et al. 1992). Patient groups were matched for age and years of duration of involuntary movements. Measures of functional disability, apathy, irritability, and cognitive function also were comparable.

As earlier positron-emission tomography studies concerning Huntington disease demonstrated, caudate, putamen, and cingulate metabolism was significantly lower in the patients compared with control subjects independent of mood state. Orbital-inferior prefrontal cortex hypometabolism, however, differentiated patients with depression from both patients with Huntington disease without depression and normal controls (Fig. 12.10).

The mechanisms for the cortical hypometabolism seen in both this and previous studies of Huntington disease again are not understood. The predominant chemical and anatomic changes occur in the striatum, but pathologic changes in cortex have not been appreciated in early cases of the disease. Both cortical atrophy (Von Sattel et al. 1985) and cell loss in the frontal cortex (Sotrel and Myers 1990), however, have been documented in more advanced cases. Nevertheless, these positron-emission tomography study findings implicate the selective involvement of paralimbic frontal cortex in the mood disorder of Huntington disease; the metabolic pattern is similar to that seen in depression associated with Parkinson disease

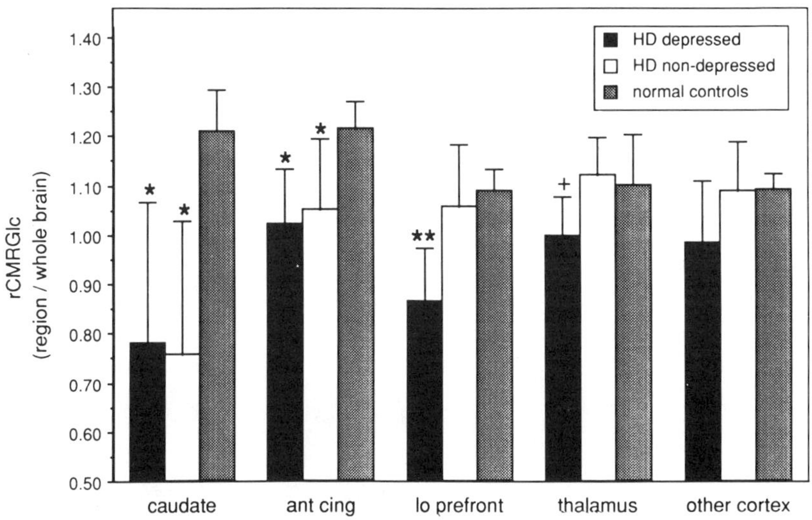

Figure 12.10. Regional glucose metabolism in Huntington disease both with and without depression. Significant hypometabolism of the caudate and anterior cingulate was seen in patients with Huntington disease independent of mood state. Orbital frontal-inferior prefontal (*lo prefront*) and thalamic hypometabolism, however, differentiated patients with HD and depression from those without depression and control subjects. **P*<0.005: all patients < controls; ***P*<0.005: depressed<controls and nondepressed; $^{+}P<0.02$: depressed<nondepressed. *Note:* nCMRGlc = regional Cerebral Metabolic Rate for Glucose; ant cing = anterior cingulate.

and suggests that the disruption of pathways linking the paralimbic frontal cortex and the basal ganglia may be integral to the development of depression in these conditions.

A UNIFYING VIEW OF DEPRESSION IN PATIENTS WITH BASAL GANGLIA DISEASE

One of the salient observations from these studies of patients with Huntington disease, Parkinson disease, and caudate strokes is the common involvement of paralimbic cortex (orbital-inferior prefrontal and temporal cortex) in patients with mood disorders independent of disease diagnosis (Figs. 12.11 and 12.12) (Mayberg and Starkstein 1991d). Based on these findings, a functional lesion-deficit map of brain areas involved in depression is proposed. The regional localization of the metabolic abnormalities matches two known pathways: the orbital frontal-basal ganglia-thalamic circuit (Alexander et al. 1986, 1990), and the basotemporal limbic circuit that links orbital frontal cortex and anterior temporal cortex via the uncinate fasciculus (Nauta 1971). The mechanisms responsible for the metabolic changes, however, have not been identified by these experiments. Hypotheses based on the known neurochemical and degenerative defects present in these disorders can be offered to account for the

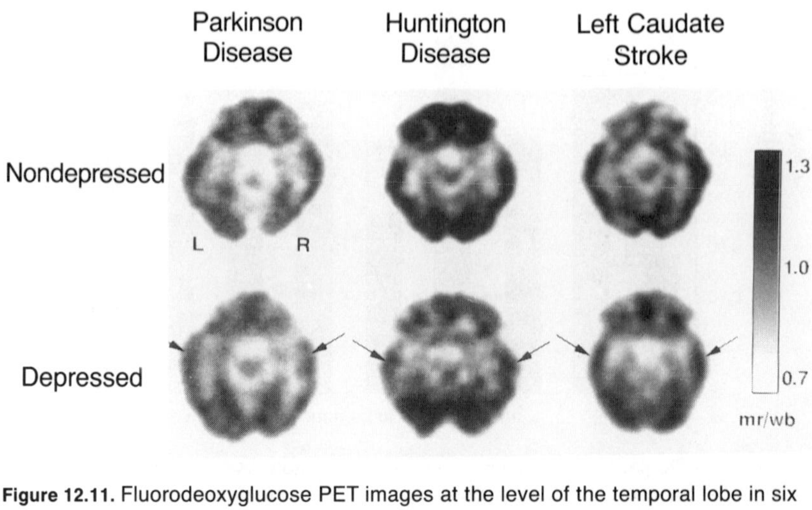

Figure 12.11. Fluorodeoxyglucose PET images at the level of the temporal lobe in six patients. Upper images show cerebral glucose metabolism in three patients without depression; there is homogeneous and symmetric temporal lobe metabolism in all. The lower images show three patients with depression and comparable neurologic impairments; there is symmetric bitemporal hypometabolism (*arrows*) independent of disease etiology. The scale is relative metabolic rate (regional absolute metabolic rate/whole brain).

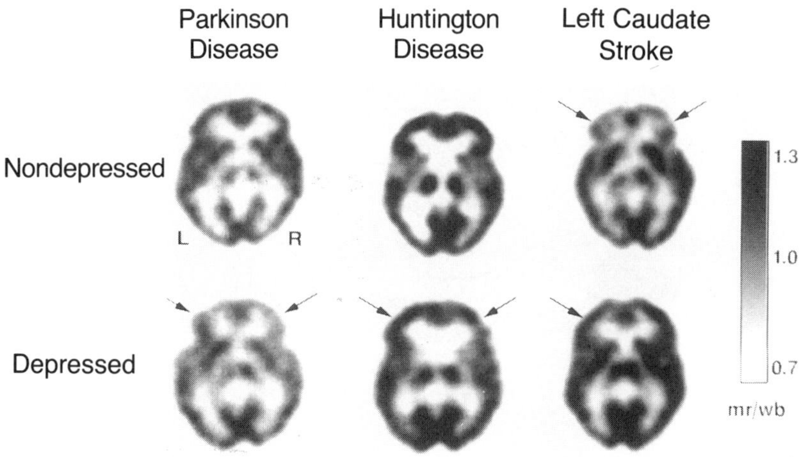

Figure 12.12. Fluorodeoxyglucose PET images at the level of the basal ganglia in six patients. Upper images show cerebral glucose metabolism in three patients without depression and the lower from three patients with depression. There is bilateral frontal lobe hypometabolism independent of disease state in all patients with depression; note however, that this area also is hypometabolic in the patient with stroke and no mood disorder. Unlike the mood-specific metabolic changes in the temporal cortex, the hypometabolism in the frontal cortex appears to be both mood and disease dependent (e.g., hypometabolism is seen with lesions of the caudate with or without mood change). The scale is relative metabolic rate (regional absolute metabolic rate/whole brain).

selective disruption of the corticostriate and basotemporal limbic pathways (Fig. 12.13), and these include:

1. cell dropout in frontal cortex, which has been reported in Huntington disease and would account for the hypometabolism seen in this region;
2. primary degeneration of the basal amygdaloid nucleus, also reported in Huntington disease (Zech et al. 1986), that has direct connections with both the orbital frontal and basotemporal areas via limbic pathways (Cassell and Wright 1986, Porrino et al. 1981);
3. anterograde or retrograde degeneration along basal ganglia-thalamic-cortical pathways secondary to caudate degeneration in either Huntington disease or stroke lesions; and
4. primary degeneration of the ventral tegmental area in Parkinson disease with disruption of dopamine projections to the mesolimbic frontal cortex (Fibiger 1984, Simon et al. 1979, Torack and Morris 1988), or secondary changes in brainstem monamines from dysfunction of the orbitofrontal cortex (the major cortical outflow to the mesencephalon) (Nauta 1981).

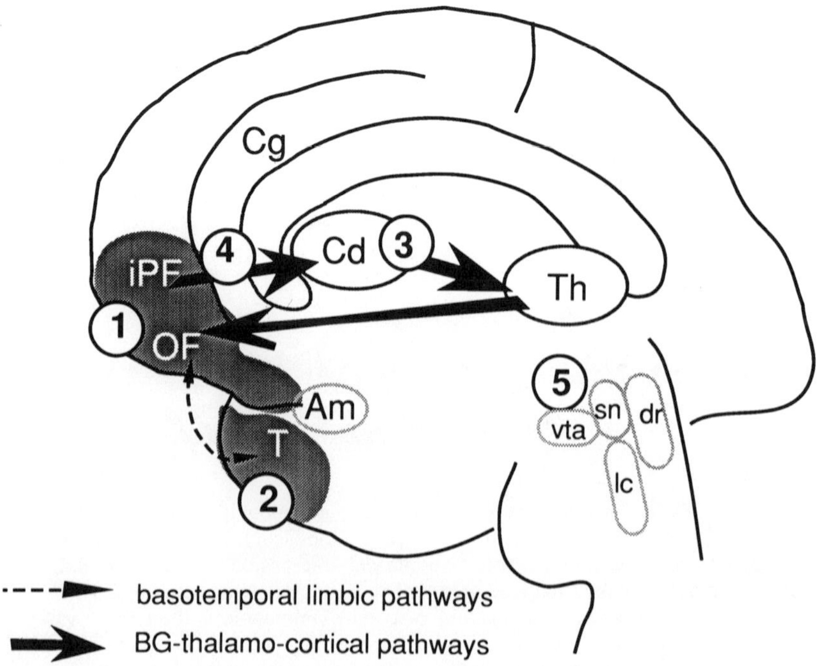

Figure 12.13. Possible mechanisms for common dysfunction of basotemporal limbic cortex in depression with three basal ganglia diseases, showing primary cell loss in frontal cortex (*1*), remote changes in basotemporal limbic regions (*2*), anterograde or retrograde disruption of BG-thalamo-cortical circuits from caudate degeneration or injury (*3, 4*), and degeneration of mesencephalic monamine neurons and their cortical projections (*5*). *Note:* Am = amygdala; Cd = caudate; Cg = anterior cingulate; dr = dorsal raphe; iPF = inferior prefontal cortex; lc = locus Ceruleus; OF = orbital frontal cortex; sn = substantia nigra; T = temporal cortex; Th = thalamus; vta = ventral tegmental area.

Disruption of connections at any point along these circuits, theoretically, might result in the characteristic metabolic defects seen in orbital frontal and temporal cortex and reconcile the presence of similar clinical symptomatology in the setting of heterogeneous disease etiologies.

Patients with depression and neurologic disease clearly are a useful model for the study of primary affective disorders. Functional imaging studies in these patients provide a focused approach to explore the biologic similarities and differences among patient groups with mood symptoms. The identification of specific in vivo neurochemical markers using positron-emission tomography in patients with depression of different etiologies will improve our understanding of the pathogenesis of these disorders, facilitate the development of more specific and effective treatments, and contribute to the elucidation of neural systems regulating normal mood and emotions.

ACKNOWLEDGMENTS

I would like to thank my collaborators, Sergio Starkstein, M.D., Robert Robinson, M.D., Carol Peyser, M.D., Susan Folstein, M.D., Thomas Preziosi, M.D., Thomas Price, M.D., and Paula Andrezejewski, M.S., who participated in the selection and examination of patients; Robert Dannals, Ph.D., Alan Wilson, Ph.D., and Hayden Ravert, Ph.D., who synthesized the positron-emission tomography radiotracers; Dean Wong, M.D., Bernard Sadzot, M.D., Dave Clough, C.N.M.T., Madge Morrell, R.N., Tina Cromwell, B.S., and Henry Wagner, M.D., who participated in the acquisition and analysis of the positron-emission tomography scans cited in this chapter. This work was supported in part by grants NS15178, MH00163, and NS15080.

REFERENCES

Albert ML, Feldman RG, Willis AL. 1974. The subcortical dementia of progressive supranuclear palsy. *J Neurol Neurosurg Psychiatry* 37:121–130.

Albin RL, Young AB, Penney JB. 1989. The functional anatomy of basal ganglia disorders. *TINS* 12:366–375.

Albin RL, Young AB, Penney JB, et al. 1990. Abnormalities of striatal projection neurons and N-methyl-D-aspartate receptors in presymptomatic Huntington's disease. *N Engl J Med* 322:1293–1298.

Alexander GE, DeLong MR, Strick PL. 1986. Parallel organization of functionally segregated circuits linking basal ganglia and cortex. *Ann Rev Neurosci* 9:357–381.

Alexander GE, Crutcher MD, De Long MR. 1990. Basal ganglia-thalamocortical circuits: parallel substrates for motor, oculomotor, "prefrontal" and "limbic" functions. *Prog Brain Res* 85:119–146.

Altshuler LL, Devinsky O, Post RM, et al. 1990. Depression, anxiety, and temporal lobe epilepsy: laterality of focus and symptoms. *Arch Neurol* 47:284–288.

Asberg M, Traskman L. 1981. Studies of CSF 5-HIAA in depression and suicidal behavior. In: Haber B, Gabay S, Issidovides MR, et al., eds. *Serotonin*. New York: Plenum Press.

Baron JC, Bouser MG, Comar D, et al. 1981. Noninvasive tomographic study of cerebral blood flow and oxygen metabolism in vivo. *Eur Neurol* 20:273–284.

Baron JC. 1985. Positron tomography in cerebral ischemia. *Neuroradiology* 27:509–516.

Baron JC. 1989. Depression of energy metabolism in distant brain structures: studies with positron emission tomography in stroke patients. *Semin Neurol* 9:281–285.

Baxter LR, Phelps ME, Mazziotta JC. 1985. Cerebral metabolic rates for glucose in mood disorders. *Arch Gen Psychiatry* 42:441–447.

Baxter LR, Schwartz JM, Phelps ME, et al. 1989. Reduction of prefrontal cortex glucose metabolism common to three types of depression. *Arch Gen Psychiatry* 46:243–250.

Beal MF, Martin JB. 1986. Neuropeptides in neurological disease. *Ann Neurol* 20:547–565.

Bear D, Fedio P. 1977. Quantitative analysis of interictal behavior in temporal lobe epilepsy. *Arch Neurol* 34:454–467.

Bear DM. 1983. Hemispheric specialization and the neurology of emotion. *Arch Neurol* 40:195–202.

Berent S, Giordani B, Lehtinen S, et al. 1988. Positron emission tomography scan investigation of Huntington's disease: cerebral metabolic correlations of cognitive function. *Ann Neurol* 23:541–546.

Blumer D, Benson DF. 1975. Personality changes with frontal and temporal lobe lesions. In: Benson DF, Blumer D, eds. *Psychiatric Aspects of Neurological Disease*. New York: Grune & Stratton, pp, 151–170.

Brown CM, Kilpatrick AT, Martin A, et al. 1988. Cerebral ischaemia reduces the density of 5HT2 binding sites in the frontal cortex of the gerbil. *Neuropharmacology* 27:831–836.

Buchsbaum MS, Wu J, DeLisi LE, et al. 1986. Frontal cortex and basal ganglia metabolic rates assessed by positron emission tomography with ^{18}F-2-deoxyglucose in affective illness. *J Affect Disord* 10:137–152.

Caine E, Shoulson I. 1983. Psychiatric syndromes in Huntington's disease. *Am J Psychiatry* 140:728–733.

Cantello R, Aguaggia M, Gilli M, et al. 1989. Major depression in Parkinson's disease and the mood response to intravenous methylphenidate: possible role of the "hedonic" dopamine synapse. *J Neurol Neurosurg Psychiatry* 52:724–731.

Cassell MD, Wright DJ. 1986. Topography of projections from the medial prefrontal cortex to the amygdala in the rat. *Brain Res Bull* 17:321–333.

Coffey CE, Figiel GS, Djang WT, et al. 1990. Subcortical hyperintensity on magnetic resonance imaging: a comparison of normal and depressed elderly subjects. *Am J Psychiatry* 147:187–189.

Comar D, Cartron JC, Maziere M, et al. 1976. Labelling and metabolism of methionine-methyl-^{11}C. *Eur J Nucl Med* 1:11–14.

Cummings JL, Victoroff JI. 1990. Noncognitive neuropsychiatric syndromes in Alzheimer's Disease. *Neuropsychiatry Neuropsychol Behav Neurol* 2:140–158.

Damasio AR, Van Hoesen GW. 1983. Emotional disturbances associated with focal lesions of the limbic frontal lobe. In: Heilman KM, Satz P., eds. *Neuropsychology of Human Emotion*. New York: Guilfore Press, pp. 85–110.

Dannals RF, Ravert HT, Wilson AA. 1990. Radiochemistry of tracers for neurotransmitter receptor studies. In: Frost JJ, Wagner HN, eds. *Quantitative Imaging: Neuroreceptors, Neurotransmitters and Enzymes*. New York: Raven Press, pp. 19–35.

Dening TR, Berrios GE. 1989. Wilson's disease: psychiatric symptoms in 195 patients. *Arch Gen Psychiatry* 46:1126–1134.

Drevets WC, Raichle ME, Fox PT, et al. 1989. Trait and state cerebral blood flow abnormalities in depression. *Soc Neurosci Abstr* 15(Part 1):30.

Eslinger PJ, Damasio AR. 1985. Severe bilateral disturbance of higher cognition after bilateral frontal lobe ablation: patient EVR. *Neurology* 35:1731–1741.

Fibiger HC. 1984. The neurobiological substrates of depression in Parkinson's disease: a hypothesis. *Can J Neurol Sci* 11(suppl 1):105–107.

Finklestein S, Campbell A, Stoll AL, et al. 1983. Changes in cortical and subcortical levels and monoamines and their metabolites following unilateral ventrolateral cortical lesions in the rat. *Brain Res* 271:279–288.
Finklestein S, Campbell A, Baldessarini RJ, et al. 1985. Late changes in cerebral monoamine metabolism following focal ventrolateral cerebrocortical lesions in rats. *Brain Res* 344:205–210.
Flor-Henry P. 1969. Psychosis and temporal lobe epilepsy. *Epilepsia* 10:363–395.
Folstein SE, Folstein MF. 1983. Psychiatric features of Huntington's disease: recent approaches and findings. *Psychiatr Dev* 2:193–205.
Folstein SE, Abbott MH, Chase GA, et al. 1983. The association of affective disorder with Huntington's disease in a case series and in families. *Psychol Med* 13:537–542.
Fox PT, Perlmutter JS, Raichle ME. 1985. A stereotactic method of anatomical localization for positron emission tomography. *J Comput Assist Tomogr* 9:141–153.
Frackowiak RSJ, Lenzi GL, Jones T, et al. 1980. Quantitative measurements of regional cerebral blood flow and oxygen metabolism in man using ^{15}O and positron emission tomography: theory, procedure and normal values. *J Comput Assist Tomography* 4:727–736.
Frost JJ. 1986. Imaging neuronal biochemistry by emission computed tomography: focus on neuroreceptors. *Trans Pharma Sci* 59 December:490–496.
Gainotti G. 1972. Emotional behavior and hemispheric side of the lesion. *Cortex* 8:41–55.
Gjedde A, Wong DF. 1990. Modeling neuroreceptor binding of radioligands in vivo. In: Frost JJ, Wagner HN, eds. *Quantitative Imaging: Neuroreceptors, Neurotransmitters and Enzymes*. New York: Raven Press, pp. 51–79.
Goldman-Rakic PS, Selemon LD. 1984. Topography of corticostriatal projections in nonhuman primates and implications for functional parcellation of the neostriatum. In: Jones EG, Peters A, eds. *Cerebral Cortex*. New York: Plenum Press, pp. 447–466.
Goodstein RK, Ferrel RB. 1977. Multiple sclerosis presenting as depressive illness. *Dis Nerv System* 38:127–131.
Gotham AM, Brown RG, Marsden CD. 1986. Depression in Parkinson's disease: a quantitative and qualitative analysis. *J Neurol Neurosurg Psychiatry* 49:381–389.
Grafman J, Vance SC, Weingartner H, et al. 1986. The effects of lateralized frontal lesions on mood regulation. *Brain* 109:1127–1148.
Hayden MR, Martin WR, Stoessl AJ, et al. 1986. PET in early diagnosis of Huntington's disease. *Neurology* 36:888–894.
Hietaharju A, Yli-Kerttula U, Hakkinen V, et al. 1990. Nervous system manifestations in Sjogren's syndrome. *Acta Neurol Scand* 81:144–152.
Holcomb HH. 1985. Parkinsonism and depression: dopaminergic mediation of neuropathologic processes in human beings. In: Lake CR, Ziegler MG, eds. *The Catecholamines in Psychiatric and Neurologic Disorders*. Boston: Butterworth Publishers, pp. 269–282.
Honer WG, Hurwitz T, Li DKB, et al. 1987. Temporal lobe involvement in multiple sclerosis patients with psychiatric disorders. *Arch Neurol* 44:187–190.
Huang SC, Bario JR, Phelps ME. 1986. Neuroreceptor assay with positron emission tomography: equilibrium versus dynamic approaches. *J Cereb Blood Flow Metab* 6:515–521.

Huntington G. 1872. On chorea. *Med Surg Reporter* 26:317–321.
Jagust WJ, Reed BR, Seab JP, et al. 1989. Clinical-physiological correlates of Alzheimer's disease and frontal lobe dementia. *Am J Physiol Imaging* 4:89–96.
Knesevich JW, Martin RL, Berg L, et al. 1983. Preliminary report on affective symptoms in the early stages of senile dementia of the Alzheimer type. *Am J Psychiatry* 140:233–235.
Kuhl DE, Phelps ME, Markham CH, et al. 1982. Cerebral metabolism and atrophy in Huntington's disease determined by 18FDG and computed tomographic scans. *Ann Neurol* 12:425–434.
Kuhl DE, Metter EJ, Riege WH. 1984. Patterns of local cerebral glucose utilization determined in Parkinson's disease by the [^{18}F]fluorodeoxyglucose method. *Ann Neurol* 15:419–424.
Kuhl DE, Metter EJ, Benson DF, et al. 1985). Similarities of cerebral glucose metabolism in Alzheimer's and Parkinsonian dementia. *J Cereb Blood Flow Metab* 5(suppl 1):S169.
Kuwert T, Lange HW, Langen K-J, et al. 1989. Cerebral glucose consumption measured by PET in patients with and without psychiatric symptoms of Huntington's disease. *Psychiatry Res* 29:361–362.
Laplane D, Levasseur M, Pillon B, et al. 1989. Obsessive-compulsive and other behavioral changes with bilateral basal ganglia lesions. A neuropsychological, magnetic resonance imaging and positron tomography study. *Brain* 112:699–725.
Lazarus LW, Newton N, Cohler B, et al. 1987. Frequency and presentation of depressive symptoms in patients with primary degenerative dementia. *Am J Psychiatry* 144:41–45.
Leenders KL, Frackowiak RSJ, Quinn N, et al. 1986. Brain energy metabolism and dopaminergic function in Huntington's disease measured in vivo using positron emission tomography. *Mov Disord* 1:69–75.
Links JM, 1990. Physics and instrumentation of positron emission tomography. In: Frost JJ, Wagner HN, eds. *Quantitative Imaging: Neuroreceptors, Neurotransmitters and Enzymes*. New York: Raven Press, pp. 37–50.
Lishman WA. 1966. Brain damage in relation to psychiatric disability after head injury. *Br J Psychiatr* 114:373–375.
Logan J, Wolf AP, Shieu CY, et al. 1987. Kinetic modeling of receptor-ligand binding applied to positron emission tomographic studies with neuroleptic tracers. *J Neurochem* 48:73–83.
Luciagnani G, Moresco RM, Fazio F. 1989. PET-based neuropharmacology: state of the art. *Cerebrovas Brain Metab Rev* 1:271–287.
Martin WRW, Beckman JH, Calne DB, et al. 1984. Cerebral glucose metabolism in Parkinson's disease. *Can J Neurol Sci* 11:169–173.
Martinot JL, Hardy P, Feline A, et al. 1990. Left prefrontal glucose hypometabolism in the depressed state: a confirmation. *Am J Psychiatry* 147:1313–1317.
Mathews WB. 1979. Multiple sclerosis presenting with acute remitting psychiatric symptoms. *J Neurol Neurosurg Psychiatry* 42:859–863.
Mayberg HS, Robinson RG, Wong DF, et al. 1988. PET imaging of cortical S_2-serotonin receptors after stroke: lateralized changes and relationship to depression. *Am J Psychiatry* 145:937–943.
Mayberg HS, Starkstein SE, Sadzot B, et al. 1989. Patterns of remote hypometabolism (FDG-PET) in subcortical strokes differentiates grey and white matter lesions. *J Cereb Blood Flow Metab* 9(suppl 1):S621.
Mayberg HS, Moran TH, Robinson RG. (1990a). Remote lateralized changes

in cortical ^{3}H-spiperone binding following focal frontal cortex lesions in the rat. *Brain Res* 516:127–131.
Mayberg HS, Starkstein SE, Sadzot B, et al. 1990b. Selective hypometabolism in the inferior frontal lobe in depressed patients with Parkinson's disease. *Ann Neurol* 28:57–64.
Mayberg HS, Starkstein SE, Morris PL, et al. 1991b. Remote cortical hypometabolism following focal basal ganglia injury: relationship to secondary changes in mood. *Neurology* 41(suppl):266.
Mayberg HS, Jeffery PJ, Wagner HN, et al. 1991a. Regional cerebral blood flow in patients with refractory unipolar depression measured with TC-99m HMPAO SPECT. *J Nucl Med* 32:S951.
Mayberg HS, Parikh RM, Morris PLP, et al. 1991c. Spontaneous remission of post-stroke depression and temporal changes in cortical S_2-serotonin receptors. *J Neuropsych Clin Neurosci* 3:80–83.
Mayberg HS, Starkstein SE. 1991d. Limbic cortex hypometabolism in depression: similarities among patients with Huntington's disease, Parkinson's disease and basal ganglia strokes. *J Cereb Blood Flow Metab* 11(suppl):S2.
Mayberg HS, Starkstein SE, Peyser CE, et al. 1992. Paralimbic frontal lobe hypometabolism in depression associated with Huntington's disease. *Neurology* 42:1791–1797.
Mayeux R, Stern Y, Rosen J, et al. 1981. Depression, intellectual impairment, and Parkinson's disease. *Neurology* 31:645–650.
Mayeux R. 1983. Emotional changes associated with basal ganglia disorders. In: Heilman KM, Satz P., eds. *Neuropsychology of Human Emotion*. New York: Guilfore Press, pp. 141–164.
Mayeux R, Stern Y, Herman A, et al. 1986. Correlates of early disability in Huntington's disease. *Ann Neurol* 20:727–731.
Mayeux R, Stern Y, Sano M, et al. 1988. The relationship of serotonin to depression in Parkinson's disease. *Mov Disord* 3:237–244.
McHugh PR. 1990. The basal ganglia: the region, the integration of its systems and implications for psychiatry and neurology. In: Franks AJ, ed. *Function and Dysfunction of the Basal Ganglia*. Manchester: Manchester University Press, pp. 259–269.
Mendez MF, Adams NL, Lewandowski KS. 1989. Neurobehavioral changes associated with caudate lesions. *Neurology* 39:349–354.
Mendez MF, Cummings UL, Benson DF. 1986. Depression in epilepsy. *Arch Neurol* 43:766–770.
Mesulam MM. 1985. Patterns in behavioral neuroanatomy: association areas, the limbic system, and hemispheric specialization. In: Mesulam MM, ed. *Principles of Behavioral Neurology*. Philadelphia: F.A. Davis, pp. 1–70.
Metter EJ, Riege WH, Kuhl DE, et al. 1984. Cerebral metabolic relationships for selected brain regions in Alzheimer's, Huntington's, and Parkinson's diseases. *J Cereb Blood Flow Metab* 4:500–506.
Metter EJ, Riege WH, Hanson WR, et al. 1988. Subcortical structures in aphasia: an analysis based of FDG, PET and CT. *Arch Neurol* 45:1229–1234.
Meyer JS, Welch KMA, Okamoto S, et al. 1974. Disordered neurotransmitter function: demonstration by measurement of norepinephrine and 5-hydroxydopamine in CSF of patients with recent cerebral infarction. *Brain* 97:655–664.
Mintum MA, Raichle ME, Kilbourn MR, et al. 1984. A quantitative model

for the in vivo assessment of drug binding sites with positron emission tomography. *Ann Neurol* 15:217–227.

Nauta WJH. 1971. The problem of the frontal lobe: a reinterpretation. *J Psychol Res* 8:167–187.

Nemeroff CB. 1989. Clinical significance of psychoneuroendocrinology in psychiatry: focus on the thyroid and adrenal. *J Clin Psychiatry* 50 (suppl):13–22.

Omdal R, Mellgren SI, Husby G. 1988. Clinical neuropsychiatric and neuromuscular manifestations in systemic lupus erythematosis. *Scand J Rheumatol* 17:113–117.

Pappata S, Tran DS, Baron JC, et al. 1987. Remote metabolic effects of cerebrovascular lesions: magnetic resonance and positron tomography imaging. *Neuroradiology* 29:1–26.

Patlak CS, Blasberg RG. 1985. Graphical evaluation of blood-to-brain transfer constants from multiple-time uptake data. Generalizations. *J Cereb Blood Flow Metab* 5:584–590.

Pearlson GD, Kubos KL, Robinson RG. 1984. Effect of anterior-posterior lesion location on the asymmetrical behavioral and biochemical response to cortical suction ablations in the rat. *Brain Res* 293:241–250.

Perini G, Mendius R. 1984. Depression and anxiety in complex partial seizures. *J Nerv Ment Dis* 172:287–290.

Perlmutter JS, Raichle ME. 1985. Regional blood flow in hemiparkinsonism. *Neurology* 35:1127–1134.

Peyser CE, Folstein SE. 1990. Huntington's disease as a model for mood disorders: clues from neuropathology and neurochemistry. *Mol Chem Neuropathol* 12:99–119.

Phelps ME, Hoffman EJ, Mullani NA, et al. 1975. Application of annihilation coincidence detection to transaxial reconstruction tomography. *J Nucl Med* 16:210–233.

Phelps ME, Huang SC, Hoffman EH, et al. 1979. Tomographic measurement of local cerebral glucose metabolic rate in humans with (F-18)2-fluoro-2-deoxy-D-glucose: validation of method. *Ann Neurol* 6:371–388.

Phelps ME, Maziotta JC, Huang SC. 1982. Studies of cerebral function with positron computed tomography. *J Cereb Blood Flow Metab* 2:113–162.

Phelps ME, Schelbert HR, Mazziotta JC. 1983. Positron computed tomography for studies of myocardial and cerebral function. *Ann Intern Med* 98:339–359.

Porrino LJ, Crane AM, Goldman-Rakic PS. 1981. Direct and indirect pathways from the amygdala to the frontal lobe in rhesus monkeys. *J Comp Neurol* 198:121–136.

Post RM, DeLisi LE, Holcomb HH, et al. 1987. Glucose utilization in the temporal cortex of affectively ill patients: positron emission tomography. *Biol Psychiatry* 22:545–553.

Rabins PV, Pearlson GD, Aylward E, et al. 1991. Cortical magnetic resonance imaging changes in elderly inpatients with major depression. *Am J Psychiatry* 148:617–620.

Raichle ME, Martin MRW, Herscovitch P, et al. 1983. Brain blood flow measures with intravenous $H_2{}^{15}O$: implementation and validation. *J Nucl Med* 24:790–798.

Reivich M, Kuhl D, Wolf A, et al. 1979. The ^{18}F-fluorodeoxyglucose method for the measurement of local cerebral glucose utilisation in man. *Circ Res* 44:127–137.

Robertson MM, Trimble MR, Townsend HRA. 1987. Phenomenology of depression in epilepsy. *Epilepsia* 28:364–368.
Robinson RG. 1979. Differential behavioral effects of right versus left hemispheric cerebral infarction: evidence for cerebral lateralization in the rat. *Science* 205:707–710.
Robinson RG, Coyle JT. 1980. The differential effect of right versus left hemispheric cerebral infarction on catecholamines and behavior in the rat. *Brain Res* 188:63–78.
Robinson RG, Kubos KL, Starr LB, et al. 1984. Mood disorders in stroke patients: importance of location of lesion. *Brain* 107:81–93.
Robinson RG. 1988. Post-stroke depression and lesion location. *Stroke* 19:125.
Robinson RG, Parikh RM, Rodriguez RA, et al. 1988. CSF monoamine metabolite measures in post-stroke depression. *Soc Neurosci Abstr* 301:S7.
Rogers D, Lees AJ, Smith E, et al. 1987. Bradyphrenia in Parkinson's disease and psychomotor retardation in depressive illness: an experimental study. *Brain* 110:761–776.
Ross ED, Rush AJ. 1981. Diagnosis and neuroanatomical correlates of depression in brain-damaged patients. *Arch Gen Psychiatry* 39:1344–1354.
Sackeim H, Greenberg MS, Weiman AL, et al. 1982. Hemispheric asymmetry in the expression of positive and negative emotions. *Arch Neurol* 39:210–218.
Sano M, Stern Y, Williams J, et al. 1989. Coexisting dementia and depression in Parkinson's disease. *Arch Neurol* 46:1284–1286.
Schildkraut JJ. 1965. The catecholamine hypothesis of affective disorders: a review of the supporting evidence. *Am J Psychiatry* 122:509–522.
Sedvall G, Farde L, Persson A, et al. 1986. Imaging of neurotransmitter receptors in the living brain. *Arch Gen Psychiatry* 43:995–1005.
Seidler GH. 1985. Psychiatrisch-psychologische aspekte des Fahr-syndroms. *Psychiatr-Prax.* 12:203–205.
Shoulson I. 1990. Huntington's disease: cognitive and psychiatric features. *Neuropsychiatry Neuropsychol Behav Neurol* 3:15–22.
Simon H, LeMoal M, Calas A. 1979. Efferents and afferents of the ventral tegmental-A_{10} region studied after local injection of [^{3}H]-leucine and horseradish peroxidase. *Brain Res* 178:17–40.
Sinyor D, Jacques P, Kaloupek DG, et al. 1986. Post stroke depression and lesion location: an attempted replication. *Brain* 109:537–546.
Sokoloff L. 1981. Localization of functional activity in the central nervous system by measurement of glucose utilization with radioactive deoxyglucose. *J Cereb Blood Flow Metab* 1:7–36.
Sotrel A, Myers RH. 1991. Morphometric analysis of prefrontal cortex in Huntington's disease. *Neurology* 41:1117–1123.
Starkstein SE, Robinson RG, Price TR. 1987. Comparison of cortical and subcortical lesions in the production of post-stroke mood disorders. *Brain* 110:1045–1059.
Starkstein SE, Robinson RG, Berthier ML, et al. 1988a. Differential mood changes following basal ganglia versus thalamic lesions. *Arch Neurol* 45:725–730.
Starkstein SE, Moran TH, Bowersox JA, et al. 1988b. Behavioral abnormalities induced by frontal cortical and nucleus accumbens lesions. *Brain Res* 473:74–80.

Starkstein SE, Brandt J, Folstein SE, et al. 1988c. Neuropsychological and neuroradiological correlates in Huntington's disease. *J Neurol Neurosurg Psychiatry* 51:1259–1263.

Starkstein SE, Preziosi TJ, Berthier ML, et al. 1989. Depression and cognitive impairments in Parkinson's disease. *Brain* 112:1141–1153.

Starkstein SE, Folstein SE, Brandt J, et al. 1989b. Brain atrophy in Huntington's disease. *Neuroradiology* 31:156–159.

Starkstein SE, Mayberg HS, Berthier ML, et al. 1990a. Mania after brain injury: neuroradiological and metabolic findings. *Ann Neurol* 27:652–659.

Starkstein SE, Preziosi TH, Bolduc PL, et al. 1990b. Depression in Parkinson's disease. *J Nerv Ment Dis* 178:27–31.

Stuss DT, Benson DF. 1986. *The Frontal Lobes*. New York: Raven Press, pp. 121–138.

Talairach J, Tournoux P. 1988. *Co-Planar Stereotaxic Atlas of the Brain*. New York: Thieme Medical Publishers.

Taylor AE, Saint-Cyr JA, Lang AE. 1986. Frontal lobe dysfunction in Parkinson's disease: the cortical focus of the neostriatal outflow. *Brain* 109:845–883.

Taylor AE, Saint-Cyr JA, Lang AE. 1988. Idiopathic Parkinson's disease: revised concepts of cognitive and affective status. *Can J Neurol Sci* 15:106–113.

Torack RM, Morris JC. 1988. The association of ventral tegmental area histopathology with adult dementia. *Arch Neurol* 45:211–218.

Van Praag HM, DeHaan S. 1979. Central serotonin metabolism and frequency of depression. *Psychiatry Res* 1:219–224.

Von Sattel JP, Meyers RH, Stevend TJ, et al. 1985. Neuropathological classification of Huntington's disease. *J Neuropathol Exper Neurol* 44:559–577.

Wolfson LI, Leenders KL, Brown LL, et al. 1985. Alterations of regional cerebral blood flow and oxygen metabolism in Parkinson's disease. *Neurology* 35:1399–1405.

Yen CK, Budinger TF. 1981. Evaluation of blood-brain barrier permeability changes in rhesus monkeys and humans using ^{82}Rb and positron emission tomography. *J Comput Assist Tomogr* 5:792–799.

Young AB, Greenamyre JT, Hollingsworth Z, et al. 1988. NMDA receptor losses in putamen from patients with Huntington's disease. *Science* 241:981–983.

Young AB, Penney JB, Starosta-Rubinstein S, et al. 1986. PET scan investigations of Huntington's disease: cerebral metabolic correlates of neurological features and functional decline. *Ann Neurol* 20:296–303.

Zech M, Roberts GW, Bogerts B, et al. 1986. Neuropeptides in the amygdala of controls, schizophrenics and patients suffering from Huntington's chorea: an immunohistochemical study. *Acta Neuropathol* 71:259–266.

Zubenko GS, Moossy J. 1988. Major depression in primary dementia. *Arch Neurol* 45:1182–1186.

Zubenko GS, Moossy J, Kopp U. 1990a. Neurochemical correlates of major depression in primary dementia. *Arch Neurol* 47:209–214.

Zubenko GS, Sullivan P, Nelson JP, et al. 1990b. Brain imaging abnormalities in mental disorders of late life. *Arch Neurol* 47:1107–1111.

13

DEMENTIA OF DEPRESSION IN PATIENTS WITH NEUROLOGIC DISEASE

Sergio E. Starkstein, M.D., Ph.D.

Several studies have demonstrated the presence of cognitive impairments in patients with depression. Madden et al. (1952) were among the first to report that cognitive deficits suggestive of dementia, such as disorientation, anterograde amnesia, and dyscalculia, may be present in such patients but "may disappear on alleviation of the psychotic picture by means of short-term intensive therapy." Kiloh (1961) later reported that patients who initially appeared to be demented were found to be suffering from a psychiatric disorder resembling a primary dementia, and several studies have shown a significant correlation between the severity of depression and the degree of cognitive impairments (Stoudemire et al. 1989). This association between cognitive impairments and depression was termed *pseudodementia*. Patients with depression may show true cognitive impairments, however, so the condition now is termed *dementia syndrome of depression* or *depression-related cognitive impairments*.

Cognitive impairments are frequent findings among patients with neurologic disorders such as stroke and Parkinson disease, and they have been related to structural brain dysfunction in these disorders. However, depression may account at least partially for these cognitive problems as well. This chapter examines the evidence supporting a phenomenon of "depression-related cognitive impairments" in patients with neurologic disorders; because little research has been carried out in other neurologic diseases, we limit our discussion to stroke and Parkinson disease.

DEPRESSION-RELATED COGNITIVE IMPAIRMENTS IN STROKE

Approximately 40% of patients with an acute stroke lesion show depression, and in several studies that included a consecutive series of patients with such lesions, we examined the association between depression and cognitive impairments using the Mini-Mental State Examination (Folstein et al. 1975). This is an 11-item examination that is reliable and valid for assessing cognitive functions in a variety of states, including dementia and brain injury. We found a significant association between cognitive impairments and depression scores, and higher depression scores correlated significantly with lower Mini-Mental State Examination scores (Robinson et al. 1986).

These findings tend to support the phenomenon of depression-related cognitive impairments, but some important limitations should be mentioned. Because lesion size and location are related significantly to cognitive impairment, the finding of significantly lower Mini-Mental State Examination scores in patients with depression may result from significantly larger lesions or the presence of lesions in critical brain areas. Aphasia is another confounding variable, and the lower cognitive performance of patients with depression may be related to its presence. Some lesion-related cognitive impairments may recover with time, so the time since stroke is another important confounding variable.

THE INFLUENCE OF DEPRESSION IN THE INTELLECTUAL IMPAIRMENT OF PATIENTS WITH STROKE

In the first study to examine empirically the relationship between intellectual deficit and post-stroke depression, we studied a consecutive series of patients with acute stroke and either major depression ($n = 11$), minor depression ($n = 10$), or no depression ($n = 17$) (Robinson et al. 1986). While there were no significant between-group differences in terms of demographic variables, neurologic findings, and social functioning, patients with major depression showed significantly lower Mini-Mental State Examination scores than both patients with minor or no depression (score $\pm$ SD = 13.0 ± 5.8, 25.0 ± 4.5, and 22.0 ± 6.0, respectively; $P < 0.05$). Moreover, patients with major depression had a significantly higher frequency of abnormal scores (i.e., scores below 24) than patients with either minor or no depression (Fig. 13.1).

Another important finding was that patients with an abnormal Mini-Mental State Examination score (i.e., below 24) had significantly larger lesion sizes than patients with a normal score. When lesion size was examined in relation to intellectual impairment, both patients with major and with no depression had a significant (nega-

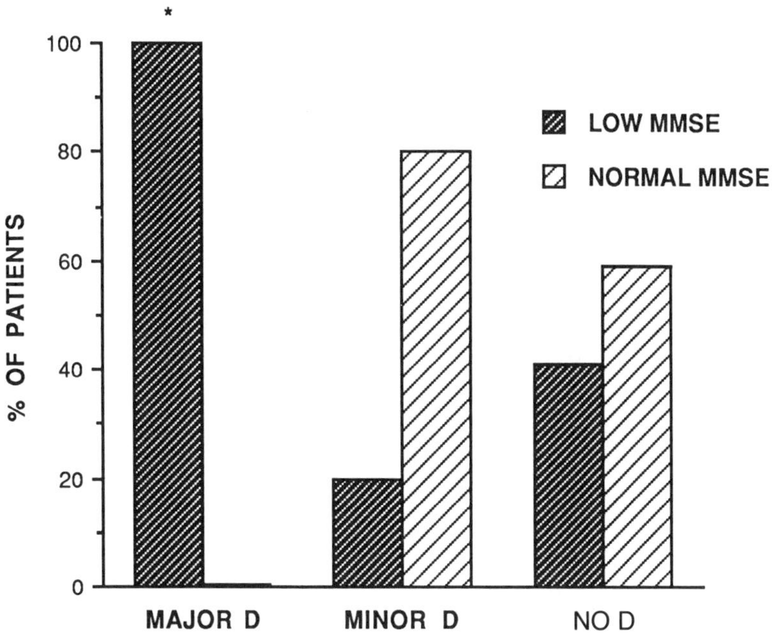

*$X^2 = 15.3$, df = 2, $P < 0.001$

Figure 13.1. Patients with major post-stroke depression (*D*) showed a significantly higher frequency of abnormal Mini-Mental State Examination (*MMSE*) scores than patients with minor or no depression.

tive) correlation between lesion size and Mini-Mental State Examination scores (i.e., the larger the lesion, the greater the intellectual impairment) ($r = -0.73$, $P < 0.01$ and $r = -0.63$, $P < 0.05$, respectively). To account for lesion size, a multiple regression analysis was carried out using these scores as the dependent variable and both lesion size and depression scores as the independent variables. Both depression scores and lesion size independently contributed to intellectual impairment; after controlling for intellectual impairment, patients with depression had significantly smaller lesion volumes than patients without depression (i.e., those without depression required a significantly larger lesion than those with depression to produce the same cognitive deficit).

In conclusion, this study provided several important findings. First, the prevalence of cognitive impairments was significantly associated with the severity of depression (i.e., all patients with major depression had abnormal Mini-Mental State Examination scores, compared with 40% of those without depression). Second, patients with intellectual deficits had significantly larger lesion sizes than patients without intellectual deficits. Third, those with major depression had greater cognitive impairments for comparable lesion sizes, and when the cognitive impairment was held constant, those with depression had significantly smaller lesion sizes than those without depression. Fourth, both lesion size and depression also were found to relate independently to cognitive impairment.

COGNITIVE IMPAIRMENTS IN PATIENTS WITH AND WITHOUT POST-STROKE MAJOR DEPRESSION MATCHED FOR SIZE AND LOCATION OF LESION

To control for lesion size and location as well as other important demographic variables, we matched a consecutive series of patients with stroke with major or no depression for length of follow-up (from time of stroke to evaluation), lesion size, lesion side (left or right hemisphere), and lesion location within the hemisphere (Starkstein et al. 1988b). Moreover, depressed and nondepressed pairs did not differ in terms of demographic variables, years of education, neurologic symptoms (including frequency and type of aphasia), and social background.

We found that patients with major depression had significantly lower Mini-Mental State Examination scores than their lesion-matched non-depressed control subjects (mean scores ± SD, 16.6 ± 7.8 [depressed], 22.4 ± 6.6 [no depression], $t = 3.21$, df = 12, $P < 0.05$). Nine of 13 patients with major depression (69%) had abnormal Mini-Mental State Examination scores, but only three of 13 patients without depression (23%) had abnormal scores ($\chi^2 = 5.5$, $P < 0.05$) (Fig. 13.2). Moreover, while 10 of the 13 patients with depression (77%) had lower scores than their respective matched controls, two had the same score and only 1 had a higher score than the respective control ($X^2 = 14.7$, $P < 0.001$). Also, because 10 of the 13 pairs had mainly cortical damage, it may be argued that these findings only apply to patients with cortical lesions; however, in another study, we found that patients with restricted subcortical lesions and abnormal Mini-Mental State Examination scores had significantly higher depression scores than patients with similar lesions but Mini-Mental State Examination scores within the normal range (Robinson et al. 1986).

While these findings demonstrate that the phenomenon of depression-related cognitive impairments is independent of lesion variables, several limitations could not be accounted for. First, 11 of the 13 pairs had left hemisphere lesions, so we could not determine

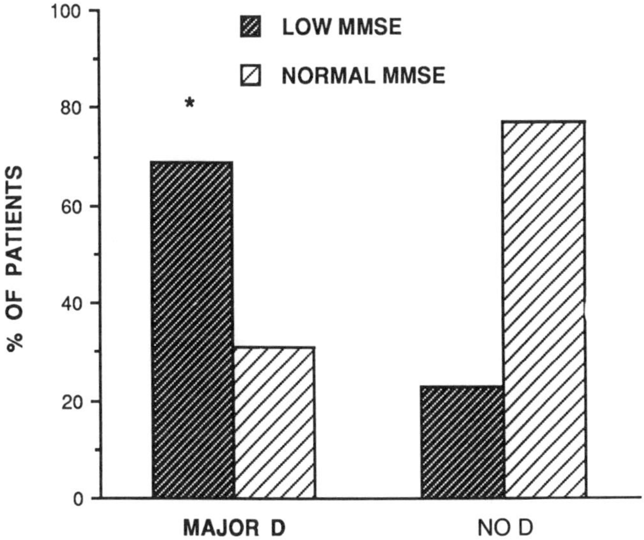

$^{*}X^2 = 5.5$, df $= 1$, $P = 0.025$

Figure 13.2. Patients with major depression (*D*) showed a significantly higher frequency of abnormal Mini-Mental State Examination (*MMSE*) scores than patients without depression who were matched for age, time since stroke, and lesion location and volume.

whether the presence of depression-related cognitive impairments also may be present among those with restricted right hemisphere lesions. Second, because the Mini-Mental State Examination is a crude measure of cognitive problems, whether intellectual deficits are more severe in specific cognitive domains also could not be determined. These factors were examined in the next study reviewed.

THE LATERALIZATION OF COGNITIVE DEFICITS IN PATIENTS WITH POST-STROKE DEPRESSION

For this study (Bolla-Wilson et al. 1989), we examined a consecutive series of patients with an acute stroke and either:

1. a left hemisphere lesion and major depression ($n = 10$),
2. a left hemisphere lesion and no depression ($n = 16$),
3. a right hemisphere lesion and major depression ($n = 8$), and
4. a right hemisphere lesion and no depression ($n = 19$).

Patients were examined with a neuropsychologic battery that included 34 subtests that were designed to assess a wide range of functional domains. These included orientation (Orientation and General Information), language (Boston Naming Test; Verbal Fluency; Months Forward; and repetition, reading, comprehension, and spontaneous speech tasks from the Boston Diagnostic Aphasia Examination and the Multilingual Aphasia Examination), remote memory (General Information and Famous Faces), verbal memory (Logical Memory, Rey Auditory Verbal-Learning Test [RAVLT], Recurrent Words, Digit Span), visual memory (Visual Reproduction), recognition tasks (recurrent words, Logical Memory, RAVLT, and Visual Reproduction), visuoperception-visuoconstruction (Block Design, Clock Drawing, Hooper Visual Organization Test), executive/motor (Alternating Fingers, Luria Motor sequences, Praxis, and finger tapping), and "frontal lobe" functions (Verbal Fluency, Alternating Fingers, and Luria Motor sequences). Patients with either a language deficit, history of alcoholism, or a metabolic disorder were excluded from this study.

No significant differences were found in demographic variables, type and severity of neurologic deficits, and lesion size and location, but the neuropsychologic evaluation revealed several important findings. A two-way ANOVA (factor 1: depression [present versus absent]; factor 2: hemisphere [left versus right]) of composite neuropsychologic scores showed a significant depression by hemisphere interaction ($F[1,42] = 6.9$, $P < 0.01$). On individual comparisons, the group with left hemisphere lesions and major depression performed significantly worse than the left hemisphere nondepressed, the right hemisphere depressed, and the right hemisphere nondepressed groups.

When patients with left hemisphere lesions, both with and without depression, were compared for performance on individual cognitive domains, patients with depression scored significantly worse on tests of orientation, language, executive/motor, and frontal lobe functions. The learning curves of the RAVLT showed that patients with depression and left hemisphere lesions had the least amount of learning over the trials, and by the fifth trial (measure of overall learning), they had learned significantly fewer words than the left hemisphere nondepressed group. In the right hemisphere group, there were no significant differences between patients with or without depression in any of the nine cognitive domains. Thus, the main finding of this study was that the significant association between post-stroke depression and neuropsychologic deficits was present only among patients with depression and left (but not right) hemisphere lesions.

The profile of cognitive deficits shown by patients with post-stroke depression and left hemisphere lesions is similar to that demonstrated by patients with functional depression (Stoudemire et al.

1989). The finding of a nonlinear learning pattern over trials on the RAVLT suggests attention/concentration difficulties and poor sequential learning that may be secondary to an inability of patients with depression to use adequate encoding strategies and organization of inputs for subsequent facilitation of recall. Coupled with the lack of significant between-group differences on cued-recall (recognition) tests, these results suggest that patients with depression may retain but not retrieve the information.

LONGITUDINAL COURSE OF POST-STROKE DEPRESSION AND INTELLECTUAL IMPAIRMENTS

In a prospective, longitudinal study, we examined eight patients without inhospital depression who remained nondepressed at 6-months post-stroke and nine patients with inhospital (major or minor) depression who remained depressed at 6-months' follow-up (Robinson et al. 1986). By the initial evaluation, patients with and without depression did not differ significantly in their Mini-Mental State Examination scores; however, at 6-months' follow-up, the nondepressed group showed improvement in their scores and the depressed group a slight decline. By the end of this 6-month period,

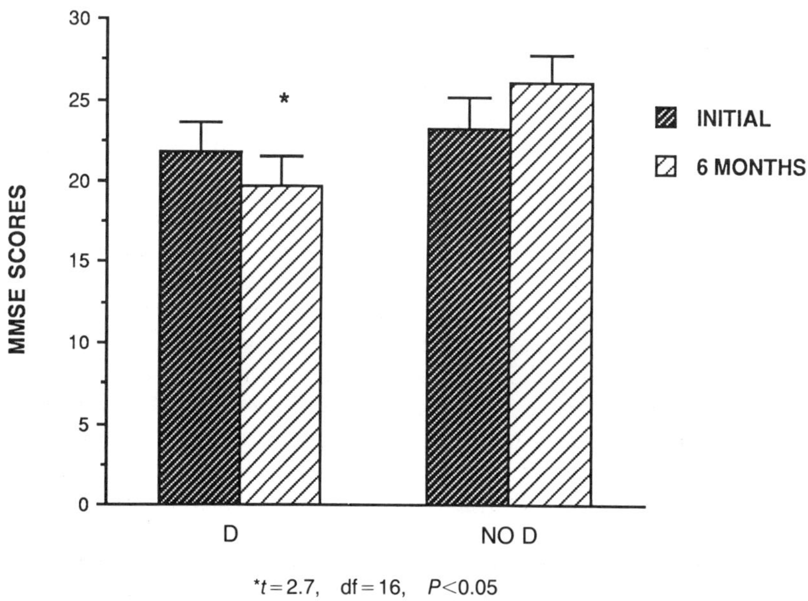

Figure 13.3. Patients with post-stroke depression (*D*) showed significantly less recovery from cognitive impairments 6-months post-stroke than patients without depression.

scores of patients with depression were significantly lower than those of the nondepressed group (Fig. 13.3). Furthermore, during the 6-months of follow-up, only one patient with inhospital depression improved spontaneously.

OVERALL FINDINGS

Several studies have demonstrated a significant association between post-stroke depression and cognitive impairments. These findings cannot be explained by demographic factors, social functioning, neurologic deficits, and lesion variables. The cognitive impairment of post-stroke depression is restricted to patients with left hemisphere lesions, and it is characterized primarily by deficits in orientation, language, executive/motor and frontal lobe functions, and verbal learning.

DEPRESSION-RELATED COGNITIVE IMPAIRMENTS IN PARKINSON DISEASE

While depression and cognitive impairments are well-known findings in patients with Parkinson disease, few studies have examined whether these disorders occur as independent phenomena or are related etiologically. To address this question, we examined a consecutive series of 105 outpatients with Parkinson disease for the presence of depression and cognitive impairment (Starkstein et al. 1990b). We found that patients with major depression ($n = 21$) had significantly lower Mini-Mental State Examination scores than those without depression ($n = 64$) (mean score ± SD = 25 ± 5.5 and 27.7 ± 3.3, respectively; $P < 0.001$); however, no significant differences were found between patients with minor depression ($n = 20$) (mean score ± SD = 28.1 ± 1.7) and those without depression.

To examine further the influence of depression on cognitive performance, a stepwise regression analysis was carried out on a subsample of patients with Parkinson disease who underwent a more detailed neuropsychologic evaluation. Mini-Mental State Examination scores were entered as the dependent variable, and age, duration of illness, age at onset, education, levodopa dosage, PSE (wing et al. 1974) depression score, North-Western Disability Scale scores (Canter et al. 1961) assessing ADLs, as well as scores of tremor, rigidity, and akinesia were entered as independent variables. The variable that accounted for most of the variance was the PSE ($R^2 = 0.17$), thus demonstrating that depression is one of the most important factors associated with cognitive impairments in Parkinson disease.

We also matched patients with major, minor, and no depression for age (± 2 years), education (± 2 years), and Hoehn and Yahr stage of illness (same stage) (Starkstein et al. 1989b). Every patient was examined with a neuropsychologic battery that included the Wisconsin Card Sorting Test (Nelson 1976), which measures the ability to develop new concepts and shift sets and also requires the subject to suppress a previously correct response and produce a new one; the Controlled Word Association Test (Benton 1968), which examines access to information with time constraint); the Trail Making Test (Reitan 1958), which examines visual, conceptual, and visuomotor tracking; the Symbol Digit Modalities (Smith 1973), which examines visuoverbal substitution speed; the Design Fluency Test, a nonverbal counterpart to the controlled Word Association Test (Jones-Gotman and Milner 1977); and the Digit Span, which examines auditory attention (Wechsler 1955).

When the 15 major-depressed and 15 non-depressed matched pairs were compared, a two-way ANOVA (Factor 1: major depression versus no depression; Factor 2: neuropsychologic test) showed a significant group effect; patients with major depression performed significantly worse than those without depression. It also showed a significant group by task interaction that was the result of a significantly poorer performance of patients with major depression on tasks classically associated with frontal-lobe dysfunction, such as the Wisconsin Card Sorting Test (Fig. 13.4), Verbal Fluency, Design Fluency, and section B of the Trail Making Test (Fig. 13.5). However, when patients having minor depression were compared with their respective matched, nondepressed group, no significant group or group by test interactions were observed.

In conclusion, our studies demonstrated that patients with Parkinson disease and major depression showed significantly more cognitive impairments than patients with PD and no depression who were matched for age, education, and stage of illness. No significant differences in cognitive performance were found between those with minor depression and those without depression, thus our findings suggest that the phenomenon of depression-related cognitive impairments is related significantly to the type of depression and consists primarily of deficits in frontal lobe–related tasks.

DEPRESSION AND COGNITIVE IMPAIRMENTS IN DIFFERENT STAGES OF PARKINSON DISEASE

The first stage of Parkinson disease (stage I of Hoehn and Yahr) is characterized by unilateral (left or right) motor symptoms. We examined patients with left or right exclusive or main unilateral symptoms (tremor, rigidity, and/or akinesia) (Starkstein et al. 1990b) and found that the right hemi-parkinsonian group (with right motor symptoms and left brain pathology) had significantly higher depres-

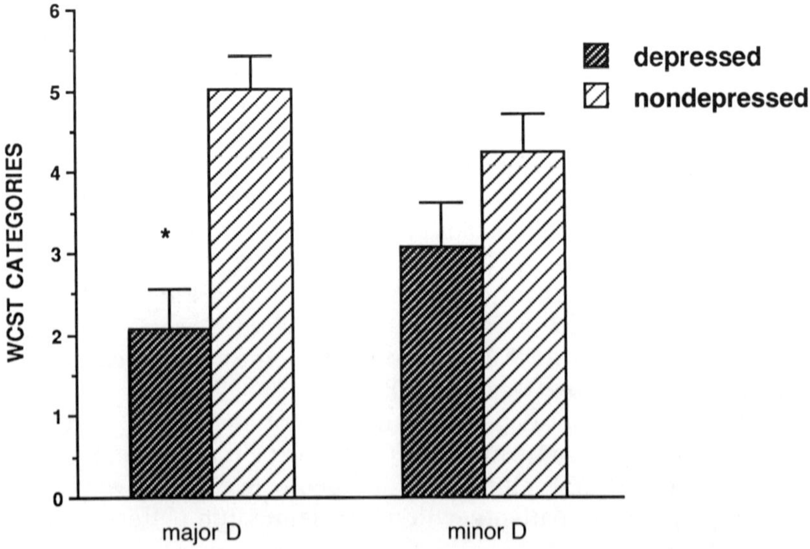

Figure 13.4. Patients with Parkinson disease and major depression (*D*) showed a significantly worse performance on the Wisconsin Card Sorting Test (*WCST*) compared with patients with Parkinson disease without depression who were matched for age, duration, and stage of illness. No significant differences were observed between patients with minor and nondepression.

sion scores and significantly lower Mini-Mental State Examination scores than patients in the left hemi-parkinsonian group (with left motor symptoms and left brain pathology). Thus, while the phenomenon of depression-related cognitive impairments already is present in the early stages of Parkinson disease, the finding is restricted to patients in the right hemi-parkinsonian group (left hemisphere dysfunction). Similar findings were reported in patients with stroke, because only those with left (but not right) hemisphere lesions showed the phenomenon of depression-related cognitive impairments (Bolla-Wilson et al. 1989).

In a comprehensive study that included 94 patients with Parkinson disease who were examined with the comprehensive neuropsychologic battery described earlier we divided patients into those with mild (stages 1 or 2), moderate (stage 3), and severe (stages 4 or 5) Parkinson disease. Each group was divided further into subgroups with and without depression (Starkstein et al. 1989a). A three-factor ANOVA (Factor 1: group [mild, moderate, severe]; Factor 2: psychi-

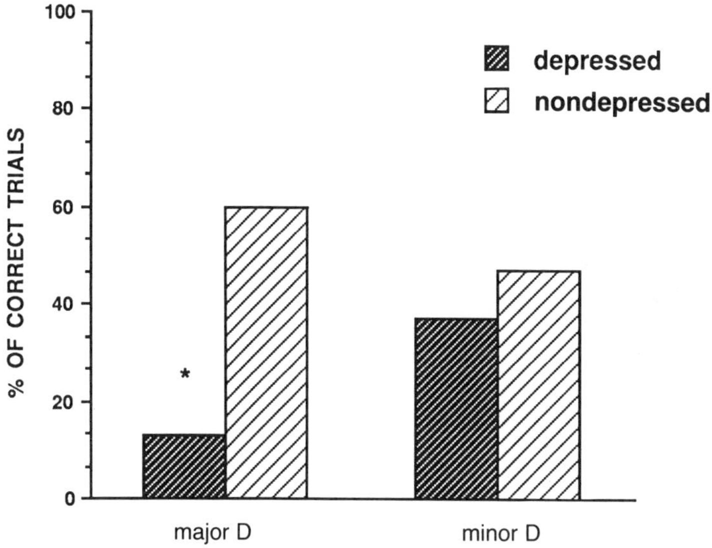

$^*X^2 = 7.03$, df = 1, $P < 0.01$

Figure 13.5. Patients with Parkinson disease and major depression (*D*) showed a significantly worse performance on Trails B compared to patients having Parkinson disease without depression who were matched for age, duration, and stage of illness. No significant differences were observed between patients with minor and nondepression.

atric status [depressed versus nondepressed]; Factor 3: neuropsychologic task) showed a significant group effect (patients with severe Parkinson disease showed significantly more cognitive impairments), a significant effect for the psychiatric status (patients with depression performed significantly worse than those without depression), and a significant group by psychiatric status interaction (patients with depression and severe PD showed significantly greater neuropsychologic impairment than the other five groups). On individual comparisons, patients with depression and severe Parkinson disease performed significantly worse on the Wisconsin Card Sorting Test (Fig. 13.6), section B of the Trail Making Test, and Symbol-Digit Modalities.

In conclusion, our studies showed that patients with Parkinson disease in the late stages of the disease had significantly greater cognitive impairments than patients in earlier stages. These intellectual deficits mainly were observed in frontal lobe–related tasks, and the finding of a significant interaction between depression and cognitive

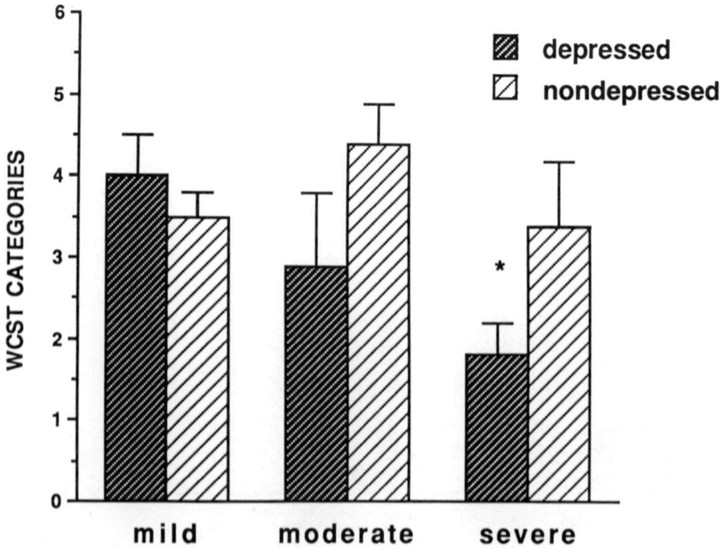

*F = 3.11, df = 5,89, $P<0.01$

Figure 13.6. Patients with depression and severe Parkinson disease showed a significantly worse performance on the Wisconsin Card Sorting Test (*WCST*) than patients with or without depression having milder Parkinson disease symptoms.

impairment restricted to late stages of the disease suggests an important interaction between the progression of the disease and the mechanisms of depression and cognitive dysfunction in Parkinson disease.

FOLLOW-UP STUDIES OF COGNITIVE IMPAIRMENT AND DEPRESSION IN PARKINSON DISEASE

The longitudinal evaluation of cognitive decline in patients with Parkinson disease either with or without depression may allow further insights into the interaction between mood changes and intellectual deficits. In our first follow-up study, we examined 49 patients with Parkinson disease on two occasions 3 to 4 years apart (Starkstein et al. 1990a). Eighteen patients showed depression and 31 patients were not depressed on the initial evaluation, and while there were no significant between-group differences in the initial Mini-

Mental State Examination scores, a two-way ANOVA with repeated measures showed a significant time effect and group by time interaction. Both groups showed significantly lower Mini-Mental State Examination scores over time, but the decline was significantly greater for those with depression (Fig. 13.7). Findings remained similar even after matching patients with and without depression for years of education, duration of illness, and severity of motor symptoms.

This study suggests that the presence of depression may be a marker of progressive cognitive decline in patients with Parkinson disease, but a structured psychiatric interview was not carried out. Patients with depression could not be classified into major or minor depression groups. Thus, we examined 92 patients and used the PSE and DSM-III criteria to diagnose depression (Starkstein et al. 1992). Patients were divided into those with major, minor, or no depression, and the 1-year outcome in terms of cognitive decline was examined. A two-way ANOVA with repeated measures for Mini-Mental State Examination scores showed a significant time effect (scores declined in all three groups), a significant group effect (patients with

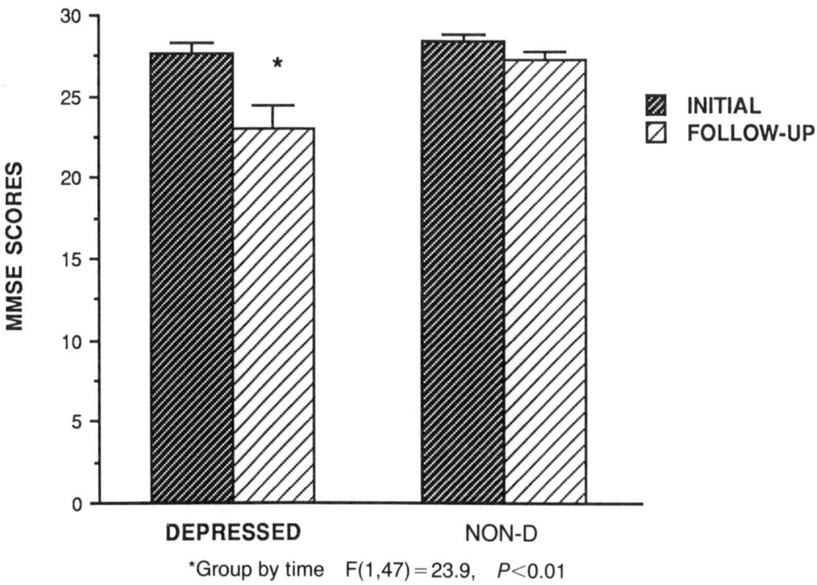

Figure 13.7. Patients with Parkinson disease and depression (*D*) showed significantly more decline in Mini-Mental State Examination (*MMSE*) scores over a 3-to-4-year period than patients without depression.

major depression had significantly lower scores), and a significant group by time interaction (patients with major depression showed a significantly greater decline in scores than patients with either minor or no depression) (Fig. 13.8). Findings remained significant even after patients were matched for duration of illness. This study not only replicated our previous finding of a significantly faster cognitive decline among patients with depression, it also showed that the phenomenon of depression-related cognitive impairments is restricted to patients with major depression.

OVERALL FINDINGS

Depression-related cognitive impairments are frequent among patients with Parkinson disease. This phenomenon is present in those with major but not in those with minor depression, and it is more evident in the late stages of the illness. Finally, the presence of a major depression may predict (at least in a subgroup of patients) a significant cognitive decline.

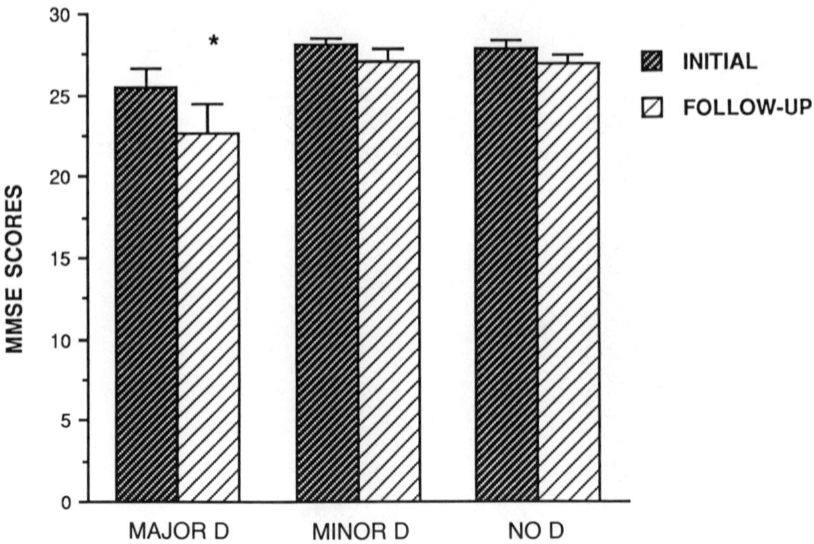

*Group by time   F = 12.6,   df = 2,89, $P<0.01$

Figure 13.8. Patients with Parkinson disease and major depression (*D*) showed significantly more decline in Mini-Mental State Examination (*MMSE*) scores over a 1-year period than patients with either minor or no depression.

COMPARISON OF DEPRESSION-RELATED COGNITIVE IMPAIRMENTS IN PATIENTS WITH NEUROLOGIC DISORDERS AND FUNCTIONAL DEPRESSION

Depression may produce cognitive changes in patients with either functional depression or neurologic disorders, but one methodologic problem is that cognitive deficit may result from the neurologic disease itself. We tried to deal with this important limitation by comparing the intellectual performance of patients with the same neurologic condition with and without depression over a range of cognitive tasks.

We used the Mini-Mental State Examination to assess cognitive performance in patients who had either cerebrovascular lesions (13 with and 13 without major depression), Parkinson disease (15 with and 15 without major depression), and both patients with depression or normal control subjects having no known neurologic disorder (12 with and 12 without major depression) (Starkstein et al. 1989c).

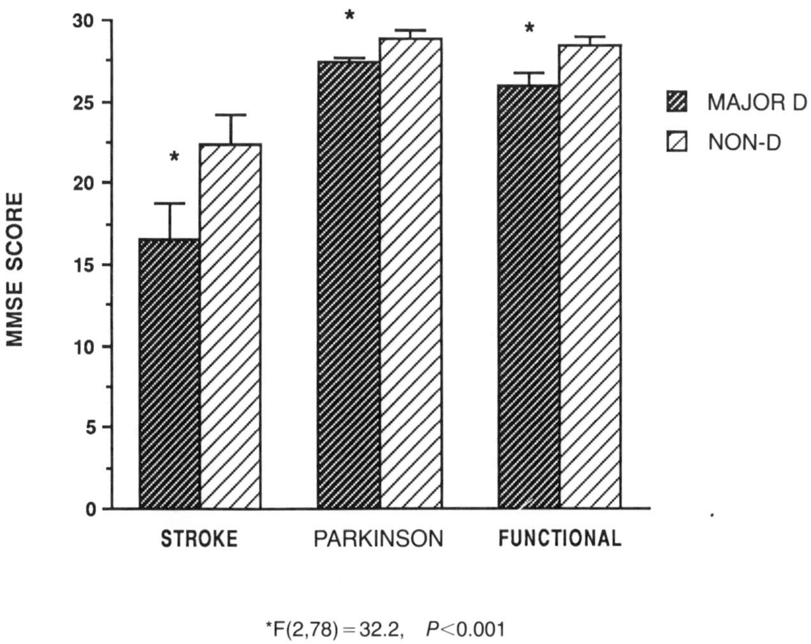

Figure 13.9. Patients with major depression (*D*) and either stroke, Parkinson disease, or functional depression showed significantly lower Mini-Mental State Examination (*MMSE*) scores than patients without depression or control subjects matched for important demographic and disease-related variables.

Group pairs were matched for the most important variables, such as age, education, and duration and stage of illness. A two-way ANOVA (Factor 1: group [stroke, Parkinson disease, functional depression]; Factor 2: psychiatric status [depressed versus nondepressed] for Mini-Mental State Examination scores showed a significant effect for psychiatric status ($F[2,78] = 32.2$, $P < 0.01$) (patients with depression showed significantly lower scores than those without depression) but no significant group by psychiatric status interaction, thus showing that the influence of depression on scores was similar across all three groups (Fig. 13.9). After a z-score transformation of scores on each Mini-Mental State Examination domain, a two-way ANOVA (Factor 1: group [major versus no depression]; Factor 2: domain) showed significantly lower scores on the delayed-recall section in all three groups of patients with major depression compared with the nondepressed groups.

In conclusions, this study showed two important findings. First, the influence of depression on cognitive functions was present in patients with major depression with and without neurologic disorders. Second, patients with depression (with or without neurologic disorders) showed the same profile of intellectual impairments, with significantly lower scores on the delayed-recall section of the Mini-Mental State Examination; this finding suggests that at least part of the cognitive impairments shown by patients with neurologic disorders such as stroke and Parkinson disease may be related to the presence of depression.

MECHANISM OF DEPRESSION-RELATED COGNITIVE IMPAIRMENTS IN PATIENTS WITH NEUROLOGIC DISORDERS

Perhaps one of the most straightforward ways to explain the presence of cognitive impairments in patients with depression is that intellectual impairments are secondary to discouragement, preoccupation with depressive themes, and poor concentration and motivation. If this is the case, however, then depressed patients with stroke lesions (regardless of lesion side) would show the phenomenon, but only depressed stroke patients with left but not right hemisphere lesions have depression-related cognitive impairments. This suggests that the mechanism is different. We hypothesize that the presence of specific asymmetric changes in biogenic amine concentrations may explain the phenomenon.

In laboratory animals, we have demonstrated that right but not left hemisphere injury leads to widespread depletion in norepinephrine and dopamine concentrations (Robinson 1979). Moreover, we also found that right but not left frontal cortical lesions may increase the turnover of dopamine in subcortical nuclei such as the nucleus accumbens (an important structure in the mesocorticolimbic dopaminergic system) (Starkstein et al. 1988a). In a study using positron-emission tomography scanning in humans, we demonstrated that right but not left hemisphere stroke lesions lead to increased binding of serotonin S_2-receptors in the uninjured temporal cortex (Mayberg et al. 1988); thus, recent studies not only have demonstrated the presence of neurologic asymmetries in the brains of laboratory animals and humans but also that focal lesions may produce biochemical changes depending on the side of lesion (i.e., right hemisphere lesions may produce specific biochemical changes while identical lesions of the left hemisphere do not result in such changes).

Several studies have demonstrated that dysfunction of the dopaminergic mesocorticolimbic system may be related to the impaired performance on delayed-recall tasks of patients with functional depression. Dysfunction of this system also has been implicated in the cognitive deficits of patients with Parkinson disease (Weingartner et al. 1981, Lees and Smith 1983). Dysfunction of the mesocorticolimbic system may account for the high frequency of depression in Parkinson disease, and we reported significant hypometabolic activity in the inferior frontal cortex (one of the main cortical afferents of dopaminergic nucleus accumbens fibers) in patients with depression and Parkinson disease (Mayberg et al. 1990). Thus, in patients with Parkinson disease, both depression and cognitive impairments may be the consequence of dysfunction of the mesocorticolimbic system. Among patients with stroke and both depression and cognitive impairments, the biochemical dysfunction of catecholaminergic pathways may involve similar frontal areas.

Few studies regarding the interaction between cognitive impairments and depression have been carried out in other neurologic illnesses. Among patients with Alzheimer disease, no association has been reported between depression and cognitive impairments; when patients with depression and Alzheimer disease were compared with patients with Alzheimer disease and no depression who were matched for duration of illness, no significant differences in the severity of cognitive impairments were observed (Reifler et al. 1986). Moreover, the successful treatment of depression in patients with Alzheimer disease did not improve the cognitive deficits (Reifler et al. 1989). However, whether patients with Alzheimer disease and depression have significantly more deficits in specific cognitive domains (such as frontal-lobe functions) has not been examined empirically.

In a study of patients with closed head injuries, we found no significant differences in Mini-Mental State Examination scores between patients with major depression and patients without depression (Fedoroff et al. 1992). This may be related to the fact that most of the patients were in their late twenties and early thirties, and the phenomenon of depression-related cognitive impairments has been reported most frequently among elderly individuals.

CONCLUSIONS

The phenomenon of depression-related cognitive impairments has been demonstrated in patients with either stroke or Parkinson disease. We found that only patients with major and not minor depression showed the phenomenon. The types of cognitive impairment are similar to findings among patients with functional depression, with deficits predominantly in frontal lobe–related tasks and anterograde memory. Dysfunction of dopaminergic and/or catecholaminergic systems may underlie the phenomenon; future studies may demonstrate the ultimate mechanism of this cognitive disturbance as well as a specific treatment for this condition.

ACKNOWLEDGMENTS

This work was supported in part by National Institute of Mental Health grant MH40355, a Young Investigator Award from the National Alliance for Research in Schizophrenia and Depression, a grant from the Institute of Neurological Research Raúl Carrea, and a grant from the Sandoz Foundation for Gerontological Research.

REFERENCES

Benton AL. 1968. Differential behavioral, effects in frontal lobe disease. *Neuropsychologia* 6:53–60.

Bolla-Wilson K, Robinson RG, Starkstein SE, et al. 1989. Lateralization of dementia of depression in stroke patients. *Am J Psychiatry* 146:627–634.

Canter GJ, de la Torre R, Mier M. 1961. A method for evaluating disability in patients with Parkinson's disease. *J Nerv Men Disord* 133:143–147.

Fedoroff JP, Starkstein SE, Forrester AW, et al. 1992. Depression in patients with acute traumatic brain injury. *Am J Psychiatry*, 149:918–923.

Folstein MF, Folstein SE, McHugh PR. 1975. Mini-Mental State: a practical method for grading the cognitive state of patients for the clinician. *J Psychiatry Res* 12:189–198.

Jones-Gotman M, Milner BM. 1977. The invention of nonsense drawings after focal cortical lesions. *Neuropsychologia* 15:653–674.

Kiloh LG. 1961. Pseudodementia. *Acta Psychiatr Scand* 37:336–351.

Lees AJ, Smith E. 1983. Cognitive deficits in the early stages of Parkinson's disease. *Brain* 106:257–270.

Madden JJ, Luhan JA, Kaplan LA, et al. 1952. Nondementing psychoses in older persons. *JAMA* 150:1567–1570.

Mayberg HS, Robinson RG, Wong DF, et al. 1988. PET imaging of cortical S_2

serotonin receptors after stroke: lateralized changes and relationship to depression. *Am J Psychiatry* 145:937–943.

Mayberg HS, Starkstein SE, Sadzot B, et al. 1990. Selective hypometabolism in the inferior frontal lobe in depressed patients with Parkinson's disease. *Ann Neurol* 28:57–64.

Nelson HE. 1976. A modified card sorting test sensitive to frontal lobe defects. *Cortex* 12:313–324.

Reifler BV, Larson E, Teri L. 1986. Dementia of the Alzheimer's type and depression. *J Am Geriatr Soc* 34:855–859.

Reifler BV, Teri L, Raskind M, et al. 1989. Double-blind trial of imipramine in Alzheimer's disease in patients with and without depression. *Am J Psychiatry* 146:45–49.

Reitan RM. 1958. Validity of the Trail Making Test as an indicator of organic brain damage. *Perceptual Motor Skills* 8:271–276.

Robinson RG. 1979. Differential behavioral and biochemical effects of right and left hemispheric cerebral infarction in the rat. *Science* 205:707–710.

Robinson RG, Bolla-Wilson K, Kaplan E, et al. 1986. Depression influences intellectual impairment in stroke patients. *Br J Psychiatry* 148:541–547.

Smith A. 1973. *Symbol Digit Modalities Test Manual.* Los Angeles: Western Psychological Services.

Starkstein SE, Bolduc PL, Mayberg HS, et al. 1990a. Cognitive impairments and depression in Parkinson's disease: a follow-up study. *J Neurol Neurosurg Psychiatry* 53:597–602.

Starkstein SE, Bolduc PL, Preziosi TJ, et al. 1989a. Cognitive impairments in the different stages of Parkinson's disease. *J Neuropsychiatry Clin Neurosci* 1:243–248.

Starkstein SE, Mayberg HS, Preziosi TJ, et al. 1992. A prospective longitudinal study of depression, cognitive decline, and physical impairments in patients with Parkinson's disease. *J Neurol Neurosurg Psychiatry* 55:377–382.

Starkstein SE, Moran TH, Bowersox JA, et al. 1988a. Behavioral abnormalities induced by frontal cortical and nucleus accumbens lesions. *Brain Res* 473:74–80.

Starkstein SE, Preziosi TJ, Berthier ML, et al. 1989b. Depression and cognitive impairment in Parkinson's disease. *Brain* 112:1141–1153.

Starkstein SE, Preziosi TJ, Bolduc PL, et al. 1990b. Depression in Parkinson's disease. *J Nerv Ment Dis* 178:27–31.

Starkstein SE, Rabins PV, Berthier ML, et al. 1989c. Dementia of depression: evidence from neurological disorders and functional depression. *J Neuropsychiatry Clin Neurosci* 1:263–268.

Starkstein SE, Robinson RG, Price TR. 1988b. Comparison of patients with and without post-stroke major depression matched for size and location of lesion. *Arch Gen Psychiatry* 45:247–252.

Stoudemire A, Hill C, Gulley LR, et al. 1989. Neuropsychological and biomedical assessment of depression-dementia syndromes. *J Neuropsychiatry Clin Neurosci* 1:347–361.

Wechsler D. 1955. *Wechsler Adult Intelligence Scale Manual.* New York: Psychological Corporation.

Weingartner H, Cohen RM, Murphy DL, et al. 1981. Cognitive processes in depression. *Arch Gen Psychiatry* 38:42–47.

Wing JK, Cooper E, Sartorius N, 1974. *Measurements and Classification of Psychiatric Symptoms.* Cambridge: Cambridge University Press.

14

CONCLUSIONS AND FUTURE DIRECTIONS

Robert G. Robinson, M.D.
Sergio E. Starkstein, M.D., Ph.D.

This text has provided a detailed account of depressive disorders associated with a wide range of neurologic conditions, including stroke, Alzheimer disease, epilepsy, multiple sclerosis, Parkinson disease, Huntington disease, traumatic brain injury, aphasia, multi-infarct dementia, and functional depression. The chapters have contained information about clinical presentation, course, and treatment of these disorders as well as discussions of their possible etiologies.

Several unifying ideas can be found, but the one that emerges most prominently from the discussions of these neurologic disorders is that depression is not a unitary phenomenon. For example, our work in patients with stroke (Chapter 3) distinguished two forms of depression, that is, major and minor depression. We also reported several studies that lent support to this distinction. We found that major, but not minor, depression was associated with a dementia of depression, failure to suppress serum cortisol following dexamethasone administration, and specific lesion locations; other authors also have distinguished different kinds of depression. Loreck and Folstein (Chapter 4) distinguished an early stage of depression in Alzheimer disease with symptoms and pathology related to the limbic system as well as a late stage related to extension of the pathology into the parietal lobe: depression is more common in the early than the late stage of Alzheimer disease. Ring and Trimble (Chapter 5) described depressive disorders related to the prodromal, peri-ictal, and interictal periods in patients with epilepsy, and Huber and Rao (Chapter 6) described both syndromic and severity-of-symptom methods for determining the existence of depression. Starkstein and Mayberg (Chapter 7) also used the distinction of major and minor depression in Parkinson disease, while Peyser and Folstein (Chapter

8) acknowledged the historical debate between the psychologic explanation of depression (a reaction to a fatal illness) and the view of the disorder as related to degeneration in the basal ganglia. These authors also described both early and late-onset depressions in the course of Huntington disease as well as unipolar versus bipolar affective disorder. The chapter on traumatic brain injury by Fedoroff, Jorge, and Robinson (Chapter 9) described both major and minor depressive disorders; however, Benson and Ardila (Chapter 10) described depressive disorders related to grief, an organic affective syndrome, and a frustration-depression-catastrophic reaction syndrome. Cummings and Sultzer (Chapter 11) acknowledged difficulties in the diagnosis of both major depression and dysthymic disorder, and they pointed out the necessity of distinguishing depressive disorder in multi-infarct dementia from pseudobulbar palsy, in which uncontrollable episodes of forced weeping occur that are associated with dysarthria, dysphasia, exaggerated gag reflex, and brisk facial reflexes. Depression in multi-infarct dementias also should be distinguished from a dementia syndrome of depression, in which elderly patients with a primary mood disorder may develop significant cognitive impairments. Finally, Rogers (Chapter 2) made the very important point that neurophysiologic causes and psychologic causes of depressive disorder are not mutually exclusive, and he pointed to evidence that suggests a link between psychologic factors such as stressful life events or other psychosocial factors and major affective disorder that is associated with both structural and biochemical abnormalities of brain. Thus, psychologic and physiologic factors must integrate with one another to produce many of the disorders discussed in this text.

Most investigators who study the phenomenon of depressive disorder associated with neurologic disease acknowledge that depression is not an unitary phenomenon; there likely are multiple types of depression within each neurologic disorder. The fundamental problem in distinguishing these various types, however, is that we remain ignorant about the etiology of these disorders. Our knowledge regarding these depressions remains at the level of clinical description and clinical correlation, but our clinical descriptions inevitably lead us to make assumptions and conclusions about the cause of these disorders. For example, in Chapter 3, the identification of a post-stroke syndromic cluster meeting DSM-III criteria for major depressive disorder, the illumination of a natural course of illness, identification of a relationship between depression and injury to specific brain areas, and demonstration of the response of depression to antidepressant medication suggest there may be a characteristic "form" to the illness. This conclusion then leads to the secondary hypothesis that the cause of these depressive disorders is related to neurochemical or neurophysiologic disturbances of the brain. However, clinical descriptions emphasizing the psychosocial effects of neurologic disease with its implication for occupational outlook, social functioning, financial stability, and family stress lead to an understanding of depression based on its "function" (i.e., an understandable response to chronic illness).

Recognition that clinical perceptions from the point of view of either form or function lead us to different etiologic assumptions about the cause of the disorders led McHugh and Slavney to describe the perspectives of psychiatry (1983). Because we lack a unified understanding of the etiology of depressive disorder, psychiatrists have adopted different ways or perspectives of viewing the same clinical material. Each perspective gives a partial insight into possible causes of the observable clinical manifestations. For example, the disease perspective is based on the underlying assumption that the cause of the clinical manifestation is related to an underlying abnormality in the brain that is manifested clinically through some neurophysiologic mechanism; the life-story perspective, however, assumes that the underlying cause of the depressive disorder is related to the individual's life circumstances and empathic connections between life events, internal mental processes, and subsequent clinical manifestations. These different views of the cause of depressive disorders naturally lead to different views on their treatment. Benson and Ardila (Chapter 10) suggest that the language therapist is the most appropriate person to treat the frustration-depression-catastrophic reaction syndrome with encouragement, avoidance of stressful tasks, and supportive care. Starkstein and Robinson (Chapter 3), however, describe a double-blind, randomized treatment study demonstrating the efficacy of nortriptyline antidepressant therapy in the treatment of major depression following stroke. These clearly reflect different views of the underlying causes of these disorders and, presumably, different types of depression.

Until a unified theory or a demonstrated etiology for these depressive disorders exists, we use these perspectives to provide partial insight and directions for further research. We invoke disease, dimensions of variation, psychologic, and social explanations for these disorders. As Rogers points out (Chapter 2), however, not only are these explanations not mutually exclusive, but ultimately, we must try to achieve an understanding of how someone's life experience might provoke biologic changes in brain. This leads to a final discussion topic, and that is future developments.

Before physicians know the etiology and mechanism of the disorders they treat, they are limited to careful clinical descriptions of the phenomenology, course, and clinical correlates of the disorder.

This is our present status regarding the understanding of depressive disorder associated with neurologic disease; this also is an area in which many years of additional work must be devoted. As pointed out by Cummings and Sultzer (Chapter 11), we do not yet understand the clinical manifestations or course of depression associated with multi-infarct dementia, nor do we understand clinical correlates, such as lesion correlates, family history, previous personal history of mood disorder, or physiologic or chemical correlates of depression. This is the case with virtually all of the disorders described in this text. Careful clinical descriptions of the symptoms of depression that are specific to each of these neurologic disorders, a study of the natural history of these disorders, and a careful description of which associated clinical findings are specific to the depressive disorder must be conducted. The need for careful clinical descriptions of these disorders brings us back to the topic with which this text was started, that is, how to diagnose depressive disorders in patients with neurologic disease. It was pointed out in the first chapter that each disorder must be studied individually for symptoms that are both specific and nonspecific to that disorder. Clearly, much additional work needs to be done in this area.

In addition to further careful clinical descriptions of these disorders, future work also must address the mechanisms of these disorders. We will never develop truly rational treatments for these disorders until we understand their etiology and mechanism, and specific interventions into the abnormalities that provoke these disorders are required for treatment to be considered truly rational. Imaging techniques as described by Mayberg (Chapter 12) may provide valuable insights into the mechanisms of these disorders. Mayberg described a mechanism involving limbic cortical and basal ganglia areas that may play a role in the production of some of these depressive disorders; this kind of intriguing hypothesis is a natural outgrowth of the combination of structural and functional imaging studies that can be performed in patients with depressive disorders and structural neuropathology. However, much future work needs to be done in this area as well as developing appropriate animal models.

Even before we know the mechanisms of these disorders, treatments still can be demonstrated to be effective. Using controlled, double-blind study methodology, empiric treatments can be developed for many of these disorders (Lipsey et al. 1984). Most depressive disorders associated with neurological disease, however, have not been evaluated for treatment efficacy using a double-blind, controlled methodology.

Many of the disorders described in this text have animal models that are useful in studying their structural and physiologic foundations. For example, Parkinson disease, Huntington disease, stroke, multi-infarct disease, and traumatic injury all have useful animal models for study in the laboratory (Zigmond et al. 1987, Schwarcz and Shoulson 1987, Parikh and Robinson 1987); the issue which has not been addressed in these animal models, however, is the possible co-existence of depression. Animal models have been used to study the mechanisms for motor systems, neuropathology, and treatment response, but only rarely have they been used to examine the mechanisms of mood syndromes such as depression. Behaviors demonstrated in these models could be utilized to study the underlying physiologic or neurochemical processes that might play an important role in the production of depressive disorders; it is likely that only through the detailed experiments performed in animals that the neural circuits, physiologic abnormalities, or chemical processes involved in the production of these disorders will be elucidated.

Although the study of depressive disorders in neurologic disease is a field containing many more questions than answers at present, this is a newly emerging field of study at the interface between neurology and psychiatry. It is an area of investigation with a promising future that is likely to benefit from rapidly expanding technology in both imaging and neuroscience. It also is a field that is wide open for investigation at any level, from clinical presentation, longitudinal course, clinical correlate, to mechanism and etiology. It is only through this kind of broad-spectrum understanding of these disorders that we ultimately will be able to identify the numerous types of depressions that may occur and either prevent or treat them with techniques aimed at specific causal factors.

REFERENCES

Lipsey JR, Robinson RG, Pearlson GD, et al. 1984. Nortriptyline treatment of post-stroke depression: a double blind study. *Lancet* i:297–300.

McHugh PR, Slavney P. 1983. *The Perspectives of Psychiatry.* Baltimore: Johns Hopkins University Press.

Parikh RM, Robinson RG. 1987. Mood and cognitive disorders following stroke. In: Coyle JT, ed. *Animal Models of Dementia: A Synaptic Neurochemical Perspective.* New York: Alan R. Liss, pp 103–136.

Schwarcz R, Shoulson I. 1987. Excitotoxins and Huntington disease. In: Coyle JT, ed. *Animal Models of Dementia: A Synaptic Neurochemical Perspective.* New York: Alan R. Liss, pp 39–68.

Zigmond MJ, Stricker EM, Berger TW. 1987. Parkinsonism: insights from animal models utilizing neurotoxic agents. In: Coyle JT, ed. *Animal Models of Dementia: A Synaptic Neurochemical Perspective.* New York: Alan R. Liss, pp 1–38.

INDEX